Positioning in Anesthesia and Surgery

Third Edition

Positioning in Anesthesia and Surgery

John T. Martin, M.D.

Professor Emeritus
Department of Anesthesiology
Medical College of Ohio at Toledo
Toledo, Ohio

Mark A. Warner, M.D.

Professor
Department of Anesthesiology
Mayo Medical School
Rochester, Minnesota

W.B. SAUNDERS COMPANY
A Division of Harcourt Brace & Company
Philadelphia London Toronto Montreal Sydney Tokyo

W.B. SAUNDERS COMPANY
A Division of Harcourt Brace & Company

The Curtis Center
Independence Square West
Philadelphia, Pennsylvania 19106

Library of Congress Cataloging-in-Publication Data

Positioning in anesthesia and surgery / [edited by] John T. Martin, Mark A. Warner.—3rd ed.

p.   cm.

Includes bibliographical references and index.

ISBN 0–7216–6674–4

1. Surgery, Operative—Positioning.   2. Anesthesia—Positioning.
   I. Martin, John T.   II. Warner, Mark A.   [DNLM: 1. Surgery, Operative.   2. Posture.
   3. Anesthesia.   WO 500 P855 1997]

RD 32.7.P67 1997   617′.91—dc20

DNLM/DLC   96–34023

POSITIONING IN ANESTHESIA AND SURGERY, third edition   ISBN 0–7216–6674–4

Printed in the United States of America.

Last digit is the print number: 9   8   7   6   5   4   3   2   1

Contributors

William Dylewsky, M.D.
Senior Staff Anesthesiologist, Department of
    Anesthesiology, Lahey Hitchcock Medical
    Center, Burlington, Massachusetts
Peripheral Nervous System

Thomas J. Ebert, M.D., Ph.D.
Professor of Anesthesiology, Medical College of
    Wisconsin; Staff Anesthesiologist, Veterans
    Affairs Medical Center, Milwaukee, Wisconsin
*Physiologic Changes Associated with the Supine
Position*

Nikolaus Gravenstein, M.D.
Professor of Anesthesiology and Neurosurgery,
    University of Florida College of Medicine,
    Gainesville, Florida
The Central Nervous System

Betty L. Grundy, M.D.
Professor Emeritus of Anesthesiology and
    Pharmaceutics, University of Florida College of
    Medicine, Gainesville, Florida
The Central Nervous System

Noel W. Lawson, M.D.
Professor and Chairman, Department of
    Anesthesiology and Perioperative Medicine,
    University of Missouri Health Sciences Center,
    Columbia, Missouri
Lateral Positions

Scott E. LeBard, M.D.
Instructor in Anesthesiology and Pediatrics, Mayo
    Medical School; Co-Director, Pediatric Intensive
    Care Unit, Mayo Clinic, Rochester, Minnesota
Pediatrics

Emilio B. Lobato, M.D.
Assistant Professor, Department of
    Anesthesiology, University of Florida College of
    Medicine, Gainesville, Florida
The Central Nervous System

**Vinod Malhotra, M.B., B.S., M.D.,
F.A.C.A.**
Associate Professor, Department of
    Anesthesiology, Cornell University Medical
    College; Clinical Director of the Operating
    Rooms, Department of Anesthesiology, The
    New York Hospital–Cornell Medical Center,
    New York, New York
Extracorporeal Shock Wave Lithotripsy

John T. Martin, M.D.
Professor Emeritus, Department of
    Anesthesiology, Medical College of Ohio at
    Toledo, Toledo, Ohio
*Introduction; General Principles of Safe Positioning;
Lithotomy Positions; Head-Down Tilt; The Ventral
Decubitus (Prone) Positions; Geriatrics*

Frederick S. McAlpine, M.D.
Anesthesia Representative, Massachusetts Medical
    Malpractice Tribunal; Senior Staff
    Anesthesiologist (Retired), Lahey Hitchcock
    Medical Center, Burlington, Massachusetts
Peripheral Nervous System

D. Joseph Meyer, Jr., M.D., Ph.D.
Assistant Professor of Anesthesiology, University
    of Missouri School of Medicine, Columbia,
    Missouri
Lateral Positions

Leslie Newberg Milde, A.B., M.D.
Professor of Anesthesiology, Mayo Medical
    School, Rochester, Minnesota; Consultant in

Anesthesiology, Department of Anesthesiology, Mayo Clinic, Scottsdale, Arizona

The Head-Elevated Positions

David A. Nakata, M.D.

Assistant Professor of Anesthesia, Department of Anesthesia, Indiana University School of Medicine, Indianapolis, Indiana

Positioning the Extremities

Timothy J. O'Brien, M.D.

Senior Resident in Anesthesiology, Medical College of Wisconsin and Affiliated Hospitals, Milwaukee, Wisconsin

Physiologic Changes Associated with the Supine Position

William Clayton Petty, M.D.

Professor of Anesthesiology, Uniformed Services University of the Health Sciences, Bethesda, Maryland; Professor and Chairman, Department of Anesthesiology and Operative Service, Madigan Army Medical Center, Tacoma, Washington

Operating Tables and Their Attachments

Bradley E. Smith, M.D.

Professor of Anesthesiology, Vanderbilt University School of Medicine, Nashville, Tennessee

Obstetrics

Robert K. Stoelting, M.D.

Professor and Chair, Department of Anesthesia, Indiana University School of Medicine, Indianapolis, Indiana

Positioning the Extremities

Marjorie Sue Vaughan, M.S.N., Ph.D.

Clinical Assistant Professor, Departments of Obstetrics/Gynecology and Health Services Research, University of North Carolina, Chapel Hill, North Carolina

Pathologic Obesity

Robert W. Vaughan, M.D.

Professor, Department of Anesthesiology, School of Medicine, University of North Carolina, Chapel Hill, North Carolina

Pathologic Obesity

Mark A. Warner, M.D.

Professor, Department of Anesthesiology, Mayo Medical School, Rochester, Minnesota

Supine Positions; Positioning the Head and Neck

Mary Ellen Warner, M.D.

Assistant Professor of Anesthesiology, Mayo Medical School; Consultant, Department of Anesthesiology, Mayo Clinic, Rochester, Minnesota

Postanesthesia Care Unit Evaluation

Kenneth J. White, J.D., B.S.J.

Principal, Jacobson, Maynard, Tuschman & Kalur Co., L.P.A., Toledo, Ohio

Medicolegal Considerations

Foreword
to Third Edition

Position is defined as "a situation that confers advantage or preference." With correct patient positioning during anesthesia and surgery, both advantage *and* preference are achieved and the patient, surgeon, and anesthesiologist are all protected and well served. Nevertheless, infrequent complications do occur and there is always more to do and learn about patient safety. Success comes slowly in the elucidation of the obscure mechanisms underlying positioning complications. The course of discovery and the advancement of knowledge are commonly measured in decades. Progress is the resolution of unsolved problems, and it is this opportunity that makes medicine a satisfying profession that attracts those who wish to extend its frontiers.

Medical history will likely record the present era as one of great and rapid advances toward the understanding and prevention of complications. For more than three decades, the senior editor of this text has thoughtfully engaged in gathering anecdotal evidence correlating complications with patient positioning. Now the process has been advanced to the clinical science of epidemiology and outcome analysis. Its result will benefit future patients. Anesthesiologists and surgeons continue to learn from this growing experience, and, increasingly, this book is recognized as the authoritative text in the field.

The editors and authors are to be commended for this third edition of *Positioning in Anesthesia and Surgery*. In it, Dr. T. Martin has responded to the suggestions of reviewers of earlier editions and has tenaciously pursued a very important area of anesthesiologic practice, one too often neglected except by risk managers, patients, and their attorneys. To his great credit, Dr. Martin's interest in accumulating data in this area preceded the time when it has become fashionable among anesthesiologists to engage in risk management, continuous self-improvement, and analyses of outcome. The addition of Dr. M. A. Warner as the associate editor assures continuance of the work in a setting in which a large database is available to pursue answers to important questions about the consequences of patient positioning.

This new third edition of *Positioning in Anesthesia and Surgery* should hasten interest in the field, stimulate inquiry into the epidemiology of its problems, and improve the outlook for our patients.

ALAN D. SESSLER, M.D.
Professor of Anesthesiology
Mayo Medical School
Rochester, Minnesota

Foreword
to Second Edition

I am honored by being invited to write these introductory words for the second edition of *Positioning in Anesthesia and Surgery.*

When it appeared in 1978, the first edition of this text was the first comprehensive coverage of a subject that must be a primary concern of every competent surgeon and anesthesiologist. The popularity and wide usage of the first edition, plus the many problems of patient positioning related to recent developments in surgical interventions, have justified this second edition.

New operations often require special positioning of the patient in order to achieve optimum access to the anatomic target. Properly arranging the patient on the operating table, in conjunction with well balanced anesthesia, should facilitate the surgical procedure while allowing only minimal interference with respiration, circulation, and neurologic function.

Nerve paralyses following anesthesia were observed shortly after the advent of ether narcosis and were attributed by some to the toxic effects of the anesthetic agent. It was soon realized, however, that these injuries were associated with the position of the patient on the operating table.

Although numerous related articles were written around the year 1900 with adequate and detailed explanations of etiology, preventable injuries have continued to occur. It is the responsibility of both the surgeon and anesthesiologist to be alert to the need for proper positioning of the patient. The greatest deterrent to careless positioning has been the increased emphasis on professional liability.

In 1942, when Dr. Harvey Slocum and I established the Department of Anesthesiology at the University of Texas Medical Branch in Galveston, Texas, we became interested in the effects of extreme positioning, physiologic deficits, and neurovascular complications from malposition on the operating table. On physiologic analysis it became evident that some patients were going into shock, not because of the anesthetic and surgical procedures per se, but because of the physiologic distress that occurred when anesthetic depression and surgical trauma were superimposed upon respiratory and cardiovascular impairment produced by improperly positioning patients on operating tables.

In 1947 and 1948, we expressed our observations in two articles entitled *Circulatory and Respiratory Distress from Extreme Positions on the Operating Table* and *Neurovascular Complications from Malposition on the Operating Table.* In 1949, when I reviewed the requests for reprints of these articles, I noticed a significant interest by surgical colleagues, by patients with residual neurological deficits, and by plaintiffs' attorneys.

Patient welfare and surgical facility will always be major concerns of the competent anesthesiologist and although every anesthesiologist and every surgeon may not obtain a copy of this book on positioning, I am confident that you may find one in the library of most plaintiffs' attorneys.

CHARLES ROBERT ALLEN, M.D.
Professor Emeritus
Department of Anesthesiology
University of Texas Medical Branch
Galveston, Texas

Preface
to Third Edition

The second edition of *Positioning in Anesthesia and Surgery* followed the first edition by nine years. Another decade has now elapsed, and sufficient new information has been developed about the problems of patient positioning to warrant the appearance of this third edition. Widespread use of the second edition in medical curricula and medicolegal confrontations confirms the innovative opinion of Dr. J.A. Aldrete, one of the original contributors to this book, that collecting the widely dispersed, somewhat sparse, and principally anecdotal data about problems of positioning surgical patients would serve a useful purpose. The identification by Meranze and Wollman[1] of *Positioning* as one of the core volumes of an acceptable anesthesiologic library underscores its value.

This new edition is constructed around a format different from its predecessors. Initially each major topic was presented individually by both a surgeon and an anesthesiologist as a means of displaying varied opinions. Despite editorial efforts to minimize duplication of information without sacrificing individuality, enough repetition remained to draw criticism from several reviewers. The surgical chapters were altered little between the first and second editions. Informal surveys of surgeons in various areas of the United States have revealed that the problems of patient positioning receive little or no formal attention in the bulk of surgical training programs.[2] Therefore, to conserve space and permit the introduction of new material, the third edition has no chapters by surgeons. Important aspects of those deleted presentations have been assimilated in the anesthesiologic chapters, and the original essays are available to the serious student in library copies of the first and second editions as well as in specific surgical textbooks. The contributions of the surgical authors to the success of previous editions of *Positioning* are recognized with respect and appreciation.

After forty-plus years of special interest in the subject of patient positioning and two decades of preoccupation with this text, my lengthening retirement from clinical anesthesiology demands that someone else should assume a leadership role in this effort. Accordingly, I am honored and delighted that my long-time friend and former student, Mark A. Warner, M.D., a graduate of Medical College of Ohio at Toledo, and now Professor of Anesthesiology at Mayo Medical School, has agreed to become Co-Editor of the third edition. His recent publications in the field[3, 4] have used the massive database at the Mayo Clinic to introduce statistical assessment of outcomes into the folklore of patient positioning and to define important risk factors for the development of positioning complications. His team is now developing prospective protocols for the evaluation of complaints alleged to be derived from positioning, an advance that will indelibly improve patient safety as time passes. Should future editions of this text be needed, Dr. Warner has agreed to be the Editor.

As with the two previous editions, the illustrations for the third edition have been created by Mr. Roy E. Schneider, the talented medical illustrator at Medical College of Ohio at Toledo. Roy began his distinguished career by converting photographs into line drawings for the first edition. Subsequently, he has received degrees from the School of Fine Arts at the University of Toledo and from the School of Medical Illustration at the University of Michigan in Ann Arbor. His growing array of medical illustrations found in articles by the MCO faculty has gained admiring attention from a widening variety of extramural sources. In view of his disconcertingly busy schedule, Roy's continued participation in this text is a matter of great personal pride and satisfaction to me.

The staff of the Division of Medical Books at the W.B. Saunders Company has been graciously helpful throughout the process of development of this new edition. Particularly cooperative and encouraging have been Ms. Lesley Day, Medical Editor, and Ms. Lisette Bralow, Vice President and Editor-in-Chief of Medical Books. Their experience and guidance have offered clear perspectives and smoothed bumps along the way. Dr. Warner and I are indebted to them for their patience and friendship.

I am very appreciative of the considerable efforts of the contributors to the third edition. The enthusiasm that they displayed when they received invitations from Mark and me to participate in a new version of the book was heartwarming. As I did in previous editions, we extend a respectful "Thank You" to each member of their families. Their coopera-tion and support during the process of producing our individual manuscripts have been a major source of strength for each author. In particular, I recognize the significant assistance of Marion Martin, my tolerant wife of half of a century, who has offered humor and enthusiasm as well as the scholarly perspective of a critical manuscript reader to the preparation of all three editions of this text.

JOHN T. MARTIN
Toledo, Ohio, 1997

REFERENCES

1. Meranze J, Wollman H: Selected list of books and journals for an anesthesiology library. Anesthesiology 62:781, 1985.
2. Martin JT: Unpublished data.
3. Warner MA, Martin JT, Schroeder DR, Offord KP, Chute CG: Lower extremity motor neuropathy associated with surgery performed on patients in a lithotomy position. Anesthesiology 81:6, 1994.
4. Warner MA, Warner ME, Martin JT: Ulnar neuropathy: Incidence, outcome and risk factors in sedated or anesthetized patients. Anesthesiology, 81:1332, 1994.

Preface
to Second Edition

When the first edition of *Positioning in Anesthesia and Surgery* was being created prior to 1978, questions arose about the style of the format as well as the usefulness of the concept that authorships should involve multiple disciplines. Happily, the reception of the book has justified the expectations of its various parents. Both the English and the Spanish versions have found effective places in the libraries of institutions, practitioners, and students.

Much of the basic information in the original volume of "Positioning" has been retained and kept current. Nevertheless, the passage of time has generated and emphasized a need to consider additional categories of patient posture. Equally important is the responsibility to include information about the causes and characteristics of newly recognized complications. Previous contributors were asked to reevaluate their chapters and to revise them where appropriate. New authors have been selected to provide fresh inclusions or to replace those authors whose personal schedules precluded their current participation. We welcome their offerings.

To provide continuity of style, most of the artwork for this edition comes from a single source. Roy Schneider, an aspiring artist who was employed in the Housekeeping Department of the Medical College of Ohio Hospital, produced line drawings for parts of the first edition. Subsequently, Mr. Schneider has graduated from the School of Fine Arts of the University of Toledo and has earned the degree of Master of Arts in medical illustration from the University of Michigan. Now a member of our department of biomedical communications, he is the medical illustrator for the Medical College of Ohio and provides a valuable new resident skill for the faculty. His participation is reported with appreciation and admiration, as a significant asset to this new volume.

Finally, the last paragraph of the preface to the first edition must be repeated in spirit, if not verbatim. The tolerance and assistance of the family of each contributor have offered strength, inspiration, and freedom from distraction to the contributor during the often isolated absenteeism necessitated by the creative efforts behind these chapters. Without their families' admirable support, an activity of this nature would be impossible. We, as a group, salute them collectively and thank them individually.

JOHN T. MARTIN
Toledo, Ohio, 1987

Preface
to First Edition

Existing literature describing the requirements, techniques, and consequences of positioning a patient for surgery is sparse, widely scattered, and difficult to assemble. It is easily overlooked, but is of vital importance to all members of the anesthesia and surgical teams. Not uncommonly, proper selection of patient posture during surgery affects the surgeon's access to the pathology as well as the patient's tolerance to anesthetic drugs and physical stresses. Thus, a clear understanding of the subject should be available to each participant if a cooperative venture such as an efficient surgical operation is to succeed.

This text addresses the task of collecting, correlating, and displaying the various fragments of knowledge about surgical positioning in a manner convenient to student, house officer, practicing physician, surgical nurse, and technician. Both surgeons and anesthesiologists have been assembled as authors, and the viewpoints represented are diverse enough to display a desirable spectrum of opinion. Techniques for establishing positions are included as suggestions and as points of departure for improvisation that will improve the patient's lot.

"Positioning" had its origins as a book early in this decade (1970s), but combinations of circumstances have produced changes of editors and style and have delayed its emergence. Credit for major portions of its evolution is due to J. Antonio Aldrete, M.D., now Professor and Chairman of the Department of Anesthesiology at the University of Colorado, and to Robert H. Smith, M.D., retired Professor of Anesthesiology at the University of California at San Francisco. Appreciation is extended to Mr. Brian C. Decker and his staff at the W. B. Saunders Company for patiently and effectively developing solutions for the various problems that emerged during the protracted incubation of this volume. Key to the eventual culmination of all of our efforts has been the admirable secretarial support of Mrs. Muriel Sindyla in the Department of Anesthesiology at the Medical College of Ohio at Toledo.

But perhaps the most meaningful contribution, meriting the most special kind of "Thank You" from each contributor, has been that of our families, who have suffered with understanding and tolerance the distractions involved in creating a durable, factual medical communication.

JOHN T. MARTIN
Toledo, Ohio, 1978

Contents

Chapter 20
Postanesthesia Care Unit Evaluation 319
Mary E. Warner

Chapter 21
Medicolegal Considerations 329
Kenneth J. White

Index 335

General Considerations

Chapter 1

Introduction

John T. Martin

BACKGROUND

Before World War II only sporadic attention was paid to disturbances in body function that were caused by positions in which the patient was placed during surgery. A thoughtful account of the effects of body position on anesthesia was published by Dutton as early as 1933.[1] However, useful interest in the subject stems from the landmark articles by Slocum and Allen and their associates at the University of Texas, Medical Branch, in Galveston. In carefully documented observations, they related circulatory and respiratory distress[2] and neurovascular complications[3] to malpositioning of the patient during anesthesia and surgery. Subsequent reviews by Henschel and associates,[4] Little,[5] Lincoln and Sawyer,[6] Britt and Gordon,[7] Courington and Little,[8] and Coonan and Hope[9] have assembled and further clarified information on this persistently consequential subject.

THE ISSUE

The term *surgical posture* denotes the body position in which a patient is placed during an operation. It serves the single purpose of offering to the surgeon the maximum acceptable access to the anatomic target. However, a specific surgical posture is sometimes less than optimum for either the surgeon or the patient. Access to the surgical target may be compromised by a patient's painful spine, excessive body bulk, or brittle physiology. Posture that compromises good exposure of the operative site usually prolongs and complicates a surgical procedure. Posture that exceeds the limits of a patient's tolerance may inflict physiologic dysfunction or physical injury on its victim. In both situations the patient suffers. When that suffering involves recognizable physical injury, legal entanglements may arise to the discomfort of the responsible physicians.

The paucity of objective signs of pain under anesthesia often allows (1) a patient to be placed in positions that would be intolerable when awake and (2) surgery to be continued beyond the limits of postural tolerance. Emphasizing the latter point, Brown and Elman[10] showed postoperative backache to be a function of the duration of surgery rather than of the type of anesthetic used. A posture that minimizes respiratory embarrassment may compromise the circulatory system and vice versa. Therefore, it is clearly within the province of the vigilant anesthesiologist to (1) participate in the selection and establishment of surgical postures, (2) evaluate the continuing effects of positioning on the dynamic physiology of the patient, and (3) advise and assist the surgeon in devising acceptable postural modifications that protect the patient while allowing the operation to be accomplished. A careful preanesthetic evaluation of a potentially compromising surgical posture may sometimes reveal the need for an alternate selection.

PERSPECTIVES

Outlining specific techniques for establishing surgical postures can be "cookbookish." Potentially, the practice implies that the reader will accept the presentation as the definitive standard for that maneuver, condemn all other alternatives, and attempt to enforce compliance thereto. Such an interpretation we neither intend nor support. An assessment of the available literature would reveal multiple instances in which experienced and responsible authors disagree about the best ways to achieve physiologically satisfactory surgical postures. One description and illustration of the kidney position in an older anesthesiology text has advocated exactly the kidney rest arrangement that most of us have long regarded as the classic example of the wrong way to establish the posture.[11] Fortunately, not all areas of disagreement are as overt.

We recognize, and specifically state, that the opinions expressed on these pages represent the acquired experience of the individual contributors and are not intended as rules or standards from which there can be no deviations. In fact, at several points the authors have deliberately chosen the often-shunned first person singular style of writing in an effort to convey information without setting standards. Our purpose is to assemble presentations that we believe to be responsibly representative of widely held opinions about the attributes and consequences of surgical postures.

The earlier editions of this book have considered anecdotes regarding the effects of positioning, either as individual case reports or as compilations thereof, from which useful general conclusions about patient care can be drawn. Unfortunately, the literature has also contained the occasional poorly drawn conclusion, based on faulty or misinterpreted evidence, that has received vigorous support, has been rarely questioned, and has not been modified or abandoned as reliable information to the contrary has accumulated. Walter Canon's espousal of head-down tilt to treat "shock" is an example.[12] Curiously, and probably because of the fervor with which the practice had been adopted by the profession, his later repudiation of that belief attracted little attention.

With the maturation of the computer age, however, anecdotal information is becoming less substantial. We are beginning to be provided with investigations that can adequately examine huge databases of information about perioperative events. An early example is the retrospective data of Warner and associates[13, 14] that permit the assembly of statistics about risk factors. Clinical experiences and laboratory investigations of the past decade have aided clinicians in developing insight into the unfortunate consequences of the additive effects of minor, expectedly inconsequential, neural trauma occurring in the presence of existing, unsuspected subclinical neuropathies (see Chapter 11).

Accumulated clinical experience has indicated that the information assembled in this text is applicable to an extensive variety of problems in surgical positioning of patients of all ages with minimal compromise of surgical access and with little probability of risk to the physiques and physiologies of the subjects. However, the practice of medicine continues to be an imprecise art that is devoid of absolutes. Whereas meticulous adherence to inherently safe routines will minimize opportunities for the appearance of unexpected problems, there is no guarantee of their complete absence. And every potential problem cannot be avoided by techniques that are generalized rather than individualized. With more intense evaluations of outcomes of patient care, future editions of this volume promise to be even more helpful in protecting our patients.

REFERENCES

1. Dutton AC: The effects of posture during anesthesia. Anesth Analg 12:66, 1933.
2. Slocum HC, Hoeflich EA, Allen CR: Circulatory and respiratory distress from extreme positions on the operating table. Surg Gynecol Obstet 84:1051, 1947.
3. Slocum HC, O'Neal KC, Allen CR: Neurovascular complications from malposition on the operating table. Surg Gynecol Obstet 86:729, 1948.
4. Henschel AB, Wyant GM, Dobkin AB, Henschel EO: Posture as it concerns the anesthesiologist: A preliminary study. Anesth Analg 36:69, 1957.
5. Little DM Jr: Posture and anesthesia. Can Anaesth Soc J 7:2, 1960.
6. Lincoln JR, Sawyer HP: Complications related to body positions during surgical procedures. Anesthesiology 22:800, 1961.
7. Britt BA, Gordon RA: Peripheral nerve injuries associated with anaesthesia. Can Anaesth Soc J 11:514, 1964.
8. Courington FW, Little DM Jr: The role of posture in anesthesia. Clin Anesth 3:24, 1968.
9. Coonan TJ, Hope CE: Cardiorespiratory effects of changes of body position. Can Anaesth Soc J 30:424, 1983.
10. Brown EM, Elman DS: Postoperative backache. Anesth Analg 40:683, 1961.
11. Collins VJ: Principles of Anesthesiology, 12th ed. Philadelphia, Lea & Febiger, 1976.
12. Porter WT: Shock at the front. Boston Med Surg J 175:854, 1916.
13. Warner MA, Martin JT, Schroeder DR, et al.: Lower extremity motor neuropathy associated with surgery performed on patients in a lithotomy position. Anesthesiology 81:6–12, 1994.
14. Warner MA, Warner ME, Martin JT: Ulnar neuropathy: Incidence, outcome and risk factors in sedated or anesthetized patients. Anesthesiology 81:1332, 1994.

General Principles of Safe Positioning

J o h n T. M a r t i n

BACKGROUND

Fundamental considerations about safe positioning can be related to the number and type of procedures done in a given surgical suite.

In large, busy institutions with reasonably constant anesthesiologic and surgical personnel, the pressure of heavy schedules requires creative teamwork to develop routines that minimize wasted time. Repetition brings educated familiarity and, with it, continuity in method and equipment. New procedures, or deviations from a basic pattern, are usually carefully introduced, and lapses in techniques are evident and correctable. Although critics might label these institutions "assembly lines" or "factories," their methodology has often provided outstanding success and safety. However, for many reasons, their techniques may not be applicable elsewhere.

By contrast, smaller facilities, with more variable case loads and major temporal inconsistencies in skill levels within the teams, may be unable to routinize less frequent procedures. Problems may be avoided only if one knowledgeable person assumes strict control of the functions of the entire team. Presuming that unusual tasks are well understood may be folly in such a setting, and only with careful training and rehearsing can materiel be assured and safe techniques be developed. An understanding of these requirements should lower morbidity and mortality statistics to the benefit of both the institution and its patients. Within this framework, specific attention given to proper positioning of the surgical patient should be demonstrably beneficial.

COMPONENTS OF SAFE POSITIONING

Knowledge, planning, teamwork, and *housekeeping*, all equally important, are the key ingredients of safe positioning of a surgical patient upon an operating table. As trite and pompous as identifying these components may seem, ignoring or being casual about any of them can easily render the care team inept, bring harm to the patient, and endanger the institution.

Knowledge

Knowledge implies theoretical and practical understanding of the general principles of arranging the posture of a patient, either unconscious or awake, for a particular operation. Specifically, this knowledge involves an appreciation of the consequences of improper or incomplete attention to the petty details of the positions involved.

Planning

Planning encompasses an understanding of the intended operation as well as of the specific problems that face either the surgeon or the anesthesiologist. Close cooperation among all members of the surgical team is an issue of overriding and inescapable importance.

Competent planning affords each team member an opportunity to assemble the necessary equipment and to know the order of procedure. Because a specific operation must be individualized to the needs of that particular patient, the major source of the necessary procedural information, and the person most heavily responsible for its dissemination, is the surgeon. The surgeon must, however, consider the problems of all team members in the planning and must help mold all into a thoughtful and cooperative working unit. For the anesthesiologist, a careful preanesthetic evaluation of the patient is a necessity.

Teamwork

Teamwork is built on having a sufficient number of personnel present to effect the patient positioning required, on having each team member either skilled or guided in the assigned duties, and on carefully coordinating the activities of those involved. Acceptable communication among team members is an inescapable necessity. Although there is no substitute for experience, there is also no excuse for avoiding "dry runs" that prove methods and train personnel should the team itself or specific members be new to critical parts of the task.

Housekeeping

Housekeeping, the most mundane aspect of safety, includes having present the devices needed for patient positioning and assuring that each part fits and functions. Once the patient is asleep and in the process of being positioned, it is too late to discover that the table will not flex, that it has no radiographic top, or that its hydraulic system is defective. Acquiring, storing, and maintaining in functional condition the various pieces of equipment needed for modern surgical procedures are costly, space-occupying, and labor-intensive endeavors. Nevertheless, either ignoring these responsibilities or accomplishing them in a haphazard fashion presents potentially life-threatening problems for the patient.

POSITIONING RESPONSIBILITY

Litigation alleging complications from patient posture during an operation frequently provokes the question of who is responsible for positioning the patient. Although responsibilities may vary between institutions, operating

suites, and surgical practices, the most comprehensive and accurate answer is "we are." That response indicates that patient positioning is a cooperative function of the operating room team. The surgeon needs to provide uncomplicated surgery. The anesthesiologist must safely anesthetize and recover the patient. Surgical nursing personnel are involved because of their responsibility to provide equipment that works.

- In some practices the surgeon assumes all of the responsibility for patient positioning, is present throughout the process, and attends personally to all of the details.
- Frequently, the anesthesiologist, knowing the intricacies of the planned procedure and the frailties of the patient, assists in positioning the patient and supervises the process before the arrival of the surgeon. In some circumstances the anesthesia care team may have full responsibility for patient positioning.
- Rarely, and probably inappropriately, positioning an anesthetized patient is left to the devices of one of the surgical nursing personnel. Although such an arrangement may be an institutional habit, it cannot be encouraged because it implies inadequate supervision. Rarely does it relieve either the surgeon or the anesthesiologist from responsibility for postural misadventures.

PERIANESTHETIC EVALUATIONS

Postural factors influence the safe conduct of a patient through an anesthetic and surgical experience in important ways, making the evaluation of potential positioning problems a vital component of the preanesthetic interview.

- Obviously, before any useful assessment of the situation with the patient can be made, the gross intentions of the surgical procedure should be known to the anesthesiologist.
- A careful inquiry should be made into positioning problems that have accompanied previous surgical procedures for the patient in question.
- Orthopnea from extreme obesity or unrelenting cardiac failure indicates the probability of ventilation and perfusion problems if the supine position is chosen or head-down tilt is demanded.

- Major increases of abdominal girth, such as seen with massive obesity, a large intra-abdominal tumor, or the late stages of pregnancy, signal that the intended prone position should be abandoned in favor of an alternative posture such as the lateral decubitus position.
- Assessing the sleeping habits or work preferences of a patient may reveal that arms cannot be placed overhead without activating a thoracic outlet syndrome that distorts the neurovascular bundle enough to produce arm pain and numbness.
- Seeking the tolerable limits of neck motion in a patient with a symptomatic protrusion of a cervical intervertebral disk helps estimate the potential for serious consequences to cervical nerve roots or the spinal cord from head extension during endotracheal intubation and neck surgery or because of head rotation when pronated.

Depending on the circumstances involved, positional problems discovered at the preanesthetic visit may need to be discussed with the patient or a responsible family member. In the record of the visit, findings that influence choices of positioning should be described succinctly, but in a careful and obvious manner. If the possibility exists of future litigation in which positional complications may be alleged, a careful description of the problem, together with deliberate documentation of perianesthetic protective measures, is usually effective in thwarting subsequent claims of negligence should complications occur despite the use of deliberate or unusual care.

In the preanesthetic holding area, as well as in the operating room, an opportunity exists to evaluate or recheck postural limitations before a patient is anesthetized. In unusual circumstances, and with patient cooperation that has been elicited by careful preliminary explanations, an attempt can be made to place the patient in the intended surgical posture to determine its suitability.

- An example is the patient who has chronic leg pain from a protruding intervertebral disk and who must have a uterine dilatation and curettage to treat bleeding. Placing her in the planned variety of lithotomy position before anesthesia can identify her tolerance for the posture, permit appropriate modifications thereof, probably avoid stress to the lumbar spine

during postinduction positioning that could exacerbate her pain postoperatively, and allow a comfortable support to be developed for her lumbar area (see Chapter 6).

Fortunately, precautions such as these are rarely indicated, but their potential assets should not be overlooked when appropriate.

Postanesthetic visits, whether in the postanesthesia care unit, an intensive care unit, or subsequently at the patient's hospital bed, are well-established sources of information about problems alleged to have been incurred during anesthesia and surgery (see Chapter 20). Because it serves their best interests, litigants frequently assert that the onset of symptoms allegedly due to a positioning problem occurred immediately on recovery from anesthesia despite the fact that the nursing records and doctors' notes contain no mention of the complaint until days later. A patient's conversational report of problems should be carefully evaluated, as should descriptions in the notes of care providers. Casual and unsupported comments by personnel who subsequently attend the alleged complications have been key factors in deciding liability. Careful record keeping during the procedure in question is strong protection against subsequent misinterpretation of events.

The acquired experience of the care team may also help identify potential problems with a given patient. Positioning complications should be added to quality assurance reviews in the same manner as are other concerns. Innovative techniques used to avoid recurrences of patient injury should be documented and widely disseminated.

Because an alleged impairment may be easily evident to lay observers, juries tend to be sympathetic to such claims. The resulting monetary awards have contributed heavily to the high cost of professional liability insurance. *Succinct documentation of methods used to minimize the potential for positioning complications is an inescapable primary responsibility of the care team.* Although some purists may scoff at such a stipulation as "defensive medicine," a more realistic and logical attitude is in the best interests of patient and physician alike.

IMPLICATIONS OF ILLNESS AND TRANSPORT

Important influences on the patient's ability to tolerate subsequent postural stresses may have begun while still in bed in the hospital room. Chobanian and associates[1] studied the metabolic and hemodynamic effects of prolonged (2 to 3 weeks) bed rest on six normal subjects. They noted negative sodium and potassium balances, reduced plasma volumes, and, when a subject was tilted to 70 degrees upright, exaggerated responses of heart rate, stroke volume, cardiac output, and peripheral resistance. If one contemplates the addition of these electrolyte and vasomotor instabilities to the expected consequences of disease or injury, the fragility of the balance mechanisms of a critically ill patient becomes easily understandable.

Rough handling of a patient can occur during shifting from bed to cart, in transport through halls and elevators to the operating suite, and on transfer from cart to operating table. The consequences can be nausea, vomiting, hypotension, confusion, severe anxiety, and even unconsciousness. Because patients are infrequently monitored during preoperative movement, few data exist regarding responses of vital signs and systems to these stresses. However, the resulting homeostatic instability may delay, complicate, or make unwise the induction of anesthesia. It may produce unanticipated intolerance to drastic surgical procedures and may even require that the operation itself be either postponed or abandoned completely. Wheelchairs, historically used to transport medicated patients to an unattended holding point within the operating suite, are now almost completely replaced by comfortable, versatile wheeled carts on which the patients can rest supine under supervision. As a result, in current practice we rarely see an incident that I encountered 40 years ago: a debilitated, heavily premedicated elderly patient, seated in a wheelchair in a poorly attended waiting area of the surgical suite, became comatose and developed positive Babinski signs due to insufficient cerebral perfusion. Nevertheless, the potential for these adversities strongly advocates careful preanesthetic surveillance of every patient. In particular, critically ill patients should be monitored during transport to encourage optimal physiologic stability when compensatory mechanisms are impaired. The posture in which a patient is placed during or after transport should be carefully selected according to the build, general condition, and reaction of each individual.

Little[2] has stressed the importance of careful manipulation of the patient in preserving homeostasis under anesthesia. He demonstrated that a rapid change from the lithotomy position to the supine position could bring about a fall in blood pressure (140/80 to 86/58 mm Hg) that had only partly recovered (to 122/76 mm Hg) 2 minutes later. If that postural change was subsequently repeated slowly after that same patient had regained vascular stability, it could be accomplished without a significant variation in blood pressure.

Movement of a patient from an operating table to a recovery bed or a cart can sometimes be disruptive, particularly if the team is hurrying to accommodate subsequent patients in the same operating room. The patient must be moved gently and by enough team members to allow proper weight distribution without injury to the handlers. Being bounced across the edge of the operating table to the adjacent cart can provoke not only decompensated perfusion but also physical injuries to the head, neck, back, and extremities. Planned use of draw sheets and body rollers, together with vigilance regarding arms, vascular lines, and monitors, promotes safe patient handling in almost any circumstance.

- A disposable body roller can be constructed by cutting away the bottom seam of a large (39 gallon or larger) unopened plastic trash bag. The resulting flattened tube is placed longitudinally under the patient's draw sheet so that it extends beyond the width of the table and onto the adjacent cart. With the use of the draw sheet, the patient can be pulled gently off of the table onto the wheeled conveyance with the slippery approximated surfaces of the trash bag rolling as an endless belt to lubricate the move.
- Mechanical patient movers and removable operating table tops have been made available from time to time but do not seem to have achieved widespread use.

THE SURGICAL TABLE

Peculiarities and potential hazards of the surgical table and its various controls should be kept firmly in mind (see Chapter 3). Tables with which the members of the surgical team are not familiar should receive a careful and detailed trial of their controls before being used. Newer models of certain tables now have tops that move horizontally in reference to their fixed pedestals. This capability improves access for the C-shaped camera arm of the portable fluoroscope. However, it also offers the possibility of shifting of the weight of a massively obese patient far enough away from the center of gravity of the table to cause the entire unit to tilt toward the floor. The disaster potential of such an occurrence is obvious.

Lateral table edges should be padded to minimize the potential for compression of nerves, vessels, tendons, and other vital structures that may rest firmly against them. All parts of the patient need to be electrically insulated from metal projections of the table. If postoperative gait impairment is to be avoided, the patient's feet should not be allowed to extend far enough beyond the caudal end of the table to compress the Achilles tendon. Fingers should be protected from table hinges.[3] Restraining straps, used to limit postural shifts when the table's attitude is altered, must be clean, intact, and placed so that damage to underlying bony prominences or neurovascular bundles will not occur. Straps should not be allowed to compromise chest expansion. Chest rolls, upon which the patient lies to free the abdomen from dorsad pressure, must be of proper length (subclavicle to pelvis) and be fixed to the contralateral edge of the table; if they shift subtly during surgery, their usefulness can be lost in an insidious, unrecognizable, and destructive manner.

Armboards are a source of both major comfort and persistent annoyance. Either padded or unpadded, they have been associated with postoperative nerve dysfunction thought to be due to compression of accessible nerve trunks. Despite the best intentions of a care team, postoperative neuropathies have not been eliminated (see Chapter 11).

- During an upper abdominal procedure a surgical team of many members may crowd an armboard cephalad sufficiently to reposition the arm into unwanted and dangerous hyperabduction. A resulting brachial plexus injury can be a tragic by-product of an otherwise successful operation.
- Two-tiered ("airplane") armboards can assist in stabilizing the patient who is in a lateral decubitus position. However, they require close attention to assure the adequacy of padding and the absence of frame pressure on the up-side axilla, the down-side arm, or the ventral chest. Trac-

tion on the up-side arm that could stretch the brachial plexus must be avoided. Plexus traction is also possible when a torso that has been stabilized in the lateral decubitus position shifts while the up-side arm is affixed to a bar or "ether screen" that is attached to the table.

When the arms need to be placed along the sides of the patient, care must be taken to stabilize intravascular lines and Doppler monitors. Lowry and co-workers[4] described the use of a tape carton or mailing tube as a circumferential arm shield for infants. The metal, toboggan-shaped Wells Arm Protector (Mercury Enterprises, North Clearwater, FL) slides under the mattress of the operating table to serve as a useful guard for the blood pressure cuff when an adult's arm is restrained alongside the trunk rather than abducted upon an armboard. Readings from an unprotected blood pressure cuff often reflect the variable pressure of the surgeon leaning upon it rather than indicating the patient's vascular pressure within the encircled arm.

A potentially dangerous part of the operating table is the elevatable bar at the middle of the table known as the "kidney rest" or "gallbladder rest." Several decades ago this attachment was routinely arranged under the supine patient at the approximate level of the first lumbar vertebra and cranked up to arch the patient's back. Supposedly, the maneuver improved exposure of the gallbladder area; however, it actually impaired ventilation, dangerously contorted the thoracolumbar spine, and threatened venous return by decreasing the caliber of the inferior vena cava that had been elongated by the arched back. Many dedicated anesthesiologists vigorously opposed the use of the gallbladder rest, believing it to be a serious threat to the physical safety of the patient. In some institutions they deliberately broke its controls. Operative cholangiography changed the concept of exposing right upper quadrant organs by demanding a flat table top for successful radiography. It taught most surgical teams that the elevated gallbladder rest was unnecessary. If flank extension in the supine position is needed, it can be accomplished by inserting several folded towels under the ipsilateral dorsal costal margin, thereby facilitating useful exposure without the structural violence of the gallbladder rest.

Currently, use of the elevatable transverse bar ("kidney rest") has reappeared as a means of arching the back of a patient whose retropubic area must be approached via a laparotomy (see Hyperlordotic Position, Chapter 8, and Fig. 8–5). With the trunk and thigh sections of the table surface angulated floorward as far as possible at their common hinge (forming a modified A-frame), the lumbar spine of the supine patient is placed over the apex of the angulation. The elevatable rest can then be raised to further exaggerate the already excessive lumbar lordosis. Adjustment of the table chassis will then lower the head of the patient to improve surgical access by moving viscera cephalad in the laparotomy incision. Thus the potential for lumbar spine distress from forced hyperlordosis has returned to the spectrum of potential positioning complications.

When the rest is used to augment lateral flexion in the kidney position, it should be raised against the down-side iliac crest and should not compress the soft tissues of the adjacent flank (see Chapter 9). Positioned cephalad to the crest, the rest restricts or actually immobilizes the down-side diaphragm, impairs ventilation, and may injure the twelfth rib.

For discussions of problems associated with various leg holders for the lithotomy position, see Chapters 3 and 6.

PROTECTIVE PADDING

Little has been written about the use of padding to protect a patient from undue pressure on vulnerable areas of the body. Because the issue seems susceptible to common sense, few authors have bothered to comment on what they consider to be the obvious. Illustrations in previous editions of this text, as well as those in other books, often have intentionally omitted the display of pads and padding that would partially obscure key points of the figures. Litigation has implied that many consider padding body parts not to be a subject meriting serious discussion. If this is true at all, such an attitude disappears when the concept becomes a major component of allegations of positioning complications suffered by a patient in whose care they participated.

Padding bony prominences is intended to disperse the pressure of a mechanical support, either the operating table surface, its edges, or one of its attachments, over a wider area of body surface and allow more nearly normal function of tissues at the points of contact. Emaciated or gnarled physiques are often susceptible to compressive forces in various areas of their skeletons that would not exist with more normal body contours. Padding can be used to align their skeletal parts in a more conventional manner or to support distorted areas that do not fit standard equipment. Neuropathies and decubitus ulcerations can result if attention is not paid to protective padding, even though padding does not guarantee the absence of problems.[5]

Historically, padding used to protect pressure points of patients positioned for anesthesia and surgery consisted of operating table mattresses, pillows, blankets, towels, and cotton batting. The batting was disposable after use, but reusable items were either scrubbed with soap products or laundered to remove contaminants. After World War II plastic materials began to appear in a wide variety of compositions and forms. Many were compressible but had excellent memories of their original shapes; consequently, they were useful as padding with which to diffuse and reduce focal pressure of the weight of a body part against a supporting surface. In addition to its native flexibility, compressible plastic foam of varying densities can be cut to shape as needed. Some types are marketed as sheets with one sticky surface that permits them to be stacked in a stable manner. Tissue sensitivity reactions to chemical components of the various plastics have developed in some patients, but the general acceptance of plastic foam padding has been excellent. Disposability permits its use in the presence of severe wound contamination.

Padding Tables and Attachments

Soft multisection mattresses that adhere by fabric locks onto the metal surfaces of operating tables are now standard parts of all surgical tables. However, table attachments, such as extremity supports and torso retainers, are usually constructed of metal that ensures durability and sanitation. Many are purchased with specially preformed, fitted and reusable pads. When that individualized padding is not available, the devices need to be well padded to prevent electrical grounding burns from stray currents as well as to distribute their contact pressure to wider areas of the patient's physique. Whereas a single towel in a metal knee crutch may prevent grounding burns, it is not sufficient to diffuse pressure. The compressible plastic foam that has one surface multiply indented in a manner similar to that of an egg carton (and known jargonistically as "egg crate") provides both insulation and padding and is a more logical choice for protecting extremities and other body surfaces from focal pressures of the table system. Folded sheeting rolled around supporting rods and taped securely in place offers similar protection for an arm retained by an over-the-table bar.

Body Parts That Need Padding

Particularly susceptible to positioning pressure insults over time are the following:

- The occiput of a supine patient
- The down-side eye and ear of a patient in a lateral position or a pronated patient whose head is rotated to rest on the down side (see Fig. 10–1)
- The elbow and its cubital tunnel of a patient in any one of the dorsal decubitus positions (see Fig. 19–2), in a lateral decubitus position (principally the up-side upper extremity), or pronated with arms alongside the head (see Fig. 10–1)
- The side of the perineal pelvis against which traction will be applied to realign fragments of a fractured femur with a patient on a fracture table (see Fig. 6–6)
- The knees of a kneeling prone patient (see Fig. 10–9)
- The down-side aspects of either lower extremity of a patient in a lateral decubitus position (particularly the area of the common peroneal nerve as it courses laterally around the head of the down-side fibula) (see Fig. 9–1)
- The heels of a patient in any one of the dorsal decubitus positions

Despite meticulous attention by members of the care team, lesions that are assumed to have been produced by pressure have appeared even in the presence of padding.[5] Although its use does not guarantee the absence of compressive injury, not providing padding that attempts to safeguard body parts from undue pressure can be interpreted as either gross carelessness or willful neglect of an implied duty to the patient. When the patient is small in stature or has a physique that is distorted by injury or disease and, as a result, does not fit the available positioning devices in the accustomed manner, padding should be carefully provided with the assumption that it is beneficial and protective.

REPOSITIONING THE PATIENT DURING ANESTHESIA

While awake, a healthy individual rapidly regulates systemic blood pressure and tissue perfusion by pressoreceptor reflexes. If the reflex is initiated by increased pressure in the carotid sinuses, aortic arch, pulmonary arteries, and major vessels cephalad to the heart, impulses ascend to inhibit the medullary vasoconstrictor center and excite the vagus nerve. The results are peripheral vasodilation, decreased heart rate, and reduced myocardial contractility.[6] Failing systemic pressure has the opposite result as the body seeks homeostasis. When mean arterial pressure falls to levels below 50 mm Hg, central nervous system ischemia produces a powerful sympathomimetic response that may sacrifice peripheral perfusion to preserve cerebral blood flow.[6] With arterial pressures in the range of 40 to 80 mm Hg systolic, the carotid and aortic chemoreceptors may sense hypoxia and cause a reflex elevation of blood pressure.[6]

In the presence of disease, injury, and anesthesia, postural changes that would not normally elicit stress are able to cause significant decreases in both arterial pressure and tissue perfusion. Hypovolemia can often be judged in the emergency department by the magnitude of hypotension and tachycardia imposed by varied degrees of head-up tilt. Drug depression blunts or accentuates these changes depending on the type and concentration of drug involved. Sympatholysis, a familiar and often intentional concomitant of many anesthetic agents and techniques, can also compromise normal vascular homeostasis.

Many patients are subjected to postural changes shortly after the induction of anesthesia. Except for a physical injury, the major hazard of repositioning relates to hypotension. As noted, compensatory mechanisms in the brain stem and myocardium are disrupted in direct proportion to the concentration of the anesthetic agents, the deficit in circulatory volume present, the reduced vigor of the patient, and the clumsiness of the posture change. Minimal levels of anesthesia, adequate volume repletion, and unhastened, gentle manipulation of the patient's body are mandatory components of any effort to establish a given new surgical posture after the start of an anesthetic.

Frequent blood pressure determinations

throughout a change in patient posture are the key indicators of its safety.

- Frequently, a minimally anesthetized patient will become somewhat hypertensive during a position change, probably as a result of tracheal and joint stimulation during the maneuver. When the cardiovascular system is placed at risk by the increased blood pressure, added analgesia, careful use of vasodilator drugs, or judicious increases in the concentrations of the anesthetic usually permit successful completion of the postural readjustment.
- If hypotension is encountered, the change in position should be delayed until normotension has been restored by an appropriate decrease in anesthetic concentration, a fluid challenge, or careful vasopressor therapy. Because most vasopressors constrict small vessels throughout the body rather than selectively in certain vascular beds, many anesthesiologists prefer to make their judicious use a last-resort therapy to be available when less anesthetic and more fluids do not correct the situation.
- When significant portions of the body are to be rendered dependent enough to promote vascular pooling and decreased venous return (e.g., the legs in either the flexed lateral or in the prone jackknife position) or are to be elevated above heart level (e.g., the lithotomy, head high, or head low positions), the new position must be established slowly enough to maintain useful blood pressure readings throughout. The same is true of the return to the horizontal supine position at the end of the surgical procedure.

If systemic perfusion cannot be sustained in the desired posture, changes must be made in either the conduct of the anesthetic or the volume of circulating blood until pressure stability is achieved. Should these maneuvers not be capable of restoring vascular stability, the position must be compromised toward a more safely tolerated alternative.

Lawson's group[7] called attention to occipital alopecia as a poorly recognized complication of cardiopulmonary bypass. Subsequently, it has been seen in prolonged use of the supine position without bypass. Apparently caused by sustained pressure on hair follicles that are compressed between the skull and the mattress, local hypoperfusion and hypo-thermia may contribute to the problem. Turning the head from one side to the other at least every 30 minutes is said to be preventive.[7] In some instances, the alopecia became permanent and was more annoying than the surgery itself.

Postural changes made later in the course of anesthetic administration or at the termination of surgery can easily be more threatening to homeostasis than was establishment of the original surgical position. Acquired but unrecognized blood volume deficits, hypothermia, electrolyte imbalances, changes in levels of spinal or epidural anesthesia, or suddenly inefficient cardiac rhythms are detrimental to circulatory stability. These abnormalities must be corrected before any change in position or their effects must be combated by judicious use of vasoactive drugs. As the supine posture is re-established before the termination of anesthesia, major changes are possible in the balance between the distribution of blood volume (head-down tilt changed to supine) and the capacity of the circulatory space (lithotomy position changed to supine). Sudden hypotension can occur despite previously consistent perfusion. If the rate of postural change is slowed and frequent blood pressure determinations are made, the appearance of hypotension can be more promptly detected and its duration minimized. When surgery must be continued subsequent to the position change, reducing the concentration of the anesthetic agent sufficiently to prevent or treat hypotension may not be practical. Sympathomimetic drugs, as well as intravascular volume adjustments, may again be necessary to support perfusion.

REFERENCES

1. Chobanian AV, Lile RD, Tercyak A, Blevins P: The metabolic and hemodynamic effects of prolonged bed rest in normal subjects. Circulation 69:551, 1974.
2. Little DM Jr: Posture and anaesthesia. Can Anaesth Soc J 7:2, 1960.
3. Courington FW: The role of posture in anesthesia. Clin Anesth 3:24, 1968.
4. Lowry RL, Lichti EL, Eggers GWN Jr: The Doppler: An aid in monitoring blood pressure during anesthesia. Anesth Analg 52:531, 1973.
5. Kroll DA, Caplan RA, Posner K, et al.: Nerve injury associated with anesthesia. Anesthesiology 73:202, 1990.
6. Guyton AC: Textbook of Medical Physiology. Philadelphia, WB Saunders, 1976.
7. Lawson NW, Mills NL, Ochsner JL: Occipital alopecia following cardiopulmonary bypass. J Thorac Cardiovasc Surg 71:342, 1976.

Chapter 3

Operating Tables and Their Attachments

William Clayton Petty

BACKGROUND

Wars have been the major source of injuries requiring surgical intervention since the advent of man's existence. At first, the earth served as an operating table. Later, as surgical procedures became more common and more complicated, the patient was elevated to the level of the surgeon's waist to improve visibility and lessen fatigue. Flat rocks, planks, doors, and other fabricated level surfaces held up by a variety of legs and bases have served as operating tables throughout the centuries.

The simple wooden table with detachable wooden trestle legs served many armies as they roamed the world in quest of power and wealth. For 1500 years dislocations and fractures were reduced on a scamnum or "luxation" table that was originally described by Hippocrates.[1] The scamnum table was a simple "thick wooden rectangular board with levers attached to stout posts, to which the patient was firmly tied. The operator then pulled the affected limb into position by means of various levers."[1]

Ambroise Paré, in the 16th century, described a wooden operating table with a back rest and a dressing bowl.[1] A separate room for surgical operating was probably introduced in hospitals in the late eighteenth century. Tables in operating rooms in the first half of the nineteenth century were wooden with an angled back rest, two steel foot rests,

and a box of sawdust underneath to catch the blood and pus. Until the advent of anesthesia in 1846, operations were very quick, rarely exceeding 10 minutes, and almost always were done as a desperate attempt to preserve life. Anesthesia enormously expanded the horizons of surgery. As surgical techniques improved and involved previously inoperable anatomic sites, accessibility demanded a variety of patient positioning. Metal was substituted for wood as the construction material for operating tables with the advent of the understanding of asepsis. Mechanical devices soon appeared that allowed fine adjustments of position. One excellent example of the transition in table design occurred in 1884 with the Trendelenburg table (Fig. 3–1), which was used for positioning the patient head down.[2]

Meyer,[2] a surgeon in New York, described his technique of achieving Trendelenburg's position before the introduction of the Trendelenburg table:

I used to fasten a strong kitchen-chair, turned upside down, on a kitchen table, and sawed off the posterior [upper] legs of the chair at the level of the cross bar. The whole inclined plane thus formed by the back of the chair was then covered with folded blankets and a sheet, held in position by a roller-bandage. On this the patient was put, pointing with the head to the window.

The Trendelenburg table was recommended for all operations inside the bladder and for laparotomies in the lower pelvis.

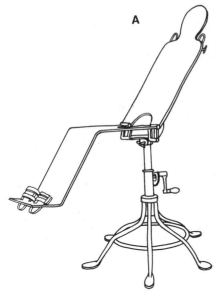
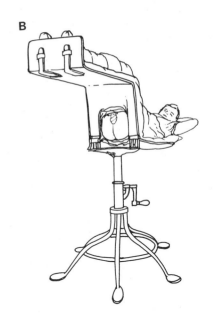

Figure 3–1

Trendelenburg table of 1890. It was designed by Dr. Trendelenburg for all bladder operations and laparotomies of the lower pelvis. The table was easy to take apart and transport to the patient's home. Features included two movable shoulder-holders, a large backrest *(A)*, height adjustment [32″ to 46″], 360-degree rotation in the vertical axis, "rapid head-down tilt", seat trap door for perineal exposure *(B)*, and a wide base for stability. (Redrawn from Meyer W: Trendelenburg's new operating table, designed for operations in the posture bearing his name. Med Record 38:658, 1890.)

In 1892, Cleveland[3] described a variant of the Trendelenburg table for use in general and gynecologic surgery. He found the best position to be an "inclined posture with both knees and thighs flexed, and the weight of the body partly sustained by the shoulders." This modified table (Fig. 3–2) was made of galvanized iron so it could "be scrubbed and deluged with water." A round cylinder supported the knees to "prevent injury to the structures in the popliteal space." Fluids were guided toward a drain pan by 2-inch guards on the sides of the table, thus preventing fluids from splashing on the floor and surgeons' clothing.

By the end of the nineteenth century, mechanical positioning devices had been introduced, metal had replaced wood, and most operating tables were similar in function. Figure 3–3 shows a table sold in 1905. It typifies the operating table design that dominated the market until the 1930s when tables began to increase positioning options as they became more streamlined, less bulky, and more space efficient. The 1905 version was made of steel for easy cleaning and durability and had removable head and feet sections, a trough cut down its center to carry drainage, combination hip and kidney elevating devices, a side wheel control for head-down and head-up tilt, and three sets of head rests.[4] Longer operations were associated with patient heat loss and prolonged recovery. To preserve body heat, hot water or steam was circulated through the tops of specially designed tables; however, the practice caused burns.[5, 6] Today we take a different approach by using warming devices, fed by hot air, on top of the patient. After World War I, the x-ray made its debut. Operating tables soon adopted radiolucent table tops, cassette tunnels, and central or eccentric bases to allow use of a camera on a C-shaped arm.

Operating table design was slow to advance. Innovations from 1940 to the present have been hydraulic lifts, electric and battery controls, improved construction material, and specialty tables. Buyers now expect an operating room table to have hand and foot controls for a reliable, smooth, fluid drive that provides an array of positions; have a floor lock system; have removable head and foot sections; have a large selection of accessories; be compatible with x-ray and image-intensification radiography; and be easy to clean. Despite these finite demands, standards have not been written for the operating table. The Association of Operating Room Nurses has

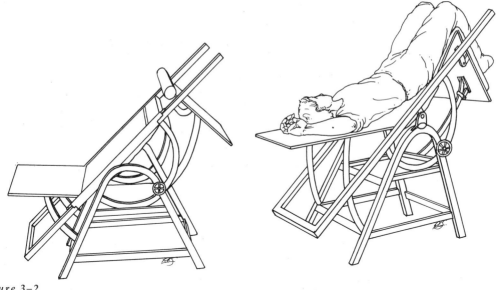

Figure 3–2

A general and gynecological table, 1892. A modification of the Trendelenburg table included several improvements: construction with galvanized iron to allow cleaning with water; a wider, more stable base; a central drain pan depression (not seen); slide guards to prevent fluid splash on the surgeon and floor; easily positioned head and foot sections; and a cylinder to support the knees. (Redrawn from Cleveland C: An operating table for general and gynaecological surgery, adapted to give the Trendelenburg posture. NY J Gyanen Obst 2:614, 1892.)

only a few referrals to the operating table in its *Standards and Recommended Practices for Perioperative Nursing*[7]:

1. Areas contaminated . . . should receive immediate attention . . . ,
2. The horizontal surfaces of furniture . . . should be cleaned with an appropriate agent,
3. The wheels and casters of furniture . . . should be pushed through the solution used for floor cleaning,
4. Furniture . . . scrubbed . . . , and
5. Wheels and casters should be cleaned and kept free of debris.

Standards exist for the electrical parts of the operating table, but none can be found for the mechanical structure and function.

BASIC OPERATING ROOM TABLES

Three basic types of surgical tables are available: (1) a general purpose table, (2) specialty tables, and (3) a fixed-base system with interchangeable table tops.

Figure 3–3

Basic operating table in 1905. Made of steel for easy cleaning, this table includes rubber-tired wheels, movable head section, detachable foot section that had counterweights to assist in positioning, center trough that emptied into the collection pan, hip and kidney elevators, side wheel control for Trendelenburg and reverse Trendelenburg, and three sets of head rests (not shown). (Redrawn from Hartley F, Murry FW: Concerning the evolution of the operating table. NY Med J 44:1276, 1911.)

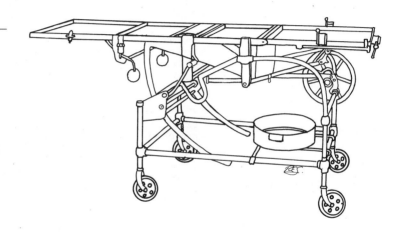

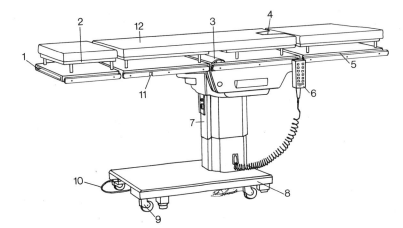

Figure 3–4

Basic features of the operating room table: 1 = x-ray cassette tunnel; 2 = removable head section; 3 = kidney elevator; 4 = perineal cut out; 5 = radiolucent top and removable foot section; 6 = hand control; 7 = electrohydraulic drive; 8 = narrow base design; 9 = locking swivel casters; 10 = power cord; 11 = side rail locking system; and 12 = pads.

The General Surgery Table

Predominantly, the general purpose surgical table is the workhorse of the operating room and the fundamental tool with which patient positioning is achieved. A basic operating table is shown in Figure 3–4, and the technical data for an average general surgery table are outlined in Table 3–1. Positioning is augmented by combining elementary positions of the operating table (Fig. 3–5) with a wide range of table accessories.

Operating tables are made of stainless steel for easy cleaning. Patients are protected from hard surfaces by some form of padding. Movement of the sections of the table top to achieve various positions is controlled either manually or by a electric or infrared hand control at the end or side of the table. The table operator selects the position of choice by pressing the appropriate button or button sequence. Electric controls are usually used to raise/lower the table, raise/lower the back section, raise/lower the foot section, lock/unlock the table base, provide right/left lateral tilt, provide head-up or head-down tilt, and turn power on/off. A "neutral function" button returns the table to the neutral horizontal position. Battery-powered tables were examined in 1974 but had only a 3-hour battery life.[8] Today the batteries that control manipulations of table surfaces are expected to last several weeks without recharging. A hydraulic system in the pedestal lowers and raises the table. The kidney elevator, a transverse bar at about the midpoint of the table surface, is usually controlled manually.

Ergomatic efficiency in the operating room begins with choosing the appropriate operating table, locating it in the correct spot, and ensuring that the patient is positioned for ideal surgical exposure. Casters allow the table to be moved easily for cleaning, positioning, and table maintenance. Pedal-operated legs can be lowered from beneath the table to elevate its base sufficiently to raise the casters off the floor and immobilize the unit.

Many operations require intraoperative radiographs. Table tops are designed to be radi-

Table 3–1

Technical Data and Features of the Operating Table*

Length of table with head plate	79–89 inches (201–225 cm)
Width of table top	20–24 inches (51–61 cm)
Height range	26–45 inches (66–114 cm)
Supports 500-lb (1100-kg) patient	
Head-down tilt range	0–33 degrees
Head-up tilt range	0–42 degrees
Lateral tilt range, either side	0–28 degrees
Back section range	Raise: 0–90 degrees
	Lower: 0–80 degrees
Head plate articulation	+15 to −30 degrees
Flex/reflex position	Flex: 0–220 degrees
	Reflex: 0–155 degrees
Leg section	Raise: 0–80 degrees
	Lower: 0–100 degrees
Kidney elevator	0–5.5 inches (14 cm)
Number of table-top sections	Up to 7
Power supply	117–120 volts, 50/60 Hz
	4–8 amperes, 300–450 watts, single phase
Battery	Several weeks without recharging

*All range limits represent composite maximum of all companies.

Actual range limits for individual tables vary with the manufacturer.

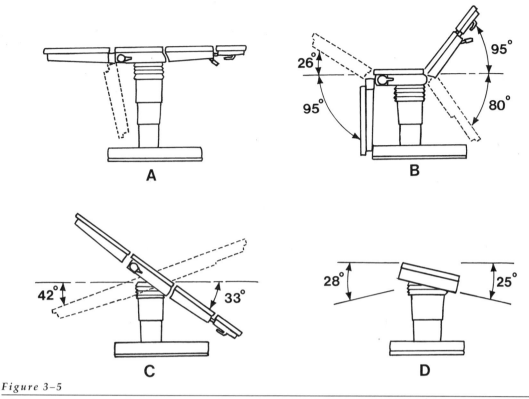

Figure 3–5

Basic positions of an operating table. *A.* Foot rest dropped through a range of 0 to 110 degrees. *B.* Foot rest raised from 0 to 28 degrees and dropped from 0 to 95 degrees. Back rest raised from 0 to 95 degrees and lowered from 0 to 80 degrees. *C.* Trendelenburg range from 0 to 33 degrees and reverse Trendelenburg from 0 to 80 degrees. *D.* Lateral tilt to right or left from 0 to 28 degrees. Limits for all positions represent the composite maximum of all companies. Individual table varies according to the manufacturer.

olucent with a space or tunnel between the table top and the platform supporting the patient that can accommodate an x-ray film cassette. Cassettes can be positioned from either the ends or sides of the tunnel and are maneuvered by detachable handles. C-arms are used frequently, so most tables are designed for maximum space beneath the table to accommodate the floor portion of the C-arm. Some tables have an eccentric pedestal at one end (Fig. 3–6) to increase the area of exposure. Other general surgery tables are made more versatile by adding a C-arm extension to the foot section of the table. Radiolucency can be increased two to three times by substituting table tops made of carbon composite material for the standard table tops.

Side rails for locking systems are essential for accessories. These rails run down both sides of the table and sometimes are present on the ends. Locking sockets and clamps of various makes, sizes, and design fit onto the side rails.

Operating room tables are durable, are expensive, and require preventative maintenance. Attention must be given to the proper assembly of the table or disaster may occur. One report describes the total collapse of the operating room table just as the patient was being transferred from the table to the transport cart after successful open-heart surgery.[9] Someone had assembled the table top backward on the pedestal.

Specialty Tables

Surgeons often have felt the need to have a special table made for their favorite operation.

- One of the first specialty tables was designed in 1911 for eye, head, ear, nose, and throat surgery.[10]
- An example of a unit intended for a specific operation is a urology microsurgery table made from wood and covered with Formica.[11] Intended to lessen fatigue, re-

A

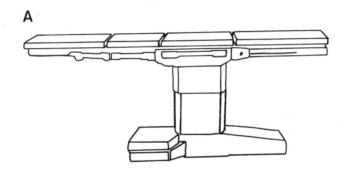

B

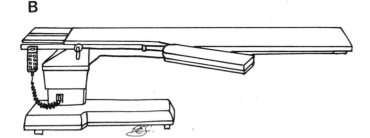

Figure 3–6

Central *(A)* and eccentric *(B)* base locations for the operating table. The eccentric base allows maximal C-arm and radiographic intervention, and more leg room is available to the sitting surgeon who is operating at the head of the table.

duce back strain, and allow better concentration, its cost was one twentieth that of a less desirable commercially available urology microsurgical table.

- Another single-purpose table was created for repairing giant retinal breaks.[12] The bed of a Stryker circular rotating table was modified to allow the patient to be moved through the longitudinal and transverse axes. Preoperatively the patient was positioned on the table to evaluate the vitreous traction on the retinal flap. During the repair of the retinal break the ophthalmologist injected an air bubble intravitreally. Subretinal fluid was forced out by the bubble to tamponade the retina against the pigment epithelium. Postoperatively intermittent changes in positioning were easily accomplished to ensure optimum bubble tamponade of the retinal break.

Urology tables are shorter than general surgery tables with emphasis on leg elevation, perineal fluid drainage, and compatibility with radiography. The capability for radiography is incorporated into the table to provide maximum fluoroscopic imaging for surgical procedures. Figure 3–7 shows a generic urology table with a perineal system, leg holders, an x-ray pedestal, and an on-line image projection screen. A typical table is about 43

inches (109 cm) long, supports a 350-lb (159-kg) patient, moves longitudinally up to 10 inches (25 cm), moves laterally up to 6 inches (15 cm), elevates from 28 to 50 inches (71 to 127 cm), tilts to 20 degrees head down and to 88 degrees head up, has a hand and foot control system, has an x-ray film cassette mechanism plus its own x-ray arm, and requires an electrical supply of 208 to 240 volts, 50/60 hertz and 30 amperes. The foot control is unique to the table and is designed to give the urologist complete control of table positioning and x-ray function during the surgery. Usual functions of the foot control include tilt, height adjustment, longitudinal and lateral movement, x-ray image system movement, fluoroscopy, and storage and recall of table position commands. Some tables come with lightweight carbon composite tops for easy cleaning and increased radiolucency.

Orthopedic tables were developed to provide countertraction for fracture reduction, hip pinning, long-bone nailing, and so on. Flexibility to accommodate the wide range of required orthopedic procedures is the basis of the orthopedic table design in Figure 3–8. C-arm access, fixation of position during surgery, and access for casting are certainly major attributes required for orthopedic surgery. Power hand control is available, but most tables are manually controlled to reduce

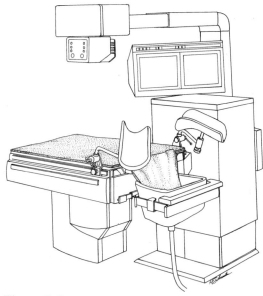

Figure 3-7

Urology table. Radiography is permanently
incorporated into the table design to provide
optimum fluoroscopic imaging. The table has leg
holders and a large perineal drain system. A single
electrical control ensures management of table
positioning and radiographic functions. Image
projection is on-line to provide rapid diagnosis and
confirm surgical success.

Optional accessories include an image ampli-
fication board that attaches to the end of the
table in place of the abductor bars, a tibial
countertraction holder, and a drape support.

Spinal surgery tables are helpful for placing
the patient in the kneeling position as well as
for imaging. Figure 3–9 (*A* and *B*) shows a
table with many built-in accessories for facilitating the kneeling position. This posture for
a surgical patient has been a favorite of many
orthopedists and neurosurgeons because it
improves fluid drainage from the surgical
field. Intra-abdominal pressure is not increased; therefore, blood is not shunted to the
vertebral venous system. The shape of the
frame allows easy C-arm access. Patients with
a cervical fracture requiring continuous traction can be placed on the table shown in *C*
and *D* of Figure 3–9. C-arm imaging is excellent. A number of surgical procedures can be
done with this table. A flat surgery table top
can be substituted for the imaging table top.

Fixed-Base System with Interchangeable Operating Table Tops

In 1923, Hirst and Van Dolsen[13] designed a
operating table top to fit both a pedestal in
the operating room and a patient transport
cart. Efficiency in handling the patient was
enhanced by placing the patient on the operating room table top in his or her room,
transporting the patient to the operating
room, and simply moving the entire table top
to a fixed pedestal base in the operating room.
Afterward the patient could be transported to
the recovery room on the same table top and
eventually transferred to the ward bed. In

costs. Table surfaces are easy to clean, a must
for open orthopedic surgery. Owing to their
unique application these tables come with a
wide variety of standard orthopedic accessories: removable leg supports, collapsible arm
extension devices, feet traction units, a transfer board for moving the patient, a nailing
support or hip rest, and traction extensions.

Figure 3-8

Orthopedic operating table.
Features include (1) standard
side rails for accessory
attachment, (2) translating
table top to ease patient
transfer and C-arm access,
(3) radiolucent sacral rest and
post, (4) foot traction boots,
(5) foot traction units, (6)
radiolucent abduction bars,
(7) positioning locks, (8)
casters, (9) foot locks, (10)
raise/lower pedal, (11) floor
lock pedal, and (12)
Trendelenburg and lateral tilt
control.

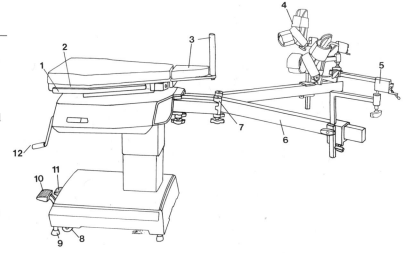

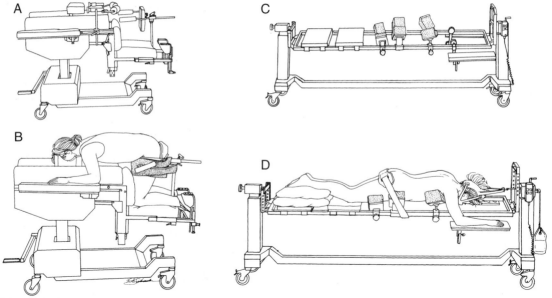

Figure 3-9

Spinal surgery tables. *A* and *B*. Patient in the prone kneeling position for decreasing intra-abdominal pressure and improving the surgical field. The body lift can be elevated. The tibial support has leg restraints to allow the patient's weight to be evenly distributed over the pretibial area. Iliac crest supports and bolster rolls help to level the lumbar spine. In *B* the patient is secured by a strap around the thighs and support frame. The feet are in bootlets, and the face is protected by a cut-out foam pad. *C* and *D*. This table is designed for imaging, surgery, and cervical traction. The degree and rotation of the patient is precisely controlled. Radiolucency is improved when a carbon composite material is used for construction. A flat surgery table top can be substituted for the imaging table top. A C-arm can easily be placed in any position for imaging and surgery. In *D* the patient is on the imaging table top in cervical traction with weights.

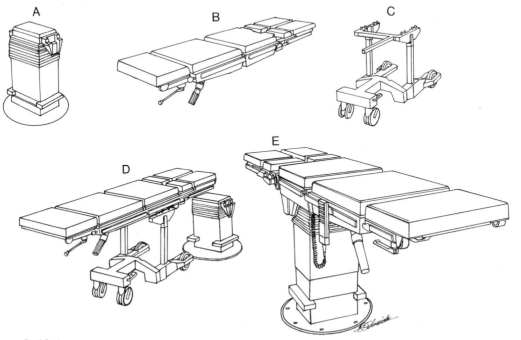

Figure 3-10

Fixed base system with interchangeable operating table tops. The pedestal *(A)* is installed in the operating room. The appropriate table top *(B)* is chosen and placed on the patient transport stretcher *(C)*. The patient is placed on the transport stretcher in the hospital ward room and taken to the operating room *(D)*. On entering the operating room, the transport stretcher is backed over the pedestal *(E)*, the table top is attached to the pedestal, the transport stretcher is removed, and the patient is prepared for surgery.

essence, the patient was moved only twice, once out of and once back to the hospital bed. This fixed-base system represents the only real change in operating room table design since the conversion of mechanically operated tables to electrically operated tables.[14] Adoption of the fixed-base system was slow. Specialized table tops for orthopedics, neurosurgery, urology, gynecology, ophthalmology, pediatrics, vascular surgery, and endoscopy were added to the armamemtarium, thus widening the choices and improving the acceptance of the system. A fixed-base table system is shown in Figure 3–10.

Some hospitals have a separate induction or preparation room adjacent to the operating room where the patients may be anesthetized and then transferred to the operating room. A fixed-base table system is ideal for these hospitals. Partial isolation from the hospital dirt and bacteria can theoretically be accomplished by transferring the table top and patient from the hospital transfer cart to an operating room transfer cart. After the operation is completed the reverse transfer takes place and the hospital transport cart and personnel never enter the aseptic portion of the operating room. Once the table top is attached to the operating room pedestal, the system operates similar to a general surgical table. Advantages of the system appear to be short set-up and take-down times, the possibility of more stringent separation of the aseptic operating room from the rest of the hospital, and a high degree of flexibility by interchanging table tops.

ACCESSORIES

Side rails and holes drilled in the ends of the operating table allow the attachment of a great variety of accessories. Without a doubt the operating table accessories are responsible for the versatility required for the finely adjusted positions that permit difficult operations. Many accessories are similar in function but of slightly different design, either to avoid patent infringement or because of the intricacies of specific operations. Because of the close similarity of multiple accessories, only a few are discussed here.

Some accessories have taken the lead in contributing to the complications of positioning. Lithotomy leg holders (Fig. 3–11) have been implicated in numerous nerve injuries. The basic cantilevered suspension-strap sup-

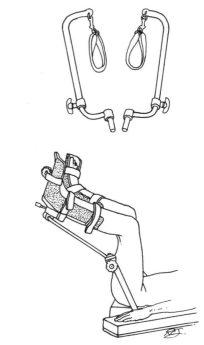

Figure 3–11

Lithotomy leg holders. *Top.* Hanging straps suspend ankles but do not immobilize extremities. *Bottom.* Padded foot and calf support unit provides versatile positioning and rigid fixation of the extremity.

port for the legs has been in operating rooms for many years. Simplicity allows height and angular adjustment and distributes pressure across the heel and foot. Design variance is marked by multiple eponyms, but leg holders basically provide flexible positioning, built-in straps to secure the leg in place, and padding to avoid leg injury.

Shoulder supports (Fig. 3–12) must be used with caution but may be necessary for a high-

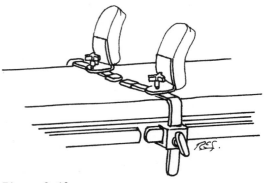

Figure 3–12

Adjustable braces used to stabilize shoulders on table tilted head-down.

angle head-down tilt. In addition to the supports attached to the table, it is prudent to use blankets, towels, and so on, to minimize pressure points, avoid skin contact, and prevent nerve injury.

Positioning the arm off the operating table or armboard requires some kind of extension device. Figure 3–13 displays a number of accessories used to support the arm, forearm, and humerus. Lateral positions requiring the arm to be out of the way of the chest or in a position to operate on the arm itself dictate some kind of special holding device. In some cases, merely placing the down-side arm on a well-padded armboard, placing two pillows between the down-side and up-side arm, and securing both arms with Velcro straps suffice. However, it is sometimes more prudent to use a device designed to protect the arm in the position of surgery.

In addition to the specialty operating table, a line of accessories is available to extend the versatility of the general surgery table to accommodate specialized orthopedic surgery.

- A complete orthopedic attachment (Fig. 3–14A) can be added to the end of the general surgery table for fracture work, nailings, and so on.
- Hip spica platforms (see Fig. 3–14B) are placed on the operating table to elevate the sacral area for casting the sacrolumbar area.
- Casting or dressing of the thoracic area is simplified by a thoracic plaster cast device (see Fig. 3–14C). The head and thoracic sections of the table are removed, and the supporting bars are placed under the patient's neck, shoulders, and thorax.
- A spinal column positioning support (see Fig. 3–14D), consisting of a seat bow with roll pad, padded lateral pelvis supports, and a padded sternal support, can be used for the kneeling position. Pressure on the abdomen is decreased, thus reducing bleeding in the operative site.
- Arthrosurgery units (see Fig. 3–14E) are available to stabilize the knee, wrist, and elbow.

Traction is very important in orthopedics and is one reason the specialized orthopedic table was designed. Devices to aid in traction and countertraction can be added to any orthopedic system to increase versatility. The traction unit assembly is attached to the abductor bars. Other devices (e.g., L-shaped and straight traction extensions, foot traction boots, traction bows, tibia countertractions devices) are then attached to the traction unit assembly or operating table.

A skull clamp (Fig. 3–15) is used to provide maximal stability of the positioned head. The clamps come in various shapes to fit different heads. Once the clamp is in place it is connected to the table attachment, the head is positioned, and the locking device is engaged. A number of adapters, supporting arms, and connecting pieces may be required for some table attachments. Figure 3–16 shows a head clamp linked to the table attachment with the patient in the supine and then the sitting position.

One very convenient item for the anesthesia provider is a hand-held infrared control unit. Features include an on/off power switch and the capability to lock/unlock the table base, raise/lower the table, raise/lower the back section, provide right or left lateral tilt or head-up or head-down tilt, and return to neutral function. Light-emitting diodes indicate the amount of charge on the main table. Foot controls for the surgeon allow height adjustment and head-up or head-down tilt of the table top.

Any direct contact between the patient and either a device or the operating table itself has the potential for injury. Pads are used to widen the pressure area and decrease the potential for focal injury. In 1973, Souther and co-workers[15] studied the effects of two types of pads on tissue ischemia and found that neither water-filled polyurethane foam pads nor standard latex rubber pads reduced pressure below mean capillary pressure. Almost any conceivable position has been used at some time in the practice of surgery. During operations, or in any circumstance in which patients are unconscious and incapable of protecting themselves, health care workers have the obligation to minimize the potential for physical injury from positioning. Standard pads can be purchased to meet the majority of positioning requirements. Special pads are available and individual requirements of patients can be supplemented with blankets, towels, and other materials. Methods and materials used for pad construction are diverse, rendering the available choices extensive. Some pads can be filled with air or other substances to individualize the fit to patient contours. Other air-filled pads are intended to be placed under the area of contact between the patient and the supporting surface and then kept in the exact anatomic contour by connection to a vacuum sys-

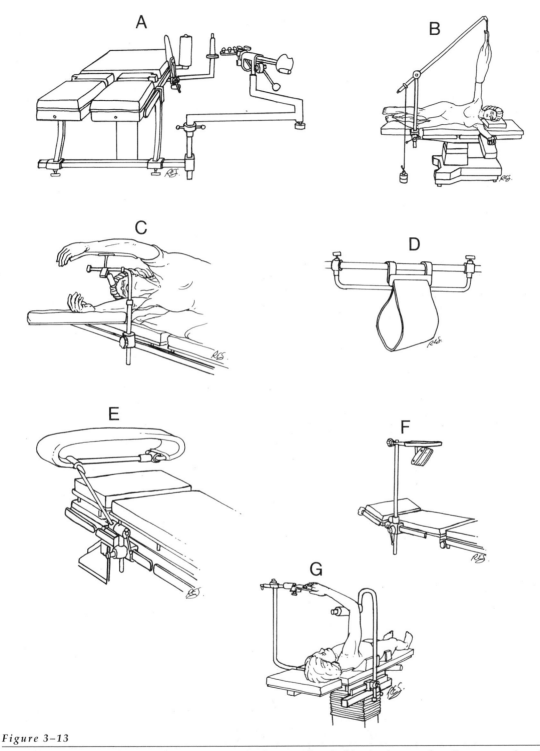

Figure 3-13

Upper extremity support systems. *A.* Arm extension device with a double pivoting arm, lateral support pad, and an axilla and elbow support. *B.* Suspension system with counterweight to keep arm upright. Height, rotation, and angle are easily adjustable. *C.* Elevating support with height and lateral adjustment. *D.* A simple cuff made from Velcro that hangs from the anesthesia screen. *E.* Cross-arm support adjustable to length and height. *F.* A forearm positioner. *G.* On the left is a humerus positioning device, and on the right is a humerus countertraction post. Unit is used to facilitate intramedullary nailing of the humerus.

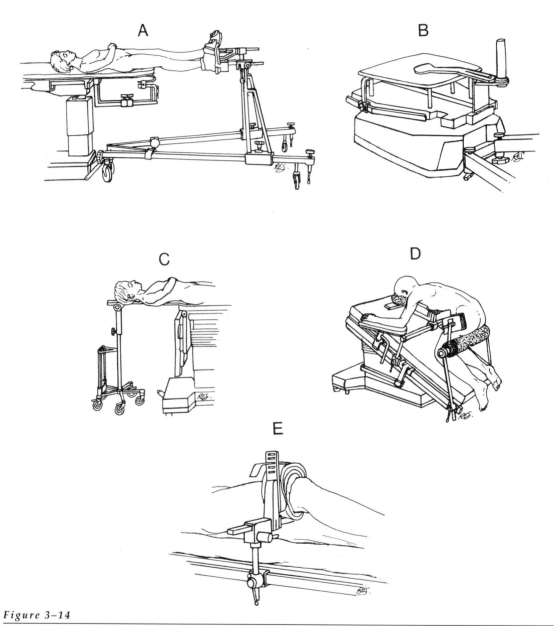

Figure 3–14

Orthopedic attachments. *A.* Complete orthopedic attachment for a general surgery table. *B.* Hip spica assembly (child version) that elevates the sacral area for casting in the sacrolumbar area. *C.* Thorax plaster casts are simplified by removing the head and back sections and placing support bars under the head, shoulders, and thorax. *D.* A spinal column positioning system consists of a seat bow with roll pad, a padded sternum support, and padded lateral pelvis supports. *E.* Positioning system for arthroscopy of the knee, wrist, and elbow.

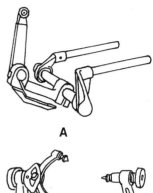

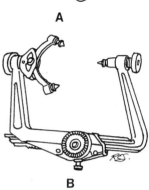

Figure 3–15

Basic skull clamping system. *A.* Mayfield frame attaches to the operating table. With local anesthesia at the points of penetration, a three-pin adjustable clamp *(B)* is attached to the skull of the patient, locked firmly in place and attached to the table frame *(A).*

A

B

tem that removes contained air and makes the pad rigid. Protective padding for a patient is limited only by the ingenuity of the operating room team.

Patients have been known to fall off operating tables during operations. For this reason alone restraint straps of some kind are justified for the majority of operations. However, severe injury has resulted from a strap that is excessively tight or is placed over the wrong anatomic area. Straps come in choices of wide/narrow or thick/thin. All are adjustable in some manner, whether with standard buckles, airplane-type quick-release buckles, or Velcro surfaces. Connections of retaining straps to the side rails of the operating table are made with a variety of clamping devices.

A

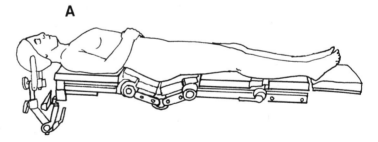

Figure 3–16

Head skull clamp and accessories being used in the supine *(A)* and the sitting *(B)* positions. Vertical, horizontal, or angular positioning and repositioning is possible. Three pins in the outer table of the skull together with a secure locking system provide excellent head fixation.

B

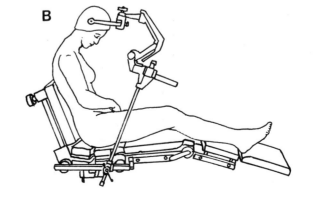

REFERENCES

1. Brian V: The operating theatre: Scenes through the centuries. Nursing Mirror 148:1, 1979.
2. Meyer W: Trendelenburg's new operating table, designed for operations in the posture bearing his name. Med Record 38:658, 1890.
3. Cleveland C: An operating table for general and gynaecological surgery, adapted to give the Trendelenburg posture. NY J Gyanen Obst 2:614, 1892.
4. Hartley F, Murry FW: Concerning the evolution of the operating table. NY Med J 44:1276, 1911.
5. Perkins JW: A hot operating table and its advantages. Int J Surg 8:283, 1895.
6. Pettit JA: Heating of operating tables. Northwest Med 7:294, 1915.
7. AORN Standards and Recommended Practices for Perioperative Nursing. Denver, Association of Operating Room Nurses, 1987.
8. Jitwauska S, Nakatani H, Kawai T, et al.: A battery powered operating table with a removable stationary column base and a detachable table top. Jpn J Surg 12:82, 1982.
9. Birch AA Jr: Collapse of an operating room table. Anesthesiology 49:62, 1978.
10. Dean LW: A table for eye, ear, nose and throat work. JAMA 47:1126, 1911.
11. Hellstrom WJG: Modifications in operating-table design for urologic microsurgery. Urol Clin North Am 17:135, 1990.
12. Peyman GA: A new operating table for the management of giant retinal breaks. Arch Ophthalmol 99:498, 1981.
13. Hirst JC, Van Dolsen WW: A new operation table, designed to avoid all lifting of the patient. JAMA 81:1098, 1923.
14. Laufman H: Trends in operating room devices. Med Instr 10:98, 1976.
15. Souther SG, Carr SD, Vistnes LM: Pressure, tissue ischemia, and operating table pads. Arch Surg 107:544, 1973.

Chapter 4

Physiologic Changes Associated with the Supine Position

Timothy J. O'Brien / Thomas J. Ebert

BACKGROUND

The focus in this chapter is on the physiologic adaptations of the cardiopulmonary system to the horizontal dorsal decubitus (supine) position. A significant portion of our life is spent supine, for a variety of reasons, and the posture is not considered to inflict significant physiologic stress. In contrast, our active life is spent primarily in the upright or seated position, both of which require considerable adaptation of the cardiopulmonary system. Interest in the adaptation to postural "stress" has led to a substantial body of knowledge regarding the physiologic adjustments to position change.[1, 2] Because the majority of anesthesia involves supine patients, a clear understanding of the impact of this position is needed to appreciate its influence on cardiopulmonary reserve.

POSITION AND THE CARDIOVASCULAR SYSTEM

One of the primary goals of the human body is to maintain cardiovascular homeostasis. The human has developed a number of neural and hormonal reflexes to assist in both the rapid and the sustained adaptation to posture changes in the face of the omnipresent force of gravity. Gravity urges both intravascular volume and the extravascular substances to sequester to the lowest point of the body. It alters the distribution of intravascular fluid, the mechanical properties of the lungs and kidneys, and the extravascular tissue forces. These effects are amplified in the human because of our biped development.

Passive Effects of Gravity on Intravascular Volume

Hydrostatic forces are always parallel to the direction of gravitational pull and are not dependent on the posture. The hydrostatic indifferent point represents the zone in which intravascular pressures and volumes stay relatively constant and is a natural reference point for hydrostatic shifts in the circulation.[1, 2] Below the hydrostatic indifferent point the vascular beds are engorged by blood draining from regions above.[3] Tissues are subject to the same gravitational forces that increase the intravascular volume below the hydrostatic indifferent point. The intravascular fluid shift that occurs with upright posture would lead to hypotension, cerebral hypoperfusion, and syncope were it not for the opposing pressure within the tissues surrounding the engorged blood vessels and for the reflex and hormonal effects within the cardiovascular system.

Veins in the legs, for example, have an intravascular pressure of 90 mm Hg erect, compared with 10 mm Hg supine. Transmural pressure (intravascular minus extravascular pressure) does not increase to the same degree because of the influence of muscle tone, venous valves, and the physical limitation of the extravascular spaces. Despite these opposing factors, the volume in the legs increases 10% to 15% after 40 minutes of standing.[4] Accordingly, it has been shown that there is a *decrease* in the calf and thigh cross-sectional areas when changing position from the upright to the supine as determined by computed tomographic scanning.[5] Other techniques to measure limb volume changes, such as circumference measurements,[6] the water displacement method,[7] and bioelectrical impedance analysis,[8] confirm this fluid loss in the lower extremities. Estimated fluid losses in the lower extremities over the first 2 to 4 hours after attaining the supine posture range from 200 to 600 mL, the total of both intravascular and extravascular fluid volume changes. In the supine position, extravascular fluids in the previously dependent regions move back into the intravascular and lymphatic systems because of a reduction in the hydrostatic force. The volume reduction in the lower extremities is distributed throughout the circulation.

Although it has never been evaluated, the fluid shift in the dependent regions has been predicted to be less in the anesthetized patient because of several factors:

- First, the administration of positive-pressure ventilation increases central venous pressure and this would presumably be transmitted to lower extremity veins, thereby opposing the movement of extravascular fluid into the intravascular space.
- Second, the loss of muscle tone during anesthesia, which is potentially greater in the paralyzed patient, lessens the forces that shift fluids into the circulation.

These effects under anesthesia are also known to predispose patients to hypotension.

Cardiovascular Reflexes Involved in Adaptation to Postural Change

Reflexes initiated by distention of the receptors located in the great veins (superior and inferior vena cava), atria, and ventricles are often referred to as the cardiopulmonary or "low-pressure" reflexes (Fig. 4–1). These sensors, in combination with the arterial baroreceptors in the aortic arch and carotid sinus, initiate reflex responses that maintain systemic blood pressure within narrow limits with a change in posture.

Cardiopulmonary Reflexes

As the body moves from the erect to the supine position, the venous return to the heart increases. The added preload results in a larger right ventricular stroke volume and a corresponding increase in the left ventricular stroke volume. Bainbridge described an increase in the heart rate during volume loading of the heart and attributed the response to baroreceptors in the great veins and right atrium.[7] Although the Bainbridge reflex has been well characterized in animal models, it has been difficult to demonstrate in humans. During volume loading of the atria, increases in heart rate occur through inhibition of vagal traffic to the sinoatrial node and possibly due to increases in sympathetic outflow.[9] Reflexes from the atria are also involved in regulation of renal sympathetic nerve activity, the regulation of plasma renin concentrations (the Henry-Gauer reflex), and the regulation of plasma levels of atrial natriuretic peptide and arginine vasopressin.[9] These reflexes contribute importantly to maintaining intravascular fluid volume, but their contribution to blood pressure homeostasis is far more gradual when compared with other atrial and ventricular reflexes that mediate rapid sympathetic responses to the peripheral vasculature.

Vagal afferent signals from the atria and ventricles of the human heart (including the venoatrial junction) appear to be tonically active and to exert a restraining effect on sympathetic outflow. When central venous pressure is increased by a change in posture to the supine position, sustained reflex decreases in sympathetic outflow to muscle and splanchnic vascular beds occur.[10, 11] These reflex changes are observed before there are any detectable alterations in heart rate or arterial pressure, suggesting that arterial baroreceptors are not involved.[9, 12] Thus, reflex sympathetic inhibition is thought to be due primarily to loading of cardiac "low-pressure" mechanoreceptors. In contrast, when blood volume is reduced, the cardiac mechanoreceptors are unloaded. This causes sympathetic excitation and is the first line of defense against hypotension. Recent support for the cardiac receptor origin of this reflex has been provided from studies in cardiac transplant patients.[13] In this model, the ventricles are denervated while neural connections to a small portion of the atria and the lungs are preserved. When nonhypotensive reductions in central blood volume are initiated, reflex

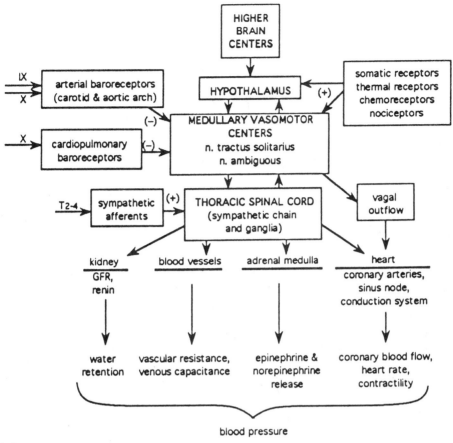

Figure 4-1

Schematic representation of the control of blood pressure. Cranial nerves IX and X provide input to the medullary vasomotor centers through the arterial and cardiopulmonary baroreceptors. This input and the input from higher brain centers, sympathetic afferents, and mechanoreceptors, thermoreceptors, and chemoreceptors control sympathetic and parasympathetic efferent activity.

forearm vasoconstriction and increases in plasma norepinephrine concentrations in transplant patients are impaired compared with normal subjects.

Ventricular receptors are believed to be involved in initiating syncopal episodes during physical exertion in patients with stenotic aortic valves. In this situation, increases in left ventricular end-diastolic pressure are thought to excite cardiac mechanoreceptors, which trigger a reflex bradycardia and hypotension.[14] A similar phenomenon may occur during excessive reductions in central blood volume. In this situation, the unloading of cardiac receptors initially elicits increases in sympathetic outflow. However, when ventricular filling is reduced beyond a "critical" level, the vigorous contractions of the empty ventricle are believed to trigger additional (or different) vagal afferents, which leads to hy-

potension through reflex sympathetic inhibition and bradycardia through enhanced vagal cardiac activity.[15]

Arterial Baroreceptor Reflexes

The increase in cardiac output caused by an increased venous return on assuming the supine position initially tends to raise the arterial blood pressure. Baroreceptors located in the walls of the aorta and the carotid arteries sense the increase. Afferent neural impulses travel in the vagus nerve from aortic baroreceptors and in the glossopharyngeal nerve from baroreceptors in the walls of the carotid sinuses to the vasomotor center in the medulla oblongata. After integration of all neural signals from the periphery and from the central nervous system, efferent sympathetic and parasympathetic outflow is established.

Inhibitory parasympathetic impulses travel to the heart through the vagus nerve to act on the sinoatrial node and the myocardium, diminishing heart rate, stroke volume, and the strength of myocardial contraction. Concurrent with this increase in parasympathetic tone, efferent sympathetic discharge to the heart and periphery is diminished. These reflex responses counteract the relative thoracic intravascular overload in the supine position and permit distribution of intravascular volume to the periphery, thereby restoring blood pressure toward baseline (see Fig. 4–1).

Combined Reflex Responses: Effects of Age, Sex, and Aerobic Training

The overall effect of the combination of cardiopulmonary and arterial reflex mechanisms when changing position from the upright to the supine has been studied by Ward and co-workers[16] and by Korner.[17] Mean arterial blood pressure, heart rate, and peripheral vascular resistance decrease whereas cardiac output and stroke volume increase (Table 4–1). The systolic blood pressure remains at about the same level, but the diastolic blood pressure decreases, leading to greater pulse pressure and lower mean pressure.

With aging, the sensitivity or gain of the neural reflexes involved in posture changes is diminished.[18] The reflex responses are further impaired by certain disease states, including diabetes, hypertension, chronic alcoholism, renal failure, recent myocardial infarction, and congestive heart failure.[19, 20] Although this impairment of reflex function has important implications for the adjustment to the

upright position,[21] and to the response to hemorrhage or hypotension, it is unlikely that it has major consequences regarding adaptation to the supine position. With reference to Table 4–1, patients with autonomic impairment who are moved from the upright to the supine position might demonstrate a greater change in mean arterial blood pressure along with a lesser change in heart rate. This would be primarily attributable to less tachycardia and a more marked decrease in blood pressure in the upright position.[19] While supine, there may be a higher resting heart rate owing to the reduction in cardiac-vagal tone that occurs with increasing age, diabetes, and other previously mentioned disease processes.

The majority of the studies on the neural control of the circulation during a change in posture have been carried out in the male population. However, one study of females indicated that they had smaller decreases in stroke volume despite apparently larger decreases in central blood volume during upright posture when compared with age-matched males.[22] Part of these differences could be accounted for by heightened reflex increases in the peripheral resistance response in females. The implications of these gender differences in the adjustment to the supine position are not known but are probably minor.

Individuals who maintain a lifestyle with a rigorous aerobic exercise component have lower resting heart rates compared with sedentary individuals and appear to have a higher incidence of syncope during upright tilt testing.[23, 24] This may be due to a higher basal cardiac-vagal tone at rest and to impaired baroreceptor reflex responses.[25, 26] In addition, while supine, a predisposition to develop presyncopal symptoms or syncope during emotionally stressful procedures such as invasive instrumentation has been noted in the endurance-trained athlete (personal observation). This response can be exaggerated if opioids are employed because of their known ability to potentiate vagal responses.[27] Admittedly, controlled studies comparing the incidence and severity of these responses in the aerobically fit versus sedentary population are lacking.

POSITION AND THE RESPIRATORY SYSTEM

Anatomy

Gravitational forces can have significant effects on the anatomy of the upper airway. An

Table 4–1

Effect of Postural Change on Circulatory Dynamics in Awake Subjects

	Supine	*Percent Change from Supine*	
	Supine	*Standing*	*Sitting*
Cardiac output (L/min)	7.07	−27.4	−9.8
Stroke volume (mL)	99.6	−45.3	−21.4
Mean arterial pressure (mm Hg)	90.2	+18.6	−2.5
Heart rate (beats/min)	71.6	+35.7	+18.6
Total peripheral resistance (dynes/cm²/sec)	1101.0	+65.3	+9.6

From Ward RJ, Danziger F, Bonica JJ, et al.: Cardiovascular effects of change of posture. Aerospace Med 37:257, 1966.

increase in soft palate thickness and area, a decrease in vertical length of the airway, and a 29% decrease in oropharyngeal area have been observed in an awake subject on going from the erect to the supine position.[28] These changes can add to the difficulty of securing an airway in select populations, albeit unlikely that instrumenting the airway in the upright position would simplify the process.

When changing from the erect to supine position in an awake subject, the anteroposterior diameter of the rib cage and abdomen decreases, with subsequent increases in the lateral diameters of both rib cage and abdomen due to gravitational forces.[29] Gravity also has effects on ventilation, perfusion, and lung volumes.

Ventilation

Regional ventilation is determined by movements of the rib cage and diaphragm and by the compliance of the lung, chest wall, and diaphragm. In the erect position, breathing is predominately a function of thoracic muscles, with those of the rib cage contributing 69% to ventilation. In the supine position, breathing is a function of abdominal or diaphragmatic movement with only a 32% contribution from the rib cage.[30, 31]

Froese[32] showed that awake supine subjects had a greater posterior, or dependent, caudad displacement of the diaphragm during tidal breathing (Fig. 4–2). Anesthetized supine subjects showed further posterior displacement of the diaphragm cephalad. Anesthetized and paralyzed supine subjects showed an even greater cephalad displacement of the posterior diaphragm. The relocation produces greater stretch of the muscle fibers of the posterior portion of the diaphragm and, therefore, allows for improved efficiency of muscle fiber shortening. Consequently, there is relatively more ventilation of the posterior portions of the lungs than the anterior portions. Since gravitational forces distribute a greater proportion of the perfusion to the posterior portions of the lung in the supine position, an improvement of the matching of ventilation and perfusion occurs.

In the average adult lung, which is 30 cm in height in the erect posture, there is a 7.5 cm H_2O hydrostatic pressure difference between the apex and the base. This pressure difference results in airways having smaller volume and being less compliant in the base than in the apex of the lung. In the erect position the base of the lung has a relatively greater increase in ventilation per unit volume than the apex of the lung, whereas there is a more uniform ventilation per unit volume of lung in the supine position.[33]

Perfusion (Circulation)

The pulmonary circulation contains 10% to 20% of the total blood volume, mostly in the pulmonary veins. The pulmonary vascular pressure is maintained at about one sixth of the systemic circulation. Regional blood flow can be determined by the vertical distance between the capillaries and the point of attachment of the pulmonary artery at the lung hilum.[34] The lung can be divided into three zones comparing pulmonary arterial pressure, pulmonary venous pressure, and pulmonary alveolar pressure.[34] Zone 1 is the nondependent portion of the lung, namely, the apex in the erect subject and the anterior lung in the supine subject. In this zone, alveolar pressure is greater than arterial pressure, which is greater than venous pressure, and

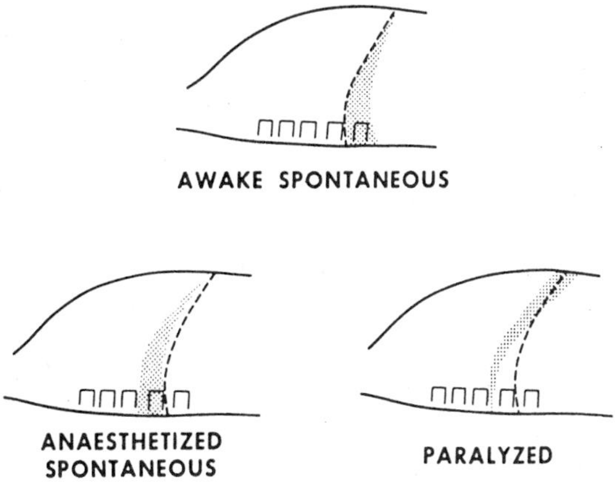

AWAKE SPONTANEOUS

ANAESTHETIZED SPONTANEOUS

PARALYZED

Figure 4–2

Diaphragm position and displacement during tidal breathing. Dashed line represents control of functional residual capacity position of the diaphragm. Stippled area represents diaphragmatic excursion during tidal breathing. (From Froese AB: Effects of anesthesia and paralysis on diaphragmatic mechanisms in man. Anesthesiology 41:242, 1974.)

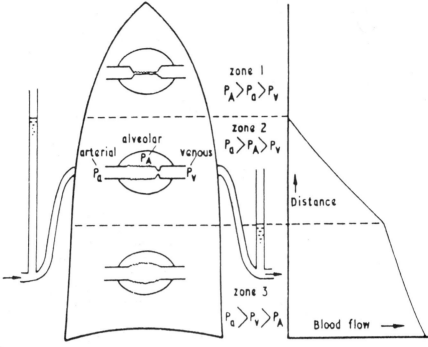

Figure 4–3

Scheme that accounts for the distribution of blood flow in the isolated lung. In zone 1, alveolar pressure (PA) exceeds arterial pressure (Pa) and no flow occurs, presumably because collapsible vessels are directly exposed to PA. In zone 2, Pa exceeds PA, but PA exceeds venous pressure (Pv). Here the flow is determined by the Pa/PA difference, which steadily decreases down the zone. In zone 3, Pv now exceeds PA and flow is determined by the Pa/Pv difference, which is constant down the lung. However, the pressure across the walls of the vessels increases down the zone, so that their caliber increases and so does flow. Note that the rates of increase down zones 2 and 3 may be quite different. (From West JB: Ventilation: Blood Flow and Gas Exchange. Oxford, Blackwell Scientific Publications, 1965.)

no pulmonary circulation will occur (Fig. 4–3). This does not occur in humans under normal circumstances. If airway pressures were increased, as occurs with large tidal volumes or high positive end-expiratory pressure, then zone 1 areas could exist.

In zone 2, arterial pressure exceeds alveolar pressure, which exceeds venous pressure. In this zone, pulmonary circulation is determined by the difference between arterial and alveolar pressure. The more dependent portions of the lungs have a greater pressure difference and, therefore, greater perfusion.

Zone 3 is characterized by an arterial pressure greater than venous pressure, which is greater than alveolar pressure. Blood flow is determined by the difference between arterial and venous pressure. Blood flow is less gravity dependent in zone 3 than in zone 2. Because of the height of the right atrium, subjects in the supine position have a majority of their pulmonary circulation in zone 3.

Lung Volumes

Going from the erect to the supine position affects the various lung volumes (Fig. 4–4). Table 4–2 presents data on changes in respiratory parameters induced by changes in posture from the upright, conscious state to the supine, both conscious and anesthetized states.

Functional Residual Capacity

Because gravitational forces on the abdominal contents pull the diaphragm down in an erect subject, the apex of the lung has a greater negative pressure than the base of the lung. This pressure gradient contributes to a greater volume in the alveoli of the apex than those of the base of the lung.[3] In the supine subject, the weight of the abdominal contents is transmitted through the diaphragm to the lungs, thus eliminating the pressure gradient.

Functional residual capacity (FRC) decreases approximately 800 mL from the erect to the

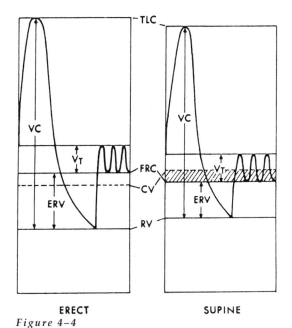

ERECT   SUPINE

Figure 4–4

Differences in lung volume between erect and supine positions. A spirometric tracing is superimposed for better understanding. The ordinate represents lung volume and the abscissa time (TLC = total lung capacity; VC = vital capacity; VT = tidal volume; ERV = end respiratory volume; RV = residual volume; FRC = functional residual capacity; CV = closing volume). In the supine position the CV is greater than FRC, and therefore VT and CV overlap (crosshatched area).

supine position.[30] The greatest decrease in FRC, approximately 20%, is observed during the first few minutes of anesthesia. There is no additional decrease in FRC in the supine, anesthetized subject who is then paralyzed.

Closing Volume

Closing volume (CV) is defined as the fraction of the total lung capacity below which a rapid increase in airway closure occurs when external pressures overcome natural elastic recoil.[35] The closure causes eventual atelectasis and, thus, increases shunting of blood from arterial to venous systems without ventilation occurring. This ventilation/perfusion mismatch occurs primarily in the lower, dependent airways in the erect subject. Airway closure is seen in awake erect subjects at about age 65 and in awake supine subjects at about age 45.[36]

The relationship between CV and FRC in erect and supine subjects can be divided into four groups (Fig. 4–5).[37] In group 1, FRC ex-

ceeds CV in both the supine and erect positions; it is seen in normal individuals without pulmonary disorders. In group 2, CV exceeds FRC only in the supine position, and an increase in alveolar-arterial oxygen tension is observed. In group 3, CV exceeds FRC in both the erect and supine positions, so that the mean alveolar-arterial oxygen tension in the erect position is similar to the value for the supine position of group 2. In group 4, CV occurs above the breathing level in both positions, and there is no significant change in the alveolar-arterial oxygen tension between the two positions.

Between ages 35 to 44 years, subjects begin to enter group 2; and about age 65, subjects enter groups 3 or 4.[36] In general, the CV/FRC relationship of subjects younger than age 7 is at best group 2.[38] The weight/height ratio in the supine position inversely affects the CV/FRC relationship to the extent that an increase in the weight/height ratio, as is seen in obese subjects, worsens their CV/FRC relationship. Smokers demonstrate an increased CV in both the supine and erect positions compared with nonsmokers.[36] Compared with nonsmokers, the FRC of smokers decreases significantly in the supine position. Arterial oxygen tensions decreased from 91 to 84 mm Hg and from 96 to 95 mm Hg in smokers and nonsmokers, respectively, on changing from erect to supine positions.[39]

Vital Capacity

Vital capacity (VC) is influenced by tidal volume, expiratory reserve volume (ERV), and

Table 4–2

Effects of Postural Change on Respiratory Parameters in Awake and Anesthetized Subjects

	Erect		Supine	
	Conscious	Anesthetized and Paralyzed	Conscious	Anesthetized and Paralyzed
FRC	Control	↓ 3%	↓ 24%	↓ 44%
IC		N/A	↑	N/A
ERV		N/A	↓	N/A
VC		N/A	↔ ↑ ↓	N/A
CC		N/A	↔ ↑ (slight)	↔ ↑ (slight)

FRC = functional residual capacity; IC = inspiratory capacity; ERV = expiratory reserve volume; VC = vital capacity.

CC = closing capacity, a measurable volume below which airway closure commences in the dependent areas of the lung.

Changes indicated as ↑ increase, ↓ decrease, ↔ unchanged; N/A = not applicable.

From Coonan TJ, Hope CE: Cardio-respiratory effects of change of body position. Can Anaesth Soc J 30:424, 1983.

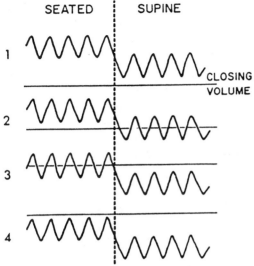

SEATED : SUPINE

CLOSING
VOLUME

Figure 4–5

Classification of subjects into groups (1–4) according
to the relationship of closing volume (CV) to
functional residual capacity (FRC) in the seated and
supine positions. In group 1, FRC exceeded CV in
both positions. In group 2, FRC exceeded CV in the
seated position only, whereas in the supine position
CV exceeded FRC. In group 3, CV occurred within
the breathing range (FRC + tidal volume) in the
seated position and exceeded it in the supine
position. In group 4, CV occurred above the
breathing range in both positions. (From Craig DB:
Closing volume and its relationship to gas exchange
in seated and supine position. J Appl Physiol 31:717,
1971.)

inspiratory capacity (IC). Studies have provided inconsistent results concerning the effect of change in posture on VC; an increase,
decrease, or no change in VC has been reported.[3] In subjects with normal lung physiology, a decrease in ERV is seen with a change
from the erect to the supine position. This
should produce a decrease in the VC. In
subjects with low ERV, as seen in chronic
obstructive lung disease, obesity, quadriplegia, or high intrathecal or epidural anesthesia,
the decrease in VC is not observed with a
change in position.[3]

Inspiratory Capacity

Inspiratory capacity (IC) increases on changing from the erect to the supine position, secondary to elevation of the diaphragm. The
function of the diaphragm is improved in the
supine position in subjects with hyperinflation of the lungs. Whether a decrease or increase in VC is observed depends on which

lung volume is affected more, the IC or the
ERV.

Forced Vital Capacity

Forced vital capacity decreases approximately
300 mL on changing from the erect to the
supine position in the awake subject, but
there are no significant changes in forced expiratory volume (FEV) during the first second
(FEV_1) or in $FEV_1/FVC\%$.[30]

Summary

The upright posture best maintains lung volume and opposes a tendency to small airway
closure, which is the main ventilatory consideration for the majority of subjects presenting
for anesthesia and surgery. The supine position increases diaphragmatic efficiency, cardiac output, and the homogeneity of distribution of pulmonary blood volume.

ENDOCRINE RESPONSES TO THE SUPINE POSITION

A number of hormones are involved in the
adaptation to postural changes. They include
atrial natriuretic peptide, arginine vasopressin, angiotensin, and aldosterone. These compounds are not involved in the acute (neural)
adjustments reviewed earlier, but rather they
gradually influence vascular smooth muscle,
renal excretory function, and fluid fluxes from
intravascular to extravascular sites. In the supine position, atrial stretch initiates the release of atrial natriuretic peptide into the circulation and may, either directly or through
neural mechanisms, inhibit the release of
arginine vasopressin and renin (from the
juxtaglomerular apparatus in the kidney).[40]
An increase in plasma atrial natriuretic peptide initiates movement of intravascular fluid
into the extravascular space and has been
associated with vasodilation, natriuresis, and
diuresis.[41] The simultaneous reduction in arginine vasopressin, angiotensin, and aldosterone levels prevents significant opposition to
the effects of atrial natriuretic peptide. The
decrease in aldosterone production after 24
hours in the supine position leads to a 25%
increase in the urinary excretion of sodium.[42]
The net effect of these gradual responses is to
reduce central blood volume by the move-

ment of fluid into the periphery, the extravascular space, and the bladder.

OTHER PHYSIOLOGIC CONSIDERATIONS FOR THE SUPINE POSITION

Blood Chemistry Values

Normal values for many serum components are different in supine and erect subjects. A significant decrease in hematocrit is observed within 5 minutes of changing from the erect to the supine position. A maximum decrease in hematocrit of 10% to 20% is seen 20 minutes after assuming the supine position.[43] A decrease in the following values is also noted on changing from supine to erect: serum calcium (-6.8%); total protein (-8.8%); albumin (-6.2%); and protein-bound iodine (-16.3%). No changes are seen in glucose or insulin levels. Colloid osmotic pressure decreases from a mean of 25.4 mm Hg in erect subjects to 21.6 mm Hg in supine subjects.[44]

Urine Flow

Because of gravitational forces, the kidneys descend by as much as 2 inches in the erect position as compared with the supine. Despite the potential for decreased renal perfusion in the upright position, urine flow appears to be increased. In addition, urine flow in the erect position is enhanced by increased uteropelvic contractions and ureteral motility, which are inhibited in the supine position.[45]

Esophageal Sphincter Tone and Gastric Emptying Time

Esophageal sphincter tone increases in the supine position.[46] This counteracts the increased propensity for esophageal reflux due to increased intra-abdominal pressure. A significant decrease in gastric emptying time is observed in erect subjects compared with those who are supine.[47] Gastric emptying of a solid meal requires an average of 49.5 minutes in the erect position compared with 62.5 minutes in the supine. A sugary fluid drink requires 41 minutes to empty in the erect position and 56 minutes in the supine position.

Uterine Blood Flow

Uterine blood flow in nonpregnant, nonanesthetized females increases 44% within 10 minutes of a shift from the erect to the supine position.[48] In 15% of pregnant females close to term, the uterus achieves a size and weight sufficient to occlude both the abdominal aorta and the inferior vena cava, producing "supine hypotension syndrome." These individuals present with hypotension, pallor, sweating, nausea and vomiting, and a decrease in both uterine and placental perfusion. This can result in fetal distress and asphyxia. A left uterine displacement of approximately 15 degrees is usually enough to prevent the appearance of a supine hypotension syndrome (see also Chapter 16).

REFERENCES

1. Gauer OH, Thron HL: Postural changes in the circulation. *In* Hamilton WF, Dow P (eds.): Handbook of Physiology. Washington, DC, American Physiological Society, 1965, p. 2409.
2. Blomqvist CG, Stone HL: Cardiovascular adjustments to gravitational stress. *In* Shepherd JT, Abboud FM, Geiger SR (eds.): Handbook of Physiology, Section 2, The Cardiovascular System. Bethesda, MD, American Physiological Society, 1982, p. 1025.
3. Coonan TJ, Hope CE: Cardio-respiratory effects of change of body position. Can Anaesth Soc J 30:424, 1983.
4. Waterfield RL: The effect of posture on the volume of the leg. J Physiol 72:121, 1931.
5. Berg HE, Tedner B, Tesch PA: Changes in lower limb muscle cross-sectional area and tissue fluid volume after transition from standing to supine. Acta Physiol Scand 148:379, 1993.
6. Nixon JV, Murray RG, Bryant C, et al.: Early cardiovascular adaptation to simulated zero gravity. J Appl Physiol 46:541, 1979.
7. Hargens AR, Tipton CM, Gollnick PD, et al.: Fluid shifts and muscle function in humans during acute simulated weightlessness. J Appl Physiol 54:1003, 1983.
8. Linnarsson D, Tedner B, Eiken O: Effects of gravity on the fluid balance and distribution in man. Physiologist 28:S28, 1985.
9. Mark AL, Mancia G: Cardiopulmonary baroreflexes in humans. *In* Shepherd JT, Abboud FM, Geiger SR (eds.): Handbook of Physiology, Section 2: The Cardiovascular System, Vol. III: Peripheral Circulation and Organ Blood Flow. Bethesda, MD, American Physiological Society, 1983, p. 795.
10. Mohanty PK, Sowers JR, McNamara C, et al.: Reflex effects of prolonged cardiopulmonary baroreceptor unloading in humans. Am J Physiol 254:R320, 1988.
11. Joyner MJ, Shepherd JT, Seals DR: Sustained increases in sympathetic outflow during prolonged lower body negative pressure in humans. J Appl Physiol 68:1004, 1990.
12. Roddie IC, Shepherd JT, Whelan RF: Reflex changes in vasoconstrictor tone in human skeletal muscle in response to stimulation of receptors in a low-pressure area of the intrathoracic vascular bed. J Physiol 139:369, 1957.
13. Mohanty PK, Thames MD, Arrowood JA, et al.: Im-

pairment of cardiopulmonary baroreflex after cardiac transplantation in humans. Circulation 75:914, 1987.

14. Mark AL: The Bezold-Jarisch reflex revisited: Clinical implications of inhibitory reflexes originating in the heart. J Am Coll Cardiol 1:90, 1983.

15. Sander-Jensen K, Mehlsen J, Stadeager C, et al.: Increase in vagal activity during hypotensive lower-body negative pressure in humans. Am J Physiol 255:R149, 1988.

16. Ward RJ, Danziger F, Bonica JJ: Cardiovascular effects of change of posture. Aerospace Med 37:257, 1966.

17. Korner PI: Integrative neural cardiovascular control. Physiol Rev 51:312, 1971.

18. Ebert TJ, Morgan BJ, Barney JA, et al.: Effects of aging on baroreflex regulation of sympathetic activity in humans. Am J Physiol 263:H798, 1992.

19. Burgos LG, Ebert TJ, Asiddao C, et al.: Increased intraoperative cardiovascular morbidity in diabetics with autonomic neuropathy. Anesthesiology 70:591, 1989.

20. Ebert TJ: Pre-operative evaluation of the autonomic nervous system. *In* Stoelting R, Barash P, Gallagher T (eds.): Advances in Anesthesia, vol. 10. St. Louis, CV Mosby, 1992, p. 49.

21. Smith JJ, Porth CM, Erickson M: Hemodynamic response to the upright posture. J Clin Pharmacol 34:375, 1994.

22. Frey MA, Tomaselli CM, Hoffler WG: Cardiovascular responses to postural changes: Differences with age for women and men. J Clin Pharmacol 34:394, 1994.

23. Denahan T, Ebert TJ: Sympathetic responses to controlled hypotension do not differ in runners and sedentary controls. Med Sci Sports Exerc 23:S5, 1991 (abstract).

24. Ebert TJ, Barney JA: Physical fitness and orthostatic tolerance. *In* Smith JJ (ed.): Circulatory Response to the Upright Posture. Boca Raton, FL, CRC Press, 1990, p. 47.

25. Smith ML, Raven PB: Cardiovascular responses to lower body negative pressure in endurance and static exercise-trained men. Med Sci Sports Exerc 18:545, 1986.

26. Smith ML, Graitzer HM, Hudson DL, et al.: Baroreflex function in endurance- and static exercise–trained men. J Appl Physiol 64:585, 1988.

27. Laubie M, Schmitt H, Vincent M: Vagal bradycardia produced by microinjections of morphine-like drugs into the nucleus ambiguus in anaesthetized dogs. Eur J Pharmacol 59:287, 1979.

28. Pae E-K, Lowe AA, Sasaki K, et al.: A cephalometric and electromyographic study of upper airway structures in the upright and supine positions. Am J Orthod Dentofac Orthop 106:52, 1994.

29. Vellody VP, Nassery M, Druz WS, et al.: Effects of body position change on thoracoabdominal motion. J Appl Physiol 45:R581, 1978.

30. Lumb AB, Nunn JF: Respiratory function and rib cage contribution to ventilation in body positions commonly used during anesthesia. Anesth Analg 73:422, 1991.

31. Wang CS, Josenhans WT: Contribution of diaphragmatic/abdominal displacement to ventilation in supine man. J Appl Physiol 31:576, 1971.

32. Froese AB, Bryan AC: Effects of anesthesia and paralysis on diaphragmatic mechanics in man. Anesthesiology 41:242, 1974.

33. Bryan AC, Bentivoglio LG, Beerel F, et al.: Factors affecting regional distribution of ventilation and perfusion in the lung. J Appl Physiol 19:395, 1964.

34. West JB, Dollery CT, Naimark A: Distribution of blood flow in isolated lung: Relation to vascular and alveolar pressures. J Appl Physiol 19:713, 1964.

35. Fairley HB: Airway closure. Anesthesiology 36:529, 1972.

36. Leblanc P, Ruff F, Milic-Emili J: Effects of age and body position on "airway closure" in man. J Appl Physiol 28:448, 1970.

37. Craig DB, Wahba WE, Don HF, et al.: "Closing volume" and its relationship to gas exchange in seated and supine positions. J Appl Physiol 31:717, 1971.

38. Mansell A, Bryan C, Levison H: Airway closure in children. J Appl Physiol 33:711, 1972.

39. Strieder DJ, Murphy R, Kazemi H: Mechanism of postural hypoxemia in asymptomatic smokers. Am Rev Respir Dis 99:760, 1969.

40. Christensen G: Cardiovascular and renal effects of atrial natriuretic factor. Scand J Clin Lab Invest 53:203, 1993.

41. Ebert TJ, Skelton MM, Cowley AW Jr: Dynamic cardiovascular responses to infusion of atrial natriuretic factor in humans. Hypertension 11:537, 1988.

42. Williams GH, Cain JP, Dluhy RG, et al.: Studies on the control of plasma aldosterone concentration in normal man: I. Response to posture, acute and chronic volume depletion and sodium loading. J Clin Invest 51:1731, 1972.

43. Ekelund LG, Eklund B, Kaijser L: Time course for the change in hemoglobin concentration with change in posture. Acta Med Scand 190:335, 1971.

44. Weil MH, Morissetto M, Michaels S, et al.: Routine plasma colloid osmotic pressure measurements. Crit Care Med 2:229, 1974.

45. McKinnon KJ, Toth J, Foote JW: The influence of position on urine transport. J Urol 109:631, 1973.

46. Babka JC, Hager GW, Castell DO: Effect of body posture on lower esophageal sphincter pressure. Am J Dig Dis 18:441, 1973.

47. Hulme-Moir I, Donnan SP, McAlister J, et al.: Effect of surgery and posture on the pattern and rate of gastric emptying. Aust NZ J Med 43:80, 1973.

48. Secher NJ, Einer-Jensen N, Juhl B: Blood flow through myometrium and endometrium in standing and supine women measured by intrauterine xenon application. Am J Obstet Gynecol 117:386, 1973.

Dorsal Decubitus Positions

Chapter 5

Supine Positions

Mark A. Warner

BACKGROUND

The surgical origins of the supine position are shrouded in antiquity. However, its use in primitive versions of treatment of injuries is all but certain. Necessary restraints for painful wound repairs could probably best be applied to a struggling victim who was supine. This position also offered good access to the mouth for therapeutic ingestion of mood-altering compounds and analgesics such as alcohol.

The horizontal supine position is the dorsal decubitus posture most commonly used by all surgical specialties today because it provides excellent surgical access to most body areas. Although there are many physiologic changes that occur when a standing patient assumes a horizontal supine position (see Chapter 4), these alterations are generally well tolerated. There are obvious exceptions to this generality, such as the potential detrimental effects in supine patients of massive obesity on respiration (see Chapter 14) or of a gravid uterus on venous return of blood volume (see Chapter 16). Overall, however, most patients tolerate the horizontal supine position as well as or better than other intraoperative positions.

VARIETIES OF SUPINE POSITIONS

The supine position has three major variations: the traditional, the contoured, and the froglegged.

- The most common version is the *traditional supine position* in which a patient lies on the back and usually has a small pillow under the head (see Fig. 5–1). The arms are either comfortably padded and restrained alongside the trunk or abducted on padded armboards. This position often places the hips and knees in extension in excess to that usually allowed by unlimbered muscles that cross the hip and knee joints. It may be poorly tolerated for prolonged periods by awake, unsedated patients. A variation of the traditional horizontal supine position, used for operations in and about the knee joint, moves the patient to situate the thigh-leg hinge of the table surface several inches cephalad of the popliteal space (see Fig. 5–2). When the leg section of the top is depressed to the vertical or removed, the lower leg hangs free, the knee joint mechanism extends beyond the caudad end of the table top, and the area about the joint is surgically accessible.
- The *contoured supine or lawn chair position* is an alternative supine position in which the hips and knees are slightly flexed into more neutral joint positions (see Figs. 5–3 and 5–4). This contoured position is similar to that assumed when resting in an adjustable reclining chair. Patients who are required to lie awake and immobile for prolonged periods in the traditional supine position usually express appreciation for the comfort provided when this alternative position is arranged.
- The *frogleg supine position* modifies the traditional supine position by flexing the hips and knees 15 to 30 degrees, externally rotating the hips and bringing the heels together in midline (see Fig. 5–5). This position is commonly used by colon-

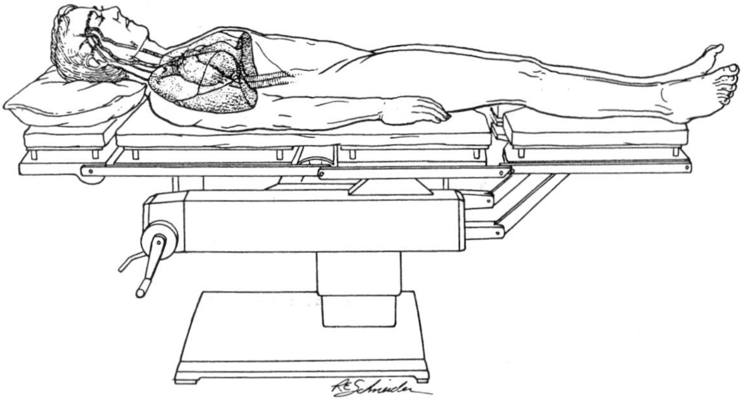

Figure 5–1

The traditional horizontal supine position, also known as "lying at attention." (From Barash PG, Cullen BF, Stoelting RK [eds.]: Clinical Anesthesia, 2nd ed. Philadelphia, JB Lippincott, 1992.)

oscopists and surgeons who require short exposures to the medial thigh, genitalia, and perineum.

ESTABLISHING THE POSITIONS

Establishing the Traditional Supine Position

The weight of a patient who is lying in the traditional supine position (Fig. 5–1) is borne by the occiput, dorsal torso and scapulae, sacrum, dorsal legs, and heels. For this reason, the operating table must be well padded with a firm supportive mattress. Additional padding may be useful under these areas. The goal of padding should be to distribute the weight along the dorsum of the body and protect bony contact points from excess weight bearing. Thoughtful but overzealous padding that fails to distribute the weight should be avoided. For example, the use of bulky padding under the legs to elevate the heels from the table and relieve them of weight bearing may result in overextension of the knees and stretching the tendons of the hamstring muscle group, the heads of the gastrocnemius muscles, and the posterior capsules of the knees.

In the traditional supine position, either the arms are padded and comfortably tucked alongside the trunk or one or both arms are abducted and secured onto padded armboards. Issues related to correct placement of the upper extremities are discussed in Chapter 11.

In many patients, great care is needed to provide comfortable arrangement and padding of the spine. Reclining into the supine position decreases the pressure inside lumbar disks by anteriorly rotating the pelvis[1] and decreasing the amount of lordotic curvature in the lumbar spine.[2] Nachemson[1] used diskometry to directly measure the pressure inside lumbar disks in volunteers who were studied in a variety of positions. A change in position from sitting erect to supine decreased pressure on the posterior part of the annulus fibrosus of lumbar and lumbosacral disks by more than 50%. Several investigative teams found that reclining reduced lumbar paravertebral muscle activity and increased intervertebral distances.[3, 4] For these reasons, the supine position (e.g., bed rest) is recommended for patients with herniated lumbar disk disease.

Loss of the normal lordotic curvature for prolonged periods, however, may cause perioperative backache. Brown and Elman[5] have concluded that the rate of postoperative backache is related to the duration of surgery. The mechanism for backache is likely perivertebral ligamentous and muscular stretch from loss of the normal lordotic curvature. Regional and general anesthetics are associated with similar rates of postoperative backache.

The supine position may result in exaggerated lumbar lordosis in patients who have large buttocks and "tight" hip flexors (i.e., iliopsoas and rectus femoris muscles). In these patients, the hip joints can be functionally hyperextended (beyond the normal stretch limitations of the hip flexors) in the supine position. Nachemson and Elfstrom[6] and others[7, 8] have noted that hyperextension at the hip can cause posterior rotation of the pelvis, increase intervertebral and paravertebral muscle activity, and increase pressure on the lumbar and lumbosacral disks. For patients with this set of characteristics, placement of a small pillow under the knees will slightly flex the hips and attenuate the increased pressure on the lumbar disks. The lawn chair (contoured supine) position provides a similar mechanical advantage by flexing the table top and depressing the foot section. Patients often express their gratitude for this small positioning and padding adjustment.

Patients with severe kyphoscoliosis, kyphosis, and other spinous degenerative disease processes present special positioning problems for the traditional supine position. Preferentially, these patients usually avoid lying supine. Attempts to provide comfort and postural stability supine by the use of appropriately placed padding should be assessed, adjusted, and confirmed before sedation is administered or anesthesia is induced.

Establishing the Supine Hanging-Leg Position

The purpose of this position is to provide surgical access to most of the circumference of a knee joint while the weight of the free-hanging lower leg keeps the joint space open. The mobile leg can be wrapped in sterile sheets and manipulated as needed by members of the surgical team during the procedure (Fig. 5–2).

After being placed supine on the operating table, the patient is drawn caudad until the hinge between the thigh and leg sections of the table top rests several inches proximal to the popliteal fossa. Subsequently, the leg section of the table top is lowered toward the vertical. As a result, the distal end of the thigh projects beyond the now-vertical surface of the leg section sufficiently for the lower leg to hang free. Importantly, the patient must be far enough caudad on the table so that the

top edge of the depressed leg section cannot impact the upper calf of either dangling lower extremity. If it does compress a dorsal lower leg, vascular complications may be produced in the compromised limb.

Establishing the Lawn Chair (Contoured Supine) Position

The *lawn chair* label was coined by Martin in earlier editions of this book.[9, 10] The following quoted passages are excerpts taken from his description in the second edition.[10]

Consider the difference between lying supine on a floor and reclining in a contour chair. While the hard floor is advocated as restful by some, the chair is preferred by most. On an unyielding flat surface the occiput, shoulders, spine, buttocks, and heels are weight bearing, and major joints are extended beyond comfortable neutral alignment. Despite the fact that a padded operating table distributes weight somewhat more equitably, joint positions are essentially unchanged. This "lying-at-attention" position (also aptly described as the rigid supine position) can, and does, rapidly contribute to discomfort for patients who are awake during protected surgical and anesthetic procedures.

In contrast, the contour chair (or lawn chair) not only distributes support along the full length of the dorsal body surface, it also permits gentle flexion at the hips and knees to put these joints into more anatomically neutral positions.

- The advantage of this arrangement can be readily demonstrated to any skeptic who first lies supine on a flat, padded operating table (Fig. 5–3A) and then has the table top flexed by three full turns of the control handle (see Fig. 5–3B) and the foot section depressed by three reverse turns of the same handle (see Fig.

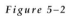

Figure 5–2

The supine position with hanging legs for access to knee joints. Note that the proximal edge of the depressed foot section of the table top is not able to impact the calf below the knee and interfere with perfusion in the posterior compartment of the leg.

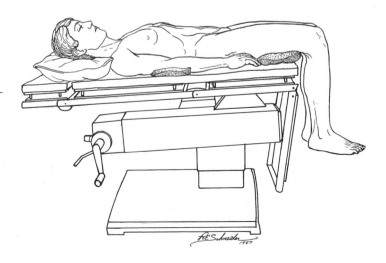

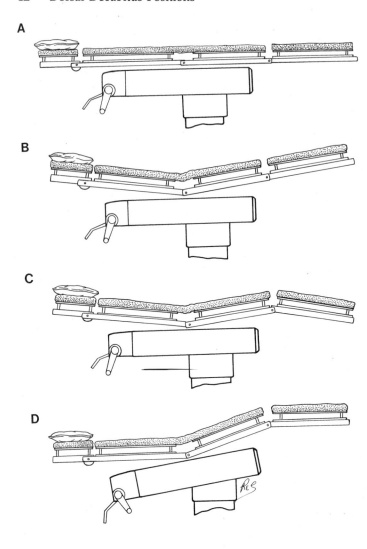

Figure 5–3

Steps in establishing the "lawn chair" or contoured supine position. *A.* Flat table top showing position selector switch and activator crank. *B.* Gentle flexion of hips obtained by three full rotations of activator crank with switch on "flex" setting. *C.* Minimal knee flexion produced by three full reverse rotations of the activator crank with switch on "foot" (or "leg") setting. *D.* Chassis tilted sufficiently head-down to level back section of table top and permit attachment of an armboard with floor-standing legs.

5–3*C*). (The surface controls of the American Sterilizer Company's model 2080 surgical table are the references for this description, et seq.) The result is that the thigh section of the table top is flexed 15 to 20 degrees on the back section, and a similar but opposite angulation is produced at the leg-thigh hinge.

- Further comfort is gained by placing a small pillow under the occiput. Not uncommonly, an audible expression of appreciation will come from the patient who experiences this change from the rigid to the contoured supine position.

When it is necessary to attach a floor-standing armboard to the back section of the table, the flexion depicted in Figure 5–3*C* renders the board one legged and unstable. This problem is easily overcome by using the chassis control to lower the cephalad end of the table until its back section is parallel to the floor, and the legs of the board are equally supportive (see Fig. 5–3*D*). The other

skeletal advantages of the contoured position are preserved, as is the comfort of the patient.

Lawn Chair Position for the Patient in Shock

A significant issue to consider in the application of the lawn chair position is its effect on an unstable cardiovascular system (Fig. 5–4).

- In the contoured supine position, the head of the patient and both lower extremities are raised gently above the long axis of the great vessels and the level of the heart.
- When cardiac output is reduced by shock, the resulting postural gradients are unlikely by themselves to lessen arterial perfusion against gravity to either the head or the legs.
- The gradients, even though small, favor gravity induced venous drainage into both the superior and the inferior venae cavae, thus aug-

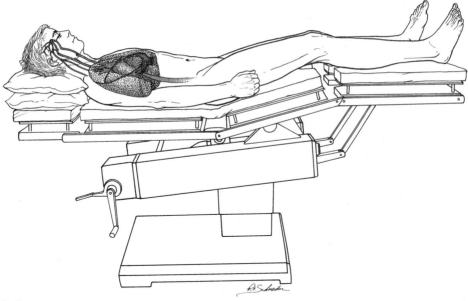

Figure 5–4

Vascular attributes of the contoured supine position. The circle of Willis and vessels in the lower extremities are slightly higher than the great vessels of the abdomen and thorax, establishing a drainage gradient in the venous system with only a slight uphill perfusion requirement for the head and limbs. (From Martin JT: The Trendelenburg position: A review of current slants about head-down tilt. *AANA Journal* 63:29–36, 1995.)

menting central blood volume, atrial filling, and ventricular output.

- Elevation of the occiput on a small pillow raises the head above the level of the atrium, lessens cerebral venous pressure, and minimizes the chances for producing or increasing cerebral edema. By contrast, the cerebral congestion produced by the head-down position has been associated with a 14 percent reduction of cerebral blood flow that threatens either to produce or to increase cerebral edema.[11]
- Because the horizontal axis of the trunk is not changed, pulmonary blood volume should not be undesirably redistributed, thereby avoiding venous congestion in poorly ventilated pulmonary apices that is a typical and detrimental aspect of head-down tilt.
- The hydrostatic indifferent point, described by Coonan and Hope (1983),[12] is maintained in its optimum position at the level of the atrium, thus maximizing cardiac filling and output.

Understandably, therefore, the lawn chair position can be viewed as approaching the ideal in the postural treatment of shock. Because the Trendelenburg position has been well documented to be a measurable insult to the patient with an impaired circulatory system,[13] the lawn chair position is a rational and strongly advocated alternative.

Lawn Chair Position and Abdominal Relaxation

An additional advantage of the lawn chair position resides in the fact that the hip flexion that it achieves slightly shortens the xiphoid-to-pubic distance, resulting in less stretching of the ventral abdominal musculature.

When the flat operating table used to facilitate a laparotomy is adjusted to the lawn chair position during closure of the abdominal wall, the relaxation so produced may often spare the need for the final increment of a curariform drug. The return of stable ventilatory sufficiency for the subsequently awakening patient may thereby be hastened.

Establishing the Frogleg Supine Position

The frogleg supine position is a modification of the traditional supine position. To expose the perineum, medial thighs, genitalia, and rectum to surgical or diagnostic procedures, the thighs are flexed and externally rotated at the hips. This movement occurs by (1) simultaneously flexing the bilateral knees and hips while the heels remain on or near the mattress, (2) separating the knees by externally rotating the hips, and (3) bringing the heels close together.

The weight of the lower extremities must be supported with blankets or pillows placed beneath the knees (Fig. 5–5*A*) or under the lateral aspects of the thighs and lower legs (see Fig. 5–5*B*) to avoid overrotation of the hips and unintended pressure on the lateral

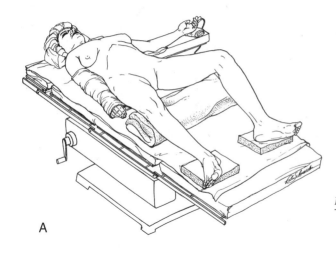

A

Figure 5–5

Variations of the frogleg position. *A*. Flexed knees separated with minimal external rotation of abducted thighs. *B*. More pronounced knee separation and external rotation of thighs with feet placed with soles together. (*B* from McLeskey CH [ed.]: Geriatric Anesthesia. Baltimore, Williams & Wilkins, in press.)

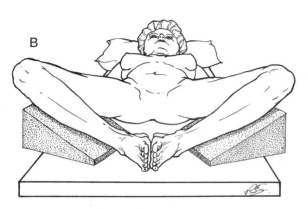

B

aspects of the knees. Depending on the mobility of the patient's skeleton, the plantar aspects of the feet may be contacting each other (see Fig. 5–5*B*). The feet then may need to be held firmly in place by carefully applied supports or restraints to prevent inadvertent extension of the knees and approximation of the thighs that would restrict surgical access to the perineum.

COMPLICATIONS

Excluding extremity injuries (see Chapter 11), there are three main complications of the supine positions: backache, pressure point reactions, and pressure alopecia.

- *Backache:* As noted earlier, patients who must lie immobile for prolonged periods in a supine position often complain of backache.[5] There are several potential causes for this finding. First, loss of the normal lumbar lordotic curvature in the supine position, especially when the effects of anesthetics and muscle relaxants have reduced or eliminated the resting tone of paraspinal muscles, may stretch those muscles and lumbar paraspinal ligaments. Second, although support of the weight of a supine body is widely distributed over a padded operating table, bony prominences, including the spine, may bear uncomfortable loads for extended periods of time in immobile patients. The uncomfortable aspects of the supine position on the spine may be augmented by immobility. Supine, motionless volunteers maintain normal distribution of tissue perfusion for approximately 1 hour.[12] Further immobility increases discomfort and restlessness. Myalgias associated with succinylcholine-induced fasciculations and other drugs are often noted in the lumbar paraspinal musculature. Any of these potential etiologies can cause backache in the postoperative period.

- *Pressure point reactions:* Tissues overlying bony prominences can develop varying degrees of ischemic changes unless padding is provided to distribute the weight bearing away from the individual prominences. During prolonged procedures in anesthetized supine patients, the heels and plantarflexor tendons are especially at risk for developing blisters and ischemic pressure areas.
- *Pressure alopecia:* The same weight-bearing forces that produce ischemic areas over bony prominences may also compress and render hair follicles ischemic. Prolonged compression of hair follicles may produce hair loss.[14] Alopecia may not occur until several days to weeks after the procedure.[15–18] The alopecia may be related to prolonged postoperative bed rest as well as prolonged surgical procedures. Hypothermia and hypotension associated with cardiopulmonary bypass may also be associated with the risk of developing alopecia.[19] Because perioperative alopecia may be related to prolonged immobilization of the occiput during the intraoperative period, it seems appropriate to frequently turn the head during lengthy operations and to use padded, soft head supports or pillows. Similar advice is also applicable in the postoperative period for nonambulatory patients, especially those who may be immobile in intensive care settings.

the potential for *supine hypotensive or aortocaval syndrome.* This syndrome is similar to the aortocaval syndrome present during term pregnancy. For mobile masses, displacement of the mass off the vena cava may improve venous return. For masses that are fixated to the abdominal wall or tethered to other intra-abdominal structures, displacement may not be possible and alternative methods of increasing cardiac preload may be needed.

- *Integrity of the spine:* Patients with severe kyphoscoliosis or kyphosis will need extra padding if positioned supine. Bony prominences of the spine should be well padded. Patients with exaggerated lumbar lordosis and pre-existing back pain may benefit from some degree of hip and knee flexion.
- *Integrity of the skin:* Patients with pre-existing cutaneous lesions of the dorsum, especially those with lesions overlying weight-bearing areas, should be carefully evaluated. Makeshift pads can be formed to alleviate excessive pressure on these areas.
- *Presence of artificial joints:* Patients with one or more total hip or knee arthroplasties may be unable to tolerate the traditional supine position or the frogleg supine variation. These patients should be positioned while awake to determine if the position places excessive stress on the hips or knees.

PREOPERATIVE EVALUATION

Although the supine positions place less stress on many parts of the body than other positions (e.g., prone and lithotomy positions), there are a number of patient-related factors to evaluate in the preanesthetic period. Often the best way to evaluate patients is to place them as nearly as is tolerable in the proposed operative position.

- *Body habitus:* There are a variety of issues related to the obese patient in a supine position (see Chapter 14). These include respiratory compromise when reclined and ability to physically fit on the operating table. Similar considerations are present for patients with increased abdominal size from ascites or large tumors. One additional issue related to the presence of large intraabdominal tumors is

REFERENCES

1. Nachemson A: In vivo discometry in lumbar discs with irregular nucleograms. Acta Orthop Scand 36:418, 1965.
2. Friberg S, Hirsch C: Anatomical and clinical studies on lumbar disc degeneration. Acta Orthop Scand 19:222, 1949.
3. Anderson BJG, Ortegren R: Myoelectric back muscle activity during sitting. Scand J Rehab Med 3:73, 1974.
4. Tannii K, Masuda T: A kinesiologic study of erectores spinae activity during trunk flexion and extension. Ergonomics 28:883, 1985.
5. Brown EM, Elman DS: Postoperative backache. Anesth Analg 40:683, 1961.
6. Nachemson A, Elfstrom G: Intravital dynamic pressure measurements in lumbar disc. Scand J Rehabil Med 1:5, 1970.
7. Stoller DW, Genant HK: Magnetic resonance imaging of the lumbar spine. *In* Weinstein JN, Wiesel SW (eds.): The Lumbar Spine. Philadelphia, WB Saunders, 1990, p. 342.
8. Clinical approach: Algorithm for the virgin back. *In* Wiesel SW, Bernini P, Rothman RH (eds.): The Aging

Lumbar Spine. Philadelphia, WB Saunders, 1982, p. 101.

9. Martin JT: General requirements of safe positioning for the surgical patient. *In* Martin JT (ed.): Positioning in Anesthesia and Surgery. Philadephia, WB Saunders, 1978, pp. 5–7.

10. Martin JT: The lawn chair (contoured supine) position. *In* Martin JT (ed.): Positioning in Anesthesia and Surgery, 2nd ed. Philadelphia, WB Saunders, 1987, pp. 37–40.

11. Shenkin HA, Scheurerman EB, Spitz EB, et al.: Effect of change of posture on cerebral circulation of man. J Appl Physiol 2:317, 1949.

12. Coonan TJ, Hope CE: Cardiorespiratory effects of change of body position. Can Anaesth Soc J 30:424, 1983.

13. Sibbald WJ, Paterson NA, Holliday RL, et al.: The Trendelenberg position: Hemodynamic effects in hypotensive and normotensive patients. Crit Care Med 7:218, 1979.

14. Wiles JC, Hansen RC: Postoperative (pressure) alopecia. J Am Acad Dermatol 12:195, 1985.

15. Courington FW: The role of posture in anesthesia. Clin Anesth 3:24, 1968.

16. Abel RR, Lewis GM: Postoperative alopecia. Arch Dermatol 81:72, 1960.

17. Patel KD, Henschel EU: Postoperative alopecia. Anesth Analg 59:311, 1980.

18. Gormley T, Sokoll MD: Permanent alopecia from pressure of a head strap. JAMA 199:157, 1967.

19. Lawson NW, Mills NL, Oschner JL: Occipital alopecia following cardiopulmonary bypass. J Thorac Cardiovasc Surg 71:342, 1976.

Chapter **6**

Lithotomy Positions

John T. Martin

BACKGROUND

Ancient physicians removed calculi from the urinary bladder and were called "lithotomists." A stone estimated to be 7000 years old was found in an Egyptian skeleton and was displayed in the Museum of the Royal College of Surgeons of England until it was destroyed during bombing of the museum in World War II.[1] Transperineal surgical extraction of a stone through the neck of the bladder was a procedure of antiquity that was reserved for young boys whose prostates were not yet large enough to block the approach. The restrained patient was held in the lap of a seated, *"strong and intelligent person who steadied the patient by pressing his* (own) *chest against his* (the victim's) *shoulder blades."*[1] That posture became known as the "lithotomy position" (Fig. 6–1). The seated arrangement apparently helped retain the stone against the bladder neck and within reach of the transperineal fingers of the surgeon. Perhaps because of its high rate of complications, heavy bleeding and common mortality, Hippocrates advocated that legitimate members of the medical profession should not perform the operation.[1]

Weyrauch found evidence of prostatectomies being accomplished as early as 490 BC and noted emphasis on the importance of proper positioning.[2] Kropp concludes that the lithotomy position was probably involved.[3]

In more recent centuries the supine posture with legs elevated and bent knees spread laterally has been called the lithotomy position. It may have been the most convenient arrangement by which to visualize the reproductive tract of the female and conduct a bimanual examination.[4] Vaginal specula have been found in the ruins of Pompeii and Her-

culaneum. Soranus reported the use of a speculum and Hippocrates described the cervices of pregnant women.[5] Ancient Egyptian physicians apparently placed medications against

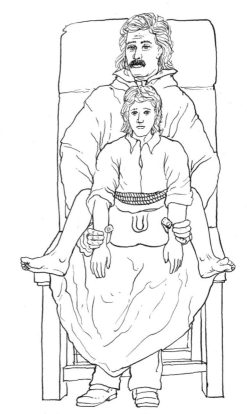

Figure 6–1

Reproduction of a woodcut showing a child being held in "lithotomy position" before having a stone removed from his urinary bladder. (Redrawn from Giannopoulos T, Kostakopoulos A, Sofras F, Dimopoulos C: The operation of lithotomy in Ancient Greece. Urol Int 42:210, 1987. S Karger, Basel.)

the cervix. Goldstein believes that use of the knee-chest and curled lateral positions for female examinations occurred much later than the advent of lithotomy positions.[5]

For more detailed discussions of the surgical uses of the lithotomy position the readers are referred to chapters in earlier editions of this text, pertinent parts of which have been incorporated in the following information.[6, 7]

VARIETIES OF LITHOTOMY POSITIONS

Classification and Terminology

Difficulties exist in accurately discussing the several types of lithotomy positions in use. Terms in the literature such as *dorsal lithotomy, semi-lithotomy,* and *modified lithotomy* are frequent, but they convey little meaning. By definition all lithotomy positions are "dorsal," and any variation can be modified: "semi" could be interpreted as meaning only one leg elevated. Classic corruptions of descriptors have occurred with the terms *inverted lithotomy*[8] and *reverse lithotomy,*[9] each coined to indicate a variation of the prone position.

Operative records frequently describe different modalities of leg elevation either in similar terms or in jargon that is inexact, inconsistent, and confusing. Antithetical opinions can be caused by a single report. The results are capable of frustrating medicolegal proceedings when complications are alleged to result from patient positioning. To obviate misinterpretation, the following simple terminology of *low, standard, high, hemi-, exaggerated,* and *tilted* is strongly recommended for standardization and general use (Fig. 6–2).[10]

Low Lithotomy (see Fig. 6–2A)

The legs of the supine patient are abducted without force until the thighs form about an 80-degree angle with each other. Each hip is gently flexed until the angle between each thigh and the table surface is about 40 degrees. The knees are bent until the lower legs roughly parallel the frontal plane of the torso and are held by the mechanical support. Separation of the thighs is sufficient to allow an operator to work at the perineum. Hip flexion is not enough to prevent an operator standing at the flank of the patient from reaching across the thigh to manipulate a surgical instrument either in the vagina or in a perineal incision. This position is most frequently re-

ferred to as *modified lithotomy,* an inexact, nondescriptive, and useless term that should be abandoned.

Standard Lithotomy (see Fig. 6–2B)

The standard or traditional lithotomy position requires that the patient's legs be separated from the midline into 30 to 45 degrees of unforced abduction and each placed in an elevated holding device. The hips are flexed until the thighs are angled between 80 and 100 degrees on the trunk with the knees being bent until the lower legs are roughly parallel to the frontal plane of the torso.

Hemilithotomy (see Fig. 6–2C)

This position is used most often to assist with the repair of a fractured femur. The nonsurgical lower extremity is elevated onto a calf rest in essentially a standard lithotomy configuration, whereas the other remains at the level of the torso (and is usually in traction). A specialized operating table with a traction attachment that realigns and maintains the position of the bony fragments in the injured extremity is required. As a primary consideration, elevating the nonoperative leg permits the C-arm of a portable fluoroscope to be placed under the raised extremity so that the camera can rotate to gain multiple views of the fracture site in the horizontal thigh without invading the sterile surgical field on its lateral surface.

High Lithotomy (see Fig. 6–2D)

This position is favored by some obstetrician-gynecologists who usually stand while operating on the perineum. The abducted thighs extend upward almost exactly at right angles to the long axis of the trunk with the knees being flexed only slightly. The high lithotomy position provides both the scrub nurse and a surgical assistant access to the perineal operating field while standing beside the shoulders of the operating surgeon.

Exaggerated Lithotomy (see Fig. 6–2E)

Well termed *exaggerated,* this version of the lithotomy position was first advocated in 1951 by Young and now bears his name.[11] The thighs are markedly flexed on the trunk and abducted enough to offer access to the suprapubic abdomen; the knees are bent; and the lower legs project almost vertically up-

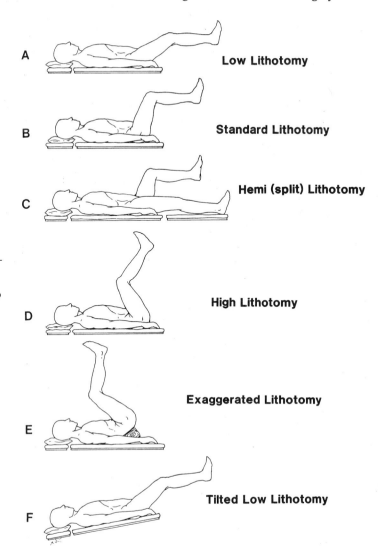

A **Low Lithotomy**

B **Standard Lithotomy**

C **Hemi (split) Lithotomy**

D **High Lithotomy**

E **Exaggerated Lithotomy**

F **Tilted Low Lithotomy**

Figure 6–2

Proposed classification and terminology for variations of the lithotomy position that is intended to end nondescriptive jargon now in use.

ward above the middle of the patient's chest. Additionally, a pad may be placed beneath the sacrum to diminish lumbar curvature. It also serves to rotate the caudal edge of the symphysis pubis ventrally far enough to improve transperineal access to retropubic structures such as the prostate.

Tilted Lithotomy (see Fig. 6–2F)

Any degree of head-down tilt can be added to any version of the lithotomy position. The posture advocated by Lloyd-Davies[12] to allow simultaneous transabdominal and transpelvic access to organs of the deep pelvis originally involved only a modest degree of head depression (see Chapter 8 and Fig. 8–4). Recently, however, some laparoscopists have required steep head-down tilt with the low lithotomy position for prolonged periods of time to avoid the surgical trauma of an open laparotomy.

Establishing Lithotomy

Table Attachments

At the junction of the thigh and leg sections of the top of a standard surgical table, or at the hinge between the trunk and foot sections of an examination table, can be located an adjustable receiver into which the vertical portion of a leg holder rod is inserted and securely clamped. After the patient is positioned, the section of the table surface beyond that junction is rotated toward the floor or removed as needed to permit access to the perineum. Before terminating the lithotomy position, the table is usually restored to its original preoperative size and contour.

Leg holders for the lithotomy positions vary in configuration despite the careless and improper tendency to refer to all varieties jargonistically as "stirrups." Each is connected to the pole that has been clamped to the side of the table. Paschal and Strzelecki[13] have published a useful review of these devices (Figs. 6–3 and 6–4).

- A "candy cane" pole (see Fig. 6–3A) suspends either the ankle and instep by a strap or the foot by a cloth boot. At the end of the curved top of the cane is a hook or clip to retain the straps of the foot holder. McQuarrie and co-workers[14] illustrated a variant that had a well-padded, short transverse bar at the top to which the sole of the foot was affixed by fabric straps. Usually this type of holder is restricted to short procedures because

the entire lower extremity is mobile and can be displaced by the body positions of the surgical team.
- A "knee crutch" (see Fig. 6–3B) supports the popliteal space but permits the foot and much of the lower leg to hang unsupported. If the crutch is ill fitting or if the extremity is unusually heavy, the effect of gravity on the unsupported lower leg and foot can cause the distal edge of the crutch to compress the calf and compromise the vasculature of the limb.
- A "calf rest" (see Fig. 6–3C and D) supports only the dorsal lower leg. Neither the foot nor the popliteal space is compressed, but the full weight of the extremity is borne by the calf.
- Several varieties of firm foot holders resemble the dorsal and/or plantar portions of a boot (see Fig. 6–4). They keep

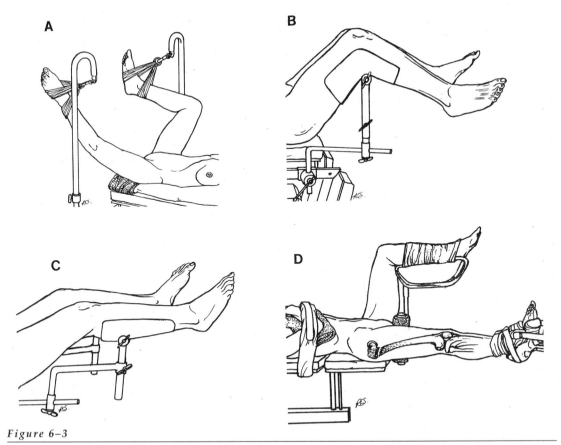

Figure 6–3

Extremity supporting devices for lithotomy position. *A.* "Candy cane" poles with cloth slings for feet. Extremities remain mobile while suspended. *B.* Knee crutch. Weight of unsupported lower leg and foot can compress calf against distal lip of crutch. *C.* Calf support. Weight of limb can compress calf if procedure is lengthy. *D.* Hemilithotomy for fracture repair during traction on injured extremity. Wrapped, elevated limb is at risk of hypoperfusion if blood pressure is low. Padding not shown for clarity. (From Martin JT: Compartment syndromes: Concepts and perspectives for the anesthesiologist. Anesth Analg 75:275, 1992.)

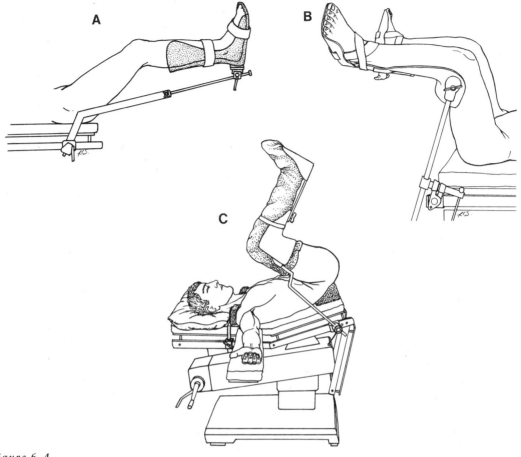

Figure 6–4

Supporting devices for relatively immobile lower extremities in lithotomy position. *A.* Cushioned dorsal boot. *B.* Adjustable knee and foot support. *C.* Unit similar to *B* retaining extremities firmly in exaggerated lithotomy position. Shoulder braces may be needed for heavy patient or tilted table top; usually the extreme hip flexion plus the metal frame of the supporting unit retain the torso against cephalad displacement. Padding not shown for clarity. (From Martin JT: Compartment syndromes: Concepts and perspectives for the anesthesiologist. Anesth Analg 75:275, 1992.)

the extremity firmly in place and free both the popliteal space and the calf from compression.

- Combinations of knee and foot supports exist (see Fig. 6–4*B* and *C*) that can be adjusted to the dimensions of a specific lower extremity.

Patient Arrangement

PRELITHOTOMY POSITION

When awake patients are first placed on the examining or operating table, they are often asked to position themselves supine in a pre-lithotomy posture in which the tip of the sacrum is situated at the break between the main table top and the section that will even-

tually be lowered or removed to permit access to the perineum. Once the lithotomy position has been established, this buttocks-to-table-end arrangement allows a vaginal or anal speculum to hang free against the perineum. However, for a patient lying supine on an operating table it may cause much of the length of the lower legs to extend beyond the distal edge of the table. The lever action of the weight of the unsupported feet and ankles can place unwanted pressure on the calves. Unless that calf compression is very brief, vascular compromise is possible, particularly for patients with significant atherosclerosis of peripheral vessels. Any lengthy induction of anesthesia with the patient in this position adds to the opportunity for a compressive vascular insult to the calves.

If not placed in the prelithotomy position before induction, the patient will need to be shifted caudad into it after anesthesia is started. This move may be accomplished with the lower extremities either extended on the table surface or placed loosely in the leg holders intended for the eventual lithotomy position. Having holders support the legs before moving the torso lessens the weight of the patient's body that positioning personnel must move, but it offers the possibility of accidentally injuring the loosely retained and relatively unattended lower extremities during the body move.

The Lower Extremities

For this description to be complete, it must incorporate some of the information already presented in the section that defined the various lithotomy positions. Several basic premises attend the establishment of any lithotomy position:

First, if both lower extremities are to be placed in holders, they should each be raised simultaneously by individual attendants. This procedure (1) minimizes the opportunity to drop and injure one extremity while manipulating the other, (2) maintains the symmetrical arrangement of the limbs, and (3) helps to avoid rotary stress on the lumbar spine that can cause disabling postoperative pain.

Second, when the need for the lithotomy position is completed, the elevated and abducted extremities are removed from their holders at the same time, one attendant handling each limb. Simultaneously, the knees are brought together in the midline, and the legs are unflexed while being lowered slowly to the level supine position. The coordinated take-down maneuver protects the relaxed lumbar spine from potentially injurious torsion in a manner similar to the simultaneous elevation of the legs. However, an even more important intention is to slow the addition of the capacitance of extremities vessels to the overall vascular circuit, thereby allowing perfusion pressure to compensate as rapidly as possible and minimizing the opportunity for the appearance of hypotension due to relative hypovolemia.

Low Lithotomy. As detailed previously when defining the position, the extremity elevation in low lithotomy is minimal compared with other versions of the posture (see Fig. 8–4). The abducted legs are held with the hips flexed only about 40 degrees or less on the trunk and the knees are bent just enough to place the lower legs roughly parallel to the floor. For transurethral surgical procedures, the amount of hip flexion should be that which the resectionist judges to produce an almost horizontal prostatic urethra for ease of handling of the resectoscope.[3] Thigh abduction is 30 to 40 degrees from the midline and is carefully unforced. When the limb is held by the mechanical supporting device, the foot section of the operating table is removed or rotated toward the floor to provide access to the perineum.

The low lithotomy position is probably the most frequent choice for a transurethral resection of the prostate. It is also applicable for other procedures because a surgeon standing alongside the flank of the patient has relatively unobstructed access across the partially elevated thigh to instruments placed through the urethra, vagina, or anus. Lloyd-Davies[12] combined the low lithotomy position with mild head-down tilt for abdominoperineal procedures in which one surgical team has transabdominal access while another operates simultaneously through the perineum (see Fig. 8–4).

The most appropriate leg holder for prolonged procedures in the low lithotomy position usually retains the foot firmly (see Fig. 6–4A) and may or may not support the popliteal fossa (see Fig. 6–4B and C). It should also resist displacement of the extremity by pressures exerted by the bodies of surgical personnel working across the thighs or between the legs of the patient.

Standard Lithotomy. The hips of the supine patient are flexed until the thighs are angled 80 to 100 degrees on the trunk with the knees being bent until the lower legs are roughly parallel to the frontal plane of the torso (Fig. 6–5). Each extremity is separated from the midline into 30 to 40 degrees of unforced abduction. Usually, the legs are externally rotated about 20 degrees in this position.

The chosen leg holder is attached securely to the edge of the table and padded as needed to prevent contact between flesh and metal as well as to minimize its pressure points on the medial, lateral, or dorsal aspects of the lower extremity. With the limbs stabilized, the foot section of the operating or examining table is

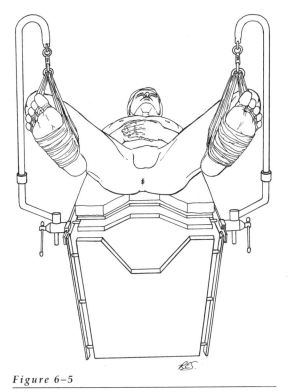

Figure 6–5

Perineal view of standard lithotomy position.

then either removed or rotated toward the floor to provide access to the perineum.

The standard lithotomy position affords excellent access to the superficial perineum, birth canal, urinary tract, and organs of the deep pelvis for an operator who is standing or seated between the elevated legs and facing the patient. It poorly accommodates simultaneous abdominal and perineal procedures because the thighs impinge on the arm motion of surgeons standing at the patient's flanks.

Hemilithotomy (Figs. 6–3D and 6–6). On a specially designed fracture table, a well-padded post is attached firmly to the table and the patient is moved to it so that the post rests against the perineum between genitalia and the intact thigh. The injured leg is bound at the ankle and foot into a rest on a worm gear that can be cranked to stretch the extremity and realign the fracture after the patient is anesthetized. The perineal pole retains the patient's pelvis and torso in position against the traction on the injured leg.

The uninjured extremity is flexed about 90 degrees at both hip and knee with the raised lower leg retained upon a padded calf rest

approximately parallel to the frontal plane of the patient's body. Portable radiographic equipment can access the fracture site by being placed under the raised leg. The patient's arm on the side of the injured leg is usually folded across the torso to exclude it from the sterile surgical field and may be loosely restrained by a nonconstrictive wristlet that ties to the opposite side of the table near the hip. The angle of the elbow in the arm retained across the torso should be as obtuse as possible to avoid a flexion alteration of the cubital tunnel that might compress the ulnar nerve. At the same time, circumduction of that arm across the torso should not be forced and stressful enough to stretch its suprascapular nerve (Schweiss JF, personal communication, 1986). Padding is placed between that arm and the ventral chest or abdomen. The arm opposite the fractured extremity is usually supinated to remove the weight of the elbow from the cubital tunnel and is extended carefully on a well-padded armboard to provide access for monitors or vascular lines.

High Lithotomy. This posture requires that the separated thighs of the patient be flexed on the trunk by at least 90 degrees, the legs be almost fully extended on the thighs, and each ankle be held by straps or booties attached to hooks atop tall vertical poles cleated to the rail at the side of the table. The lower extremities, minimally flexed at the knees, extend upward almost exactly at right angles to the long axis of the trunk. Frequently, the leg holder chosen is a "candy cane" that is extended almost to its full height. Abduction tends to be less than in the standard or low lithotomy positions because the elevated extremities are more out of the way of personnel at the patient's perineum.

Exaggerated Lithotomy. Young's position requires that the patient have a flexible skeleton. The thighs are flexed until the knees are almost directly above the middle of the chest, the knees are separated sufficiently to avoid pressure on the abdomen or flanks, and the lower legs extend almost vertically upward (see Figs. 6–4C and 6–7). Add to this a pad under the sacrum, plus possible flexion of the thigh-trunk hinge of the table top, and the patient is almost curled up. The intent is to rotate the caudal edge of the symphysis pubis ventrally far enough to allow improved transperineal access to retropubic structures in the deep pelvis such as the prostate. When properly placed for surgical access, the previously

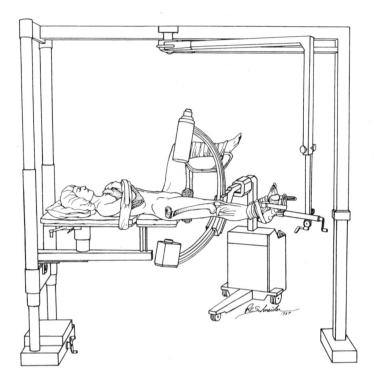

Figure 6–6

Hemilithotomy position on fracture table. Note position of arm across chest, presence of perineal pole, and potential perfusion problems for nonsurgical lower extremity that is elevated on calf rest to provide access for radiologic equipment.

Figure 6–7

Exaggerated lithotomy position. Note potential brachial plexus threat from shoulder braces and potential perfusion problems with elevated lower extremities.

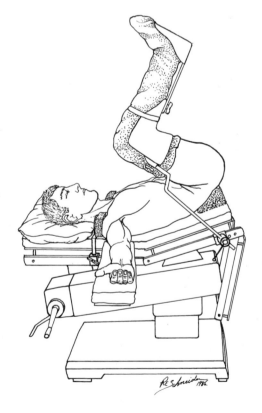

vertical face of the perineum is nearly parallel to the floor.

Each lower extremity must be retained in a holder that firmly maintains the position against cephalad slippage initiated by the sacral pad. Usually the anchored lower leg and knee prevents movement of the femur, the rigid caudal thrust of which steadies the pelvis through the hip joint. To retain the position of a heavy patient or one with a gnarled physique, a brace may be needed over the cap of each shoulder if tilt is added. As can be surmised, skeletal stress from the posture can be significant. Some authors have termed it the *extreme lithotomy position*. Angermeier and Jordan reported a retrospective review of 177 procedures done in the exaggerated lithotomy position.[15] They analyzed patient age, height, weight, and time in position. Although they noted a 15.8% incidence of common peroneal neuropathies, statistical analysis failed to show any relationship between nerve dysfunction and the factors evaluated.

Tilted Low Lithotomy. With the possible exception of the specialized fracture table used for the hemilithotomy position, some degree of head-down tilt, usually minimal (15–20 degrees or less), can be added to any version of the lithotomy position.

With the patient in position and the legs elevated, the padded leg holders are adjusted to the dimensions of the extremities and the legs are retained by one or more straps that hold without compressing the limb.

Compressing Elevated Legs

Goldstein[5] refers to Sigel and associates'[16] advocacy of using compressive wrappings or elastic stockings to combat venous stasis in the legs of patients who will be in lithotomy position for more than 15 minutes. Despite the fact that venous stasis is unlikely with the legs elevated, this injunction has often been adopted and followed without evidence of its efficacy. The external compression of the wraps or stockings raises compartmental pressures and opposes the arterial driving pressure needed to successfully perfuse the tissues of raised extremities.[17] Some compression of the extremity may be unavoidable because of the straps or wraps needed to retain it in either a knee crutch or a calf support. But deliberate application of compressive wraps to avoid the remote possibility of vascular stasis in the raised leg encourages compartment syndromes, particularly in the presence of hypotension and/or peripheral vascular disease, and is almost impossible to justify.

Lachman and colleagues[18] have implicated an intermittent pneumatic compression device, placed on each lower leg as a prophylaxis against phlebitis, as a cause of a compartment syndrome in a patient in a lithotomy position. Such an instrument needs documented periodic maintenance to assure that it decompresses completely between inflation cycles and does not become a chronically constrictive perfusion hazard.

Obstetric Variants of Lithotomy Positions

In earlier editions of this text, Goldstein[5] discussed the use of position change to free the shoulders of a large fetus that is wedged in the birth canal after delivery of a small head. The mother is taken out of the routine lithotomy position and her thighs are strongly flexed on her abdomen. The result is the supine form of a severe squatting posture in which the area of her pelvic outlet can be increased. Pressure applied to the anterior shoulder of the infant assists vaginal extraction by the obstetrician and completes the delivery.

Walcher, a German obstetrician, examined women in the lithotomy position with their thighs flexed firmly on their torsos.[19] In that position he calibrated the intravaginal diagonal conjugate manually and became convinced that descent and extension of the legs enlarged the posterior diameter of the pelvis and facilitated delivery. Goldstein[5] indicated that this dangling legs position, given scientific validity by Walcher and bearing his name, had been used for centuries by midwives attending difficult births. Because modern forceps and vacuum extractors cannot be applied in the Walcher position, it is rarely used today.

The Arms

In any variant of the lithotomy position the patient's arms can be (1) supinated and abducted laterally on armboards, (2) retained alongside the flanks roughly parallel to the long axis of the torso, (3) flexed across the abdomen or chest (see Fig. 6–6), or (4) suspended at about 90 degrees to the frontal plane of the body on some type of an elevated bar or rest.

- Elbows of abducted, supinated arms should rest upon the olecranon process of the ulna so as to avoid pressure on the cubital tunnel and its contained ulnar nerve. The effectiveness of placing additional padding about the elbow to protect the ulnar nerve is under debate because Kroll and associates[20] have reported the occurrence of postoperative ulnar neuropathies despite such padding. Abduction of the extremity should be less than 90 degrees to avoid thrusting the head of the humerus into the axillary neurovascular bundle with the possibility of stretching or compressing its contents.
- Arms retained alongside the flanks usually rotate out of supination and result in palms resting against the thighs and the weight of the extremity being borne in part by the cubital tunnel at the medial aspect of the elbow. As noted earlier, the use of padding about the elbow to protect the ulnar nerve from compression has not been totally effective even though it is generally applied when the arm is retained at the side.
- Arms crossed over the abdomen or chest are usually retained in place by some type of nonconstrictive wristlet fixed to the opposite side of the table or by a strap across the table that is not tight enough to restrict diaphragmatic excursions (see Fig. 6–6). Severe flexion of the elbows should be avoided because it can decrease the size of the cubital tunnel in some patients and compress the ulnar nerve.[21, 22] The elbow regions can be padded in such a way that there is no external pressure on the cubital tunnel. If a wristlet is used, pulses must be checked periodically to ensure that it has not become constrictive. This method of arm retention adds weight to the ventral chest or abdomen and usually requires some amount of added inspiratory pressure to produce adequate lung expansion.
- Arms affixed to elevated rests are intended to be out of the ventral operating field. The rests must resist relocation by body pressures of the surgical team. The musculature about each axilla must be relaxed and radial pulses should be checked periodically to assure that the head of the humerus is not compromising the axillary neurovascular bundle.

PHYSIOLOGY OF LITHOTOMY POSITIONS

In general, the physiology of a patient in a lithotomy position is not different from that of a supine patient except for the elevated legs. Because the details of postural physiology are dealt with elsewhere in this volume, comments here are restricted to issues specific to the raised lower extremities.

Circulatory System

Vascular Calculations

If a healthy person 6 feet tall is placed supine and horizontal, the mean arterial pressure (MAP) at the atrium should be essentially the same as the MAP either at the lateral malleolus of the ankle or at the circle of Willis. Using the calculations of Enderby,[23] indicating that the MAP at a measurement site varies 2 mm Hg with each vertical inch (2.5 cm) that the site lies above or below the atrium, that mythical person would have become accustomed to ankle MAPs in the range of 190 mm Hg when standing (Fig. 6–8). This can easily be confirmed with a normotensive, healthy volunteer of appropriate size.

In the low lithotomy position, the pressure values in Figure 6–9 can be derived convincingly. If the foot is raised 12 inches above the atrium, an average distance for that position, an MAP that was 90 mm Hg at the atrium would fall to 66 mm Hg at the ankle. Add 15 degrees of head-down tilt and the ankle is now 23 inches above the atrium with an MAP of 44 mm Hg.

Without head-down tilt, but with higher elevation of the foot (standard lithotomy, 22 inches; high lithotomy, 36 inches), the MAP at the ankle will fall further as the distance above the atrium is increased. Thus in a standard lithotomy the MAP is $90 - (2 \times 22 = 44) = 46$ mm Hg; in a high lithotomy it is $90 - (2 \times 36 = 72) = 18$ mm Hg (Fig. 6–10).

If the driving pressure into the elevated extremity is compromised by the vasoconstrictive hypotension of blood loss, by the myocardial depression that accompanies various types of anesthesia, by external compression wraps or devices applied to the leg, by the use of controlled hypotension, or by combinations of these factors, the MAP at the ankle will be dangerously lower. Figure 6–6 demonstrates that hypotension causing atrial MAPs of about 60 mm Hg would allow ankle

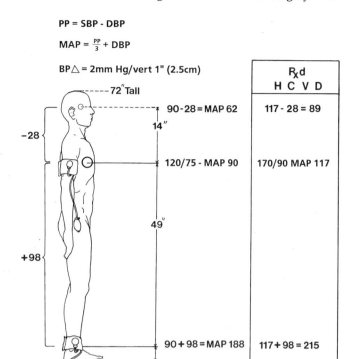

$$PP = SBP - DBP$$

$$MAP = \frac{PP}{3} + DBP$$

$$BP\triangle = 2mm\ Hg/vert\ 1"\ (2.5cm)$$

Figure 6–8

Blood pressure calculations at circle of Willis, heart, and ankles of healthy normotensive erect subject compared with same measurements in treated hypertensive subject of same size. (From McLeskey CH [ed.]: Anesthesia. Baltimore, Williams & Wilkins, in press.)

MAPs of only about 13 mm Hg in the low lithotomy position. That pressure over an extended period of time is an invitation to inadequate perfusion of the lower leg, particularly in the presence of compressive wraps. The importance of maintaining acceptable perfusion pressure when extremities are elevated becomes obvious, as does the fact that using vasoconstrictive therapy rather than judicious volume replacement to maintain satisfactory blood pressure numbers at a traditional measurement site imposes its own risk of periph-

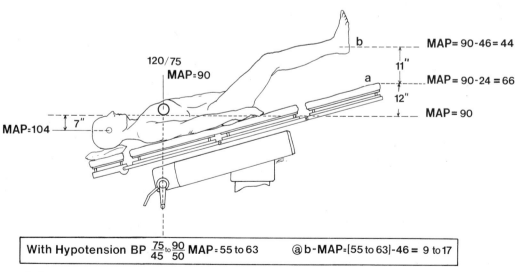

Figure 6–9

Blood pressure calculations in low lithotomy position with 15 degrees head-down tilt. Box at bottom indicates values calculated for the presence of intraoperative hypotension of the degree indicated. (From Martin JT: Compartment syndromes: Concepts and perspectives for the anesthesiologist. Anesth Analg 75:275, 1992.)

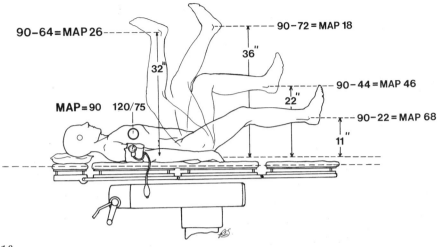

Figure 6-10

Effect of leg elevation in various lithotomy positions on calculated mean arterial pressures (MAP) at the ankle in the presence of a stable atrial MAP in a normotensive subject. (From McLeskey CH [ed.]: Geriatric Anesthesia. Baltimore, Williams & Wilkins, in press.)

eral hypoperfusion. A pragmatic, widely used way of assessing the pressure at a point above the heart is to place an arterial line, usually as a catheter in a radial artery that is retained in the lateral plane of the torso, and position the transducer at the level of the elevated site in question.

Vascular Capacitance Changes and Volume Shifts

As the legs are elevated, a significant amount of intravascular volume shifts downhill to augment the central circulation and the functional vascular capacitance of the lower extremities is diminished until the posture is terminated. In the normovolemic patient with healthy circulatory and autonomic nervous systems, baroreceptors on great vessels in the thorax and neck may regard the added volume as an overload and activate vasodilative reflexes to ease the central congestion. Initially, the enlarged blood volume in the central vasculature is capable of increasing intracranial blood volume by elevating atrial filling pressures, increasing cardiac output, and aiding internal carotid flow while simultaneously creating caval congestion and decreasing intracranial venous drainage. Normal vascular compensatory reflexes tend to make these changes transient in a healthy circulatory system. In disease states, however, these changes may persist in a manner that is detrimental to the cranial contents.

Cardiovascular Measurements

Kopman and Sandza[24] measured the hemodynamic effects of the head-down lithotomy position in 12 patients with coronary artery disease. Initial data were collected with the patients supine, and measurements were repeated after 10 minutes with the patients in the lithotomy position with 10 degrees of head-down tilt. Tilt increased venous return. Patients with good myocardial contraction responded to the increased filling pressure by an increase in cardiac output and systolic pressure. One patient had no significant change. Two patients with low ejection fractions were unable to adjust to the increased filling pressures and had significant decreases in their cardiac outputs. Half of the patients in their study had elevations of pulmonary capillary wedge pressures to levels above 18 mm Hg that are consistent with the onset of pulmonary congestion, increased left ventricular end-diastolic pressure, increased left ventricular wall tension, and increased myocardial oxygen demands. Because their study time for each patient was short, they did not see ST segment changes; however, they postulated that subendocardial ischemia could have occurred. They concluded that this category of patients withstands tilted lithotomy poorly and deserves capable hemodynamic monitoring when the position is required by a surgical lesion.

Five years later Kubal and associates[25] found the same detrimental effects of mild head-down tilt in awake patients with coronary artery disease who were having central catheters placed through the jugular system for monitoring and therapy before cardiopulmonary bypass procedures. Thus, little support should remain for the notion that minimal head-down tilt in patients with cardiovascular impairment is a casual and harmless addition to a surgical posture.

Respiratory Tract

The effect of the lithotomy position on tidal volume was measured by Jones and Jacoby[26] and by Henschel and associates.[27] Lithotomy by itself caused a 3% decrease in tidal volume; with 10 degrees of head-down tilt the value was 14%; with 20 degrees of tilt, it was 15%. Supported ventilation can easily counteract these changes.

In normal human volunteers, the exaggerated lithotomy position forces the contents of the abdomen against the diaphragm and hinders respiratory movement. Giesecke and associates[28] examined elderly patients with pulmonary disease and found that their preoperative timed forced vital capacities increased 9% in the exaggerated lithotomy position under spinal anesthesia. They thought that the improvement was the result of the weight of abdominal viscera and the compression of flexed thighs acting on the diaphragm to improve its resting position. Inspiratory reserve was increased, and force was added to a maximum expiratory effort. Although this finding is fortuitous, it does not establish the posture as therapeutic for patients with pulmonary disease, and any surgical procedure should be accomplished as expeditiously as possible.

Gastrointestinal Tract

Lower Esophageal Sphincter

Responding to contentions that the risk of gastroesophageal reflux is increased during pregnancy and that anesthesia for pregnant surgical patients should not be induced in the lithotomy position, Jones and associates[29] measured gastric pressure, lower esophageal sphincter pressure, and barrier pressure in the supine and lithotomy position in 17 healthy women undergoing termination of pregnancy in the first trimester. General endotracheal anesthesia was used with a standardized protocol. Nonpregnant controls were not in-

cluded. Values when supine were those of nonpregnant patients published by others. In the lithotomy position, both the lower esophageal pressures and the barrier pressures were significantly reduced without changes in intragastric pressure. They concluded that the risk of regurgitation was increased by the lithotomy position during early pregnancy.

Nervous System

Tilt with Central Nervous System Disease

In Chapter 8 the physiology and complications of head-down tilt are detailed. Suffice it to say here that the casual addition of head-down tilt to versions of the lithotomy position for the purpose of improving transabdominal or transperineal access to the surgical target is not a universally safe practice. Normal physiques can withstand the process satisfactorily. However, pulmonary, cardiac, intraocular, and intracranial pathology are adversely affected by tilt. Figure 6–8 shows an increase of MAP at the circle of Willis in the presence of minimal head-down tilt. The magnitude of the insult depends on the nature and intensity of the pathologic changes and is undoubtedly influenced by the degree and duration of the head-down tilt. Tilt should be avoided in the presence of a pathologic process that it could worsen. When tilt is mandatory in the presence of compromising disease, the general rule should be to use the least amount that is effective and to continue it for the shortest possible period of time.

Musculoskeletal System

Loss of Lumbar Curvature

Low back pain invokes muscle spasm to stabilize and protect the spine. During the muscular relaxation that attends either regional or general anesthesia, the patient who is placed in a lithotomy position loses much of the normal lordotic curvature of the lumbar spine.[30] Postoperatively, this may appear as a backache of varied severity and duration or it may provoke the recurrence of a previously symptomatic lumbar disk.

COMPLICATIONS OF LITHOTOMY POSITIONS

Circulatory System

Compartment Syndromes

Anatomic compartments are relatively rigid osseofascial subdivisions of the human musculoskeletal system. They contain muscular, nervous, vascular, connective, and adipose tissues. Normal tissue pressures within a compartment of a supine lower extremity range from 9 to 15 mm Hg.[31] Therefore, a certain minimum perfusion pressure is needed to nourish the contents. If the compartment is compressed by outside forces (casts, tight dressings), or if its contents expand against its boundaries (edema, bleeding, the muscle hypertrophy of exercise), the intracompartmental pressure rises (46–65 mm Hg)[31] above minimum perfusion pressure, and, to prevent ischemia, the vascular driving pressure needed for adequate perfusion must increase accordingly. Ashton[32] found that tissue circulation ceased when compressive compartmental pressures reached 64 mm Hg in the forearm or 55 mm Hg in the calf. If the compartment pressure remains normal but the perfusion pressure diminishes (regional or systemic hypotension, arterial spasm, vascular obstruction), ischemia threatens.

A compartment syndrome, per se, entails hypoxic, ischemic, or absent perfusion of the compartment; hypoxic disruption of capillary boundaries; extravasation of intravascular fluid and formed elements into adjacent tissues when reperfusion occurs; edema of compartmental contents; elevated compartment pressures and worsening ischemia; tissue necrosis with myoglobinuria, lung damage, and nephrotoxicity; complicated and persistent fluid and electrolyte upsets; local and systemic infection; remote organ compromise or failure; and a high potential for a fatal outcome.[17] Suggestions that circulation in the lower extremity should be monitored during the lithotomy position to detect the onset of compartment syndromes are flawed by the fact that the pathologic process happens at the level of tissue perfusion. Larger peripheral vessels are not affected unless the cause is systemic hypotension or a remote perfusion failure such as retractor obstruction of a pelvic vessel.[17]

Compartment syndromes have been associated with prolonged use of the lithotomy position, probably most often with tilted low lithotomy used for combined or simultaneous abdominopelvic operations. Reported cases have occurred with lithotomy positions lasting more than 5 hours.[17]

Controversy has arisen about the potential for postoperative epidural opioid pain control impairing the diagnosis of a compartment syndromes. Strecker and colleagues[33] re-ported a patient in whom they believed that the recognition of a compartment syndrome was obscured by the use of postoperative epidural opioid analgesia for pain control. However, Montgomery and Ready[34] presented two instances of unilateral compartment syndromes after prolonged use of the lithotomy position in which the diagnosis was not hindered by the presence of postoperative epidural morphine analgesia. They believe, however, that a high index of diagnostic suspicion should be maintained for patients at risk of developing a compartment syndrome while receiving postoperative epidural analgesia.

Respiratory System

The respiratory complications of the lithotomy positions are those of other dorsal decubitus positions unless there is restriction to the descent of the diaphragm from severely flexed thighs or steep head-down tilt.

Nervous System

Cubital Tunnel and Arm Position

The issue of arm positioning and compression of the ulnar nerve at the elbow is examined in detail elsewhere in this text (see Chapters 11 and 19). However, all of the precautions applied to arm positioning for the supine positions should be practiced with lithotomy positions. Of importance is the fact that ulnar nerve conduction defects have been demonstrated in the clinically normal opposite arms of patients with symptomatic postoperative ulnar neuropathies.[22] The cubital tunnel is narrowed by elbow flexion in some people.[21] Patients with a history of chronic hand use with flexed elbows (e.g., drivers, carpenters, chefs) may have an increased risk of developing postoperative ulnar neuropathies.[22] Unfortunately, ulnar dysfunction has occurred postoperatively despite meticulous, documented attention to elbow padding and positioning.[20]

The reader is referred to Chapter 11 for an important and applicable discussion of the double crush syndrome and related concerns.

Persistent Motor Neuropathies

In a retrospective, controlled study of persistent postoperative motor neuropathies of the lower extremities, Warner's group[35] examined the histories of 198,461 consecutive patients who underwent surgical procedures historically involving the lithotomy position at the Mayo Clinic. Persistent motor neuropathies, defined as lasting for more than 3 months, were identified in 55 patients for an occurrence rate of 1:3608. Patient characteristics that constituted risk factors were (1) low body mass index (less than 20 kg/m^2); (2) increasing age (55% greater for each decade of life); (3) smoking within 1 month of the surgical procedure (a 15-fold increase over nonsmokers or those who quit more than 1 month before surgery); and (4) pre-existing diabetes or vascular disease or both (25% of the cases). The only important nonpatient variable was the duration of the procedure (more than 4 hours). Involved nerves were the common peroneal (43/55), sciatic (8/55), and femoral (4/55). No obturator motor neuropathies were found, and no nerve injury was bilateral. Although their retrospective study had the advantage of a massive and unique data base (1,412,116 surgical procedures between January 1, 1957, and December 31, 1991), it did not permit identification of less prolonged motor neuropathies, postoperative sensory deficits, varieties of the lithotomy position involved, or the type of leg holder used.

Obturator Neuropathies

The obturator nerve arises from L2, L3, and L4 nerve roots and leaves the bony pelvis through the obturator foramen to innervate adductor muscles and transmit cutaneous sensation centrally from a diffuse area of the inner thigh above the knee. Weakness of adduction and thigh rotation are signs of obturator dysfunction and can be assessed by having the patient attempt to adduct the thigh against the examiner's hand. Although frequently dissected during radical surgery within the pelvis, obturator nerve injuries are rarely encountered postoperatively and none was found in the study by Warner's group.[35] However, obturator nerve injuries have been found after obstetric procedures performed in a lithotomy position. Nearly all are transitory, and a significant proportion are bilateral. Both of these findings suggest direct trauma to the obturator nerves by compression as the fetus passes through the birth canal. Whether forceps-assisted deliveries have a higher risk of obturator nerve injuries is not clear (Warner MA, personal communication, 1995).

Femoral Neuropathies

Arising from L2, L3, and L4 roots and passing along the anterolateral border of the psoas muscle, the femoral nerve exits the pelvis under the inguinal ligament (Fig. 6–11) to innervate principally the quadriceps femoris muscle but also flexors, adductors, and rotators of

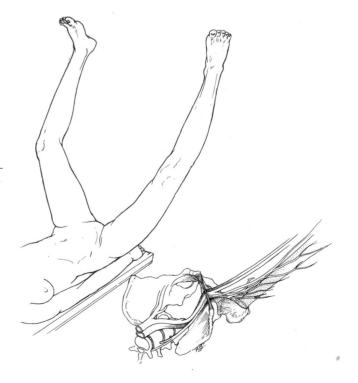

Figure 6–11

Leg elevation angulating femoral nerve and contents of femoral canal under a tight inguinal (Poupart's) ligament. (From McLeskey CH [ed.]: Geriatric Anesthesia. Baltimore, Williams & Wilkins, in press.)

the thigh.[36] Injury weakens or prevents knee extension (quadriceps), obliterates knee jerk, impairs stair climbing (flexors), and produces anesthesia in the anterior thigh and medial leg.

Although rare today, Vargo's group[37] noted that, at the beginning of this century, postpartum femoral neuropathies occurred after 4.7% of deliveries (4700 per 100,000). Apparently the symptoms resolved within the first few weeks after delivery. By contrast, Vargo and associates reviewed 143,019 live births at a large maternity hospital between 1971 and 1987 and found that the current incidence of postpartum femoral neuropathies was only 2.8 per 100,000. They attributed that dramatic change to a shorter duration of labor in modern practice and an increased incidence of cesarean sections. The earlier high incidence puzzled them because the nerve does not traverse the true pelvis and should be relatively unaffected by processes of childbirth that can traumatize the lumbosacral trunk and sciatic nerve. They did not speculate about the neuropathic potential of labor and delivery in the lateral position of Sims (see Chapter 9), a practice that was in vogue early in the 1900s.

Tondare and associates[38] reported three patients who had subarachnoid analgesia for vaginal hysterectomies in the lithotomy position. Straight rod leg supports with swing stirrups were used and the procedures lasted for 2½ hours. Postoperatively, the patients developed solitary unilateral peripheral femoral neuropathies. These patients recovered fully within 8 to 10 weeks. The authors deemed the cause to be extreme abduction of thighs with external rotation at the hip that kinks the contents of the femoral canal under the inguinal ligament and causes ischemia of the nerve (see Fig. 6–11). They thought that the complication could be prevented by using lateral thigh supports to limit the degree of abduction of the lower extremity while in the lithotomy position.

Extreme angulation of the contents of the femoral canal can be postulated to occur in patients with tight inguinal ligaments whose hips are flexed considerably beyond 90 degrees and abducted when they are placed either in high or exaggerated lithotomy positions. Whether this potential problem can be detected preoperatively is not clear. Few patients will be able to assume such a test position while awake, and the signs of a positive test for short-term femoral canal compression are uncertain.

Five instances of femoral mononeuropathy in young women who underwent uncomplicated vaginal deliveries (3/5) or laparoscopies (2/5) while in the lithotomy position were reported by al Hakim and Katirji.[39] The lesions were localized to the inguinal ligament and had an excellent prognosis. They believed that causative factors were compression of the nerve at the inguinal ligament or its being stretched by excessive abduction and external rotation of the thigh.

Sciatic Neuropathies

The sciatic nerve arises from nerve roots L4 through S3 of the lumbosacral plexus, traverses the thigh, and splits into the common peroneal and tibial nerves in the popliteal space. Injuries to the thigh portion of the nerve disrupt flexion of the leg; peroneal nerve dysfunction produces footdrop and inversion of the foot; tibial nerve injuries abolish ankle jerk.[40]

McQuarrie's group[14] reviewed 1000 consecutive vaginal hysterectomies in patients in lithotomy positions performed by 10 different gynecologic surgeons in one hospital and reported four postoperative unilateral sciatic nerve dysfunctions (0.4%). The nerve is known to be susceptible to injury during obstetric delivery and gynecologic surgery. Postulated causes have been stretching of the nerve,[41] hyperflexion of the back,[14] nerve compression during vaginal delivery,[42] and neural contusion during laparoscopy.[43]

Romfh and Currier[44] have suggested that the hip flexion of the lithotomy position might cause the nerve to be compressed as it passes through the sciatic notch and that its accompanying blood supply could be compromised sufficiently to produce an ischemic neuropathy (Fig. 6–12). Either the sciatic artery or the arteria comitans nervi ischiadici, a tiny branch of the gluteal artery that supplies only the sciatic nerve, would be the affected vessel.

Reinstein[45] reported a patient who developed a sciatic neuropathy after 30 minutes in the lithotomy position during general anesthesia. She had a history of intramedullary nailing of a midshaft fracture of the femur 7 years earlier. Postoperative radiographs showed a large heterotopic ossification above the greater trochanter of the femur on the side of the neuropathy. Apparently that bony mass had already stretched its adjacent sciatic nerve and, in the lithotomy position, postero-

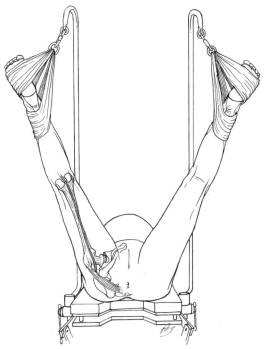

Figure 6–12

Leg elevation showing potential for piriformis muscle to compress sciatic nerve in the sciatic notch as it leaves the pelvis near the head of the femur. The nerve is fixed at the point that it leaves the pelvis through the sciatic notch and also where it passes around the neck of the femur. Rotation of the shaft of the femur may stretch the nerve between the notch and the femoral neck.

medial shift of the ossification increased the neural stretch/compression sufficiently to produce the neuropathy.

Femoral Cutaneous Nerves

The femoral cutaneous nerves supply sensation to variable portions of the lateral, ventral, and medial thigh. The lateral femoral cutaneous nerve arises from the second and third lumbar roots, emerges from the lateral border of the psoas major muscle, and runs retroperitoneally to enter the thigh under and through Poupart's ligament just medial to the anterior-superior iliac spine. It serves the proximal portion of the anterolateral thigh almost to the knee. The anterior femoral cutaneous nerve arises in the femoral triangle and supplies sensation to the middle portion of the lower two thirds of the ventral thigh and the area of the knee.[46]

In a prospective study of 412 consecutive postpartum patients in a single hospital, O'Donnell and associates found fresh neurop-

athies in 21% of patients overall; 97% of the lesions were sensory and 66% were unilateral.[47] Thirty-eight percent of the neuropathies involved lateral femoral cutaneous nerves whereas 14% affected anterior femoral cutaneous nerves. Ninety-four percent of the lesions in the overall group resolved within 40 days, but 6% had not cleared by 6 months. Their study detected no specific neuropathic effect of regional anesthesia. However, cesarean delivery, either with or without undergoing prior labor, correlated with an increased incidence of paresthesias. Included in the patient factors contributing to postpartum neuropathies was an increased duration of pushing (increased intra-abdominal pressure) in lithotomy position with or without stirrups.

Common Peroneal Nerve

The common peroneal nerve is a terminal branch of the sciatic nerve that arises in the popliteal fossa and courses laterally around the neck of the fibula to split into superficial and deep branches. The major muscle innervated by the common peroneal nerve is the tibialis anterior that dorsiflexes the foot. Depending on where the common peroneal nerve divides, either it or the superficial peroneal nerve will lie in a position that is easily palpated, particularly in a thin patient, on the lateral aspect of the lower leg just distal to the fibular neck. At this point it is vulnerable to any pressure that compresses it against the fibula.[48, 49] A prominent sign of common peroneal nerve dysfunction is footdrop.

When a "candy cane" leg holder is placed lateral to a leg of a patient in a lithotomy position and the attachment to the holder is either a cloth ankle/foot sling or a laced cloth boot, the entire lower extremity is mobile and floppy. Lateral displacement of the thigh is possible either from the weight of the limb or from crowding by a member of the surgical team. Limitation of any lateral shift of the thigh is usually produced by pressure of the leg, just below the knee where the common peroneal nerve is most vulnerable to compression, against the immobile vertical pole of the holder (Fig. 6–13A).

Anesthesia of a small area of the posterior and lateral aspect of the lower leg just below the knee[48] or the lateral aspect of the lower leg and the dorsum of the foot[49] is characteristic. Footdrop, the inability to dorsiflex the foot, is a usual motor accompaniment. Padding of the vertical pole, or the use of a more reten-

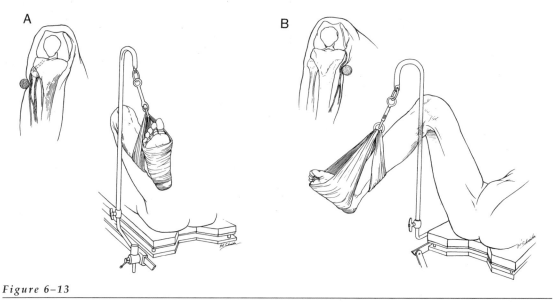

Figure 6–13

Raised lower extremity pressed against an unpadded leg support. *A.* Lateral support compresses common peroneal nerve just caudad to the head of the fibula. *B.* Medial support compresses saphenous nerve in the region of the medial condyle of the tibia.

tive type of leg holder, is the recommended prophylaxis.

Herrara-Ornelas and associates[50] reviewed 11 instances of common peroneal palsies that followed careful low lithotomy positioning using a well-padded combined knee crutch and foot support. The surgical procedures involved intrapelvic malignancies and lasted from 4½ to 13 hours. Some degree of intraoperative hypothermia was present in most patients, but hypotension did not occur. Blame was placed on mechanically faulty metal leg supports in over half of the cases; consequently, their group has subsequently switched to the plastic calf-foot boot fixed to an adjustable metal rod as their usual leg holder. Intraoperative removal of tumor tissue from a lumbosacral plexus was required in only one patient. They deemed the duration of surgery to be an important causative factor for the peroneal neuropathies and thought that not all of the neuropathies associated with lesions requiring prolonged, meticulous surgical dissections may be preventable.

In a retrospective study of 177 patients operated on in the exaggerated lithotomy position, Angermeier and Jordan[15] found that common peroneal neuropathies were the most frequent neural complication of the series.

Tibial Nerve

The tibial nerve passes through the midportion of the popliteal space and descends through the dorsomedial leg to pass around the medial malleolus of the tibia and enter the foot.[49] Although the nerve can be anticipated to be one of the structures susceptible to damage by pressure in the popliteal space from a knee crutch or by a compartment syndrome involving the dorsal lower leg, reports of tibial nerve dysfunction after use of the lithotomy position are scarce.

Saphenous Nerve

The saphenous nerve, a branch of the femoral nerve, lies just deep to the sartorius muscle on the inner aspect of the mid thigh, crosses the medial aspect of the knee joint and continues down the inner portion of the lower leg to the medial side of the foot, supplying sensation to its area below the knee.[36]

If the vertical pole of a "candy cane" leg holder is placed against the medial aspect of the lower extremity of a patient in a lithotomy position to help separate the thighs, its lateral pressure against the mid thigh or knee has been thought to have contributed to postoperative dysfunction of the saphenous nerve (see Fig. 6–13B).[51] The lesion produced is anesthesia of the medial aspect of most of the lower leg, the heel, and the foot to the base of the great toe.[36] The pole must be well padded to distribute its pressure if the medial surface of the elevated lower extremity must rest against it. For a lengthy procedure another type of extremity holder would seem to be a better choice.

Urinary Tract

Rhabdomyolysis and Myoglobinuria

Two reports document the postoperative appearance of acute renal failure caused by rhabdomyolysis after use of the exaggerated lithotomy position:

Guzzi and coworkers'[52] patient was obese, remained in the exaggerated lithotomy position with 15 degrees of head-down tilt for 6½ hours, was hypotensive when returned to the supine position, developed oliguric renal failure with high serum myoglobin levels, had no evidence of compartment syndromes, and continued to break down muscle for the first 2 days. Dialysis lasted for 20 days. No postoperative neuropathies developed.

The patient reported by Ali and colleagues[53] was in the exaggerated lithotomy position for 6 hours with a wedge under the sacrum. On awakening he complained of severe bilateral lower back pain, lower extremity pain, and numbness. Pulses in the lower limbs were intact, but he had ecchymoses over his lower back. Postoperatively, he developed acute renal failure, believed to be due to rhabdomyolysis secondary to ischemia of lumbar and pelvic muscles that were compressed by the exaggerated lithotomy position. A whole-body bone scan with technetium-99m on the third postoperative day showed intense uptake in the posterior spinal, psoas, and gluteal muscles; 2½ weeks later the scan was normal. Unspecified peripheral neuropathies in the lower extremities slowly improved during the first postoperative year.

Although these accounts are only anecdotal, they imply that heavy patients who are in the exaggerated lithotomy for long periods may be at risk of muscle damage in the lower torso as a result of the position. Whereas the pathophysiology is probably that of a compartment syndrome, the location is unusual.

Posture-induced postoperative rhabdomyolysis was first reported by Gordon and Newman[54] in 1953 and concerned the prone tuck position. A prospective study was done by Targa's group involving 36 patients who were operated upon either in lateral (13/36), prone (13/36), or supine (10/36) positions.[55] Screen-ing tests did not suggest the susceptibility of a given patient to the appearance of rhabdomyolysis. They concluded that the major risk factors for rhabdomyolysis were the lateral position and the duration of surgery. Although the incidence is low, to that list should be added concern for heavy patients who are in exaggerated lithotomy for lengthy periods.

Musculoskeletal System

Lumbar Pain and Diskogenic Symptoms

The lumbar relaxation associated with anesthesia flattens the normal lumbar curvature and frequently produces a postoperative backache.[56-59] Although not associated with a particular type of anesthetic, Brown and Elman[57] noted that backache increased in occurrence and intensity as the duration of surgery lengthened. Lumbosacral trauma may also be caused by elevating only one lower extremity at a time into the lithotomy position.

In patients with a history of lumbar disk disease who are currently relatively asymptomatic, exposure to only a short interval of anesthesia in the lithotomy position may cause an acute flare-up of lumbar distress. This has occurred in asymptomatic patients who have been placed in a standard lithotomy position gently while awake and who were comfortable in the posture before the careful induction of anesthesia.

Clarke and co-workers[60] have published a prospective study of 101 women whose hysterectomies were done in either the supine[53] or the lithotomy[51] positions. Twenty percent of the supine group and 14% of those in lithotomy developed postoperative backache with a mean duration of symptoms of 7 months. The authors concluded that postoperative backache occurred equally between the two positions and was an underrecognized postoperative complication.

One hundred fifty-five patients without histories of backache were studied by O'Donovan during surgery in either the supine or the lithotomy positions.[61] The test group had an inflatable wedge placed under their lumbosacral curvatures; the controls did not. Postoperative backache appeared in 38% of the control group but in only 8.5% of the wedge group, an almost fivefold difference! The wedge used was a plastic 3-L urologic irrigation bag to which had been attached a bulb pump and an aneroid manometer. In the supine position the wedge was inflated to 25 mm Hg pressure; in the lithotomy the inflation pressure was 30 mm Hg. Both values had been established as mean pressures that produced comfort in awake volunteers during an initial pilot study by the same investigators. Lincoln and Sawyer[58] had previously reported good results using the bladder of a blood pressure cuff as the lumbar wedge (Fig. 6–14).

Frequently, small superficial focal points that are tender when pressed upon, so-called trigger points, exist over bony prominences, muscles, and tendons. When these trigger points are present among the musculature of the lower back, the presence of a lumbar wedge may activate pain in the tender spots and will not be well tolerated by the patients.

Lumbosacral Plexus Stretch

Three instances of postoperative leg weakness after relatively brief (4, 2¼, and 2 hours) urologic procedures done in the low lithotomy position were reported by Flanagan and associates.[62] In each instance the lumbosacral plexus was out of the operative field. Electromyographic evaluation implicated a plexus injury in each patient, and the conclusion was that the femoral and sciatic nerves had been stretched by hyperabduction of the hip while the lower extremities were elevated in the lithotomy position.

Skeletal Rigidity

Frail, elderly or arthritic patients are often markedly osteoporotic with stiff skeletons and long bones that are susceptible to stress fractures. Damage to their knees, hips, and femurs may occur if positioning is careless. During minor surgery in the lithotomy position, such a patient may benefit from having the legs held in moderate degrees of abduction and flexion by one or a pair of attendants while the operative procedure is accomplished swiftly. Those holding the extremities can respond to demonstrated limits of movement better than can mechanical support devices.[5]

Fingers

Courington and Little[63] reported finger injuries in a young woman who was placed in the lithotomy position for a brief gynecologic procedure. Apparently her arms were long enough when retained along her sides to allow her fingers to protrude into the crevice between the thigh section and the depressed foot section of the operating table (Fig. 6–15, inset; see also Fig. 8–4, inset). When the foot section of the table surface was elevated to the horizontal before terminating the lithotomy position, the scissoring action of the two approximating metal edges of the sections amputated several of her fingers. This potential catastrophe lurks in all operating suites

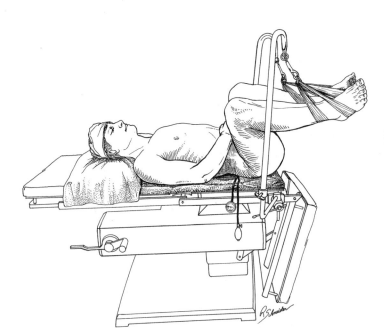

Figure 6–14

Use of an expandable support to counteract flattening of the lumbar curvature in the lithotomy position. A large blood pressure cuff or a large plastic bag intended for irrigation fluids can be inflated as needed. See text.

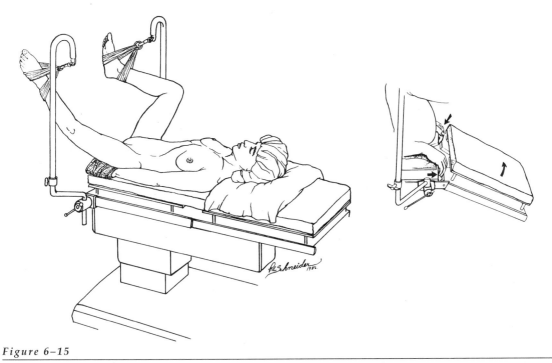

Figure 6–15

Potential damage to fingers from scissor action of elevating depressed leg section of operating table at end of a procedure requiring lithotomy position. Wrapped hand prevents extension of fingers over the end of the table mattress.

on a daily basis, and persistent vigilance is required to avoid it. Welborn[64] has advocated wrapping the fisted hand of the patient in a surgical towel to make a mitten that will keep the fingers out of the gap between the sections of the table top (see Fig. 6–15).

Miscellaneous

Perineal Pole for Hemilithotomy

In the hemilithotomy position, the perineal pole that retains the pelvis against traction placed on the fractured extremity can be a serious hazard to the patient's perineum (see Fig. 6–6). Unless it is placed initially against intact pubic rami on the side opposite the fractured femur, the traction force may draw the perineum across the pole and damage genitalia. Padding on the pole should be abundant to distribute pressure against the rami and minimize the risk of compression of the pudendal nerve. After the patient has been placed in position, the location of the pole must be checked to see that labia, or scrotum and penis, are free from compression. While traction is being applied, the perineal relationships between the pole and the genitalia must remain unchanged. In the pres-

ence of a crushed, unstable pelvis, use of the perineal pole may be undesirable.

Body Habitus

Warner and associates[35] identified a body mass index of less than 20 kg/m^2 as an important factor in predicting risk of postoperative neuropathies of the lower extremity after use of the lithotomy position. Thin or emaciated physiques have less protective tissue over bony prominences and around nerve sheaths. The implication for protective external padding is clear, even though padding elbows is known not to be totally effective in protecting ulnar nerves.[20]

The problems of positioning the obese patient are discussed in Chapter 14. Folding obese thighs onto a massive abdomen can add resistance to lung expansion during intermittent positive-pressure inspiration. In the exaggerated lithotomy position that detriment becomes more pronounced, particularly in the presence of visceral shifts produced by head-down tilt.

Duration of Lithotomy Position

In a review of available literature, Martin[17] found that compartment syndromes that oc-

Table 6–1

Approximate Proportional Risk of Lower Extremity Neuropathy After Surgery on Patients in the Lithotomy Position

Risk Factor	No. of Procedures	No. of Cases	Proportional Risk
None present	141,150	8	1:17,640
Body mass index >20 kg/m^2	4400	5	1:880
+ Smoker, or	1500	11	1:140
+ Duration >4 h	50	3	1:20
Smoker	46,950	16	1:3560
+ Duration >4 h	1500	3	1:500
Duration >4 h	4400	0	—
All factors present	50	9	1:10

— = Not able to be calculated by itself. All patients in the study who were in lithotomy more than 4 hours and who developed neuropathies were smokers, had body mass indices less than 20, or both.

From Warner MA, Martin JT, Schroeder DR, et al.: Lower extremity motor neuropathy associated with surgery performed on patients in a lithotomy position. Anesthesiology 81:6, 1994.

curred after use of the lithotomy position had been associated with several different types of leg holders but in no instance had the complication appeared in less than 5 hours of lithotomy time.

Warner and co-workers[35] noted that each hour that the patient remained in the lithotomy position increased the likelihood of motor neuropathies in the lower extremity by nearly 100-fold. The largest proportion of their persistent postoperative motor neuropathies developed in cases in which the patient was in lithotomy for more than 4 hours.

Each of these observations indicates that some degree of planning should be applied to lengthy operations in which the lithotomy position is not needed for the entire procedure. Whether it is better to restrict the use of lithotomy to specific stages of a given procedure or whether it is more advisable to occasionally remove a patient briefly from lithotomy and then re-establish the posture is a debate that cannot be solved at this time. Each practice has built-in hazards, and neither can be a clear choice. However, interrupting and re-establishing the use of lithotomy while an abdominoperineal wound is open and capable of being contaminated is a complicated undertaking that would need major justification.

PREANESTHETIC EVALUATION

Enough information now exists for a preanesthetic interviewer to be able to identify risk factors for potential complications resulting from use of the lithotomy positions. The following items require evaluation, and any positive findings should be considered to increase the risks of perioperative complications.

- Patients who continue smoking within 1 month of surgery
- Very thin patients with body mass indices of 20 kg/m^2 or less and severely obese patients who may not be able to be flexed into the desired lithotomy position
- The presence of diabetes mellitus or vascular diseases
- Lumbosacral discomfort or neuropathic symptoms suggestive of a protruded lumbar intervertebral disk
- Cardiorespiratory or intracranial pathology that might be worsened by head-down tilt
- Procedures expected to exceed about 4 hours in lithotomy

Proportional risk factors for some of the variables were calculated by Warner and co-workers[35] and are shown in Table 6–1. Important to note is the astonishing magnitude of increase in risk produced by combinations of factors (from 1:17,640 to 1:10!). Whereas all patients deserve the same relative degree of maximum care, more than the usual amount of perioperative attention should be focused on those patients with the greatest opportunities for complications from the indicated operation.

REFERENCES

1. Giannopoulos T, Kostakopoulos A, Sofras F, Dimopoulos C: The operation of lithotomy in Ancient Greece. Urol Int 42:210, 1987.

2. Weyrauch HM: Surgery of the Prostate. Philadelphia, WB Saunders, 1959.
3. Kropp KK: The lithotomy position: Surgical aspects: Urology. *In* Martin JT (ed.): Positioning in Anesthesia and Surgery, 2nd ed. Philadelphia, WB Saunders, 1987, chap. 7.
4. Graham H: Byzantine midwifery. *In* Eternal Eve. New York, Doubleday, 1951.
5. Goldstein PJ: The lithotomy position: Surgical aspects: Obstetrics & gynecology. *In* Martin JT (ed.): Positioning in Anesthesia and Surgery, 2nd ed. Philadelphia, WB Saunders, 1987, chap. 6.
6. Martin JT: Positioning in Anesthesia and Surgery. Philadelphia, WB Saunders, 1978, chap. 8.
7. Martin JT: Positioning in Anesthesia and Surgery, 2nd ed. Philadelphia, WB Saunders, 1987, chaps. 6–8.
8. Campbell JG: Inverted lithotomy. Dis Colon Rectum 29:772, 1986.
9. Lehman T, Bagley DH: Reverse lithotomy: Modified prone position for simultaneous nephroscopic and ureteroscopic procedures in women. Urology 36:529, 1988.
10. Martin JT, Warner MA: Patient positioning. *In* Barash PG, Cullen BF, Stoelting RK (eds.): Clinical Anesthesia, 3rd ed. Philadelphia, JB Lippincott, 1995, chap. 27.
11. Young HH: Tumors of the prostate. In Lewis' Textbook of Surgery. Hagerstown, MD, WF Prior, 1951.
12. Lloyd-Davies OV: Lithotomy-Trendelenburg position for resection of rectum and lower pelvic colon. Lancet 2:74, 1939.
13. Paschal CR Jr, Strzelecki LR: Lithotomy positioning devices. AORN J 55:1011, 1992.
14. McQuarrie HG, Harris JW, Ellsworth HS, et al.: Sciatic neuropathy complicating vaginal hysterectomy. Am J Obstet Gynecol 113:223, 1972.
15. Angermeier KW, Jordan GH: Complications of the exaggerated lithotomy position: A review of 177 cases. J Urol 151:866, 1994.
16. Sigel B, Edelstein AL, Felix WR, Memhardt CR: Compression of the deep venous system of the lower leg during inactive recumbency. Arch Surg 106:38, 1973.
17. Martin JT: Compartment syndromes: Concepts and perspectives for the anesthesiologist. Anesth Analg 75:275, 1992.
18. Lachman EA, Rook JL, Tunkel R, Nagler W: Complications associated with intermittent pneumatic compression. Arch Phys Med Rehabil 73:482, 1992.
19. Brill HM, Danelius G: Roentgen pelvimetric analyses of Walcher's position. Am J Obstet Gynecol 42:821, 1941.
20. Kroll DA, Caplan RA, Posner K, et al.: Nerve injury associated with anesthesia. Anesthesiology 73:202, 1990.
21. Feindel W, Stratford J: The role of the cubital tunnel in tardy ulnar palsy. Can J Surg 1:287, 1958.
22. Miller RG: The cubital tunnel syndrome: Diagnosis and precise localization. Ann Neurol 6:56, 1979.
23. Enderby GEH: Postural ischaemia and blood pressure. Lancet 1:185, 1954.
24. Kopman EA, Sandza JG Jr: Hemodynamic effects of head-down lithotomy position in patients with coronary artery disease. Obstet Gynecol 53:273, 1979.
25. Kubal K, Komatsu T, Sanchala V, et al.: Trendelenburg position used during venous cannulation increases myocardial oxygen demand. Anesth Analg 63:239, 1984 (abstract).
26. Jones JR, Jacoby J: The effect of surgical positions on respirations. Surg Forum 5:686, 1955.
27. Henschel AB, Wyant GM, Dobkin AB, Henschel EO: Posture as it concerns the anesthesiologist: A preliminary study. Anesth Analg 36:69, 1957.
28. Giesecke AH Jr, Cale JO, Jenkins MT: The prostate, ventilation and anesthesia. JAMA 203:389, 1968.
29. Jones MJ, Mitchell RWD, Hindocha H, James RH: The lower esophageal sphincter in the first trimester of pregnancy: Comparison of supine with lithotomy positions. Br J Anaesth 61:475, 1988.
30. Schleyer-Saunders E: Prevention of backache in women. BMJ 1:28, 1954.
31. Reneman RS: The Anterior and the Lateral Compartment Syndrome of the Leg. Paris, Mouton, 1968.
32. Ashton H: Critical closing pressure in human peripheral vascular beds. Clin Sci 22:79, 1966.
33. Strecker WB, Wood MB, Bieber EJ: Compartment syndrome masked by epidural anesthesia for postoperative pain. J Bone Joint Surg Am 68:1447, 1986.
34. Montgomery CJ, Ready LB: Epidural opioid analgesia does not obscure diagnosis of compartment syndrome resulting from prolonged lithotomy position. Anesthesiology 75:541, 1991.
35. Warner MA, Martin JT, Schroeder DR, et al.: Lower extremity motor neuropathy associated with surgery performed on patients in a lithotomy position. Anesthesiology 81:6, 1994.
36. deGroot J, Chusid JG: Correlative Neuroanatomy, 20th ed. Los Altos, CA, Lange Medical Publications, 1988, plate 6–24.
37. Vargo MM, Robinson LR, Nicholas JJ, Rulin MC: Postpartum femoral neuropathy: Relic of an earlier era? Arch Phys Med Rehabil 71:591, 1990.
38. Tondare AS, Nadkarni AV, Sathe CH, Dave VB: Femoral neuropathy: A complication of lithotomy position under spinal anesthesia. Can Anaesth Soc J 30:84, 1983.
39. al Hakim M, Katirji B: Femoral mononeuropathy induced by the lithotomy position: A report of 5 cases with a review of the literature. Muscle Nerve 16:891, 1993.
40. deGroot J, Chusid JG: Correlative Neuroanatomy, 20th ed. Los Altos, CA, Lange Medical Publications, 1988, plate 6–28.
41. Burkhart FL, Daly JW: Sciatic and peroneal nerve injury: A complication of vaginal operations. Obstet Gynecol 28:99, 1966.
42. Johnson EW Jr: Sciatic nerve palsy following delivery. Postgrad Med 30:495, 1961.
43. Loffer RD, Pent D, Goodkin R: Sciatic nerve injury in a patient undergoing laparoscopy. J Reprod Med 21:371, 1978.
44. Romfh JH, Currier RD: Sciatic neuropathy induced by the lithotomy position. Arch Neurol 40:127, 1983 (letter).
45. Reinstein L, Eckholdt JW: Sciatic nerve compression by preexisting heterotopic ossification during general anesthesia in dorsal lithotomy position. Arch Phys Med Rehabil 64:65, 1983.
46. Netter FH: The Ciba Collection of Medical Illustrations. Vol I: Nervous System; Section VI, Plate 11. West Caldwell, NJ, Ciba Geigy, 1983, p 123.
47. O'Donnell D, Rottman R, Kotelko D, et al.: Incidence of maternal postpartum neurologic dysfunction. Anesthesiology 81:A1127, 1994 (abstract).
48. deGroot J, Chusid JG: Correlative Neuroanatomy, 20th ed. Los Altos, CA, Lange Medical Publications, 1988, plate 6–29.
49. Netter FH: Atlas of Human Anatomy. Summit, NJ, Ciba Geigy, 1989.

50. Herrera-Ornelas L, Tolls RM, Petrelli NJ, et al.: Common peroneal nerve palsy associated with pelvic surgery for cancer: An analysis of 11 cases. Dis Colon Rectum 29:392, 1986.
51. Slocum HC, O'Neal KC, Allen CR: Neurovascular complications from malposition on the operating table. Surg Gynecol Obstet 86:729, 1948.
52. Guzzi LM, Mills LM, Greenman P: Rhabdomyolysis, acute renal failure, and the exaggerated lithotomy position.
53. Ali H, Nieto JG, Rhamy RK, et al.: Acute renal failure due to rhabdomyolysis associated with the extreme lithotomy position. Am J Kidney Dis 22:865, 1993.
54. Gordon BS, Newman W: Lower nephron syndrome following prolonged knee-chest position. J Bone Joint Surg Am 35:764, 1953.
55. Targa L, Droghetti L, Caggese G, et al.: Rhabdomyolysis and the operating position. Anesthesia 46:141, 1991.
56. Magill IW: Postoperative care: Anaesthetic aspects. Practitioner 138:247, 1937.
57. Brown EM, Elman DS: Postoperative backache. Anesth Analg 40:683, 1961.
58. Lincoln JR, Sawyer HP: Complications related to body positions during surgical procedures. Anesthesiology 22:80, 1961.
59. Healy TEJ, Wilkins RG: Patient posture and the anaesthetist. Ann R Coll Surg Engl 66:56, 1984.
60. Clarke AM, Stillwell S, Paterson ME, Getty CJ: Role of the surgical position in the development of postoperative low back pain. J Spinal Disord 6:238, 1993.
61. O'Donovan N, Healy TEJ, Faragher RG, Hamilton AA: Postoperative backache: The use of an inflatable wedge. Br J Anaesth 58:280, 1986.
62. Flanagan WF, Webster GD, Brown MW, Massey EW: Lumbosacral plexus stretch injury following the use of the modified lithotomy position. J Urol 134:567, 1985.
63. Courington FW, Little DM Jr: The role of posture in anesthesia. Clin Anesth 3:24, 1968.
64. Welborn SG: The lithotomy position: Anesthesiologic consideration. *In* Martin JT (ed.): Positioning in Anesthesia and Surgery, 2nd ed. Philadelphia, WB Saunders, 1987.

Chapter 7

The Head-Elevated Positions

Leslie Newberg Milde

BACKGROUND

The head-elevated positions discussed in this chapter include the sitting position, used primarily for neurosurgical procedures; the low sitting position, used for neck dissections or dental procedures, and its variant, the reclining shoulder position, intended for procedures about the shoulder; the head-elevated prone positions, used for neurosurgical procedures; and the head-elevated supine position (jargonistically referred to as "reverse Trendelenburg"), used for thyroidectomies and laparoscopic procedures in the upper abdomen.

An operative site is deliberately elevated above the level of the heart to improve drainage of body fluids (blood and cerebrospinal fluid [CSF]) away from the surgical site, thus decreasing bleeding in the surgical field and reducing intracranial pressure, and/or to provide excellent visual and instrumental access for the surgeon. The actual degree of head elevation varies with the type of surgery and the experience of the surgeon. The choice of patient position is usually decided on by the surgeon in consultation with the anesthesiologist. It is based on (1) assessment of the technical demands of the surgical approach, (2) efforts to obtain optimum operating conditions, (3) consideration of the physical status of the patient with regard to the presence of any cardiopulmonary disease and problems of airway management, and (4) the risk of complications.

THE SITTING POSITION

Preliminary Considerations

The sitting position (Fig. 7–1) has been in vogue for surgery since the 1800s when it was used routinely for head and neck procedures and for dental operations. Harvey Cushing used it for neurosurgical procedures, believing that elevation of the head reduced venous pressure in the surgical field, minimized blood loss, and improved exposure at the operative site.

In 1913 the sitting position[1] was advocated for posterior fossa surgery because it promoted venous drainage, offered the surgeon eye-level access to the contents of the posterior fossa, and, compared with the prone position, offered minimal restriction to ventilation at a time when all patients breathed spontaneously during anesthesia. The structures of the posterior fossa to which surgical access is gained by means of the sitting position are presented in Table 7–1. In the past, the sitting position has provided access to mass lesions located in the superior zone of the posterior cranial fossa; an infratentorial, supracerebellar approach to the pineal region[2]; an intraluminal approach to the apex of the fourth ventricle and aqueduct; and access to the cervical spine.

Surgical advantages of the sitting position include the following:

- Improved surgical exposure with direct access to the operative site and good visual alignment with critical anatomy

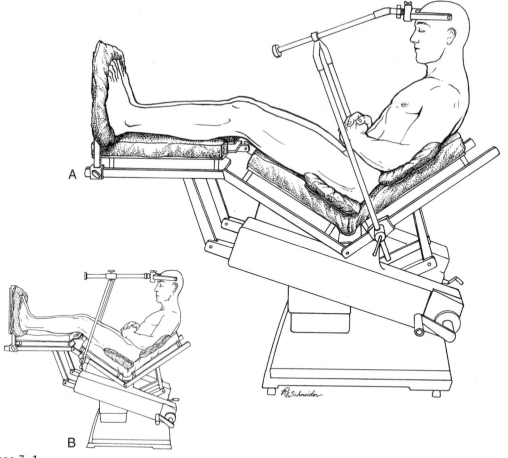

Figure 7-1

A. Conventional neurosurgical sitting position. The legs are at approximately the level of the heart and gently flexed on the thighs; the feet are supported at right angles to the legs; subgluteal padding protects the sciatic nerve. The frame of the head holder is *properly* clamped to the side rails of the back section of the table so that the patient's head can be lowered simply and rapidly by lowering the back section in the event of hemodynamically significant air embolism. *B. Improper* attachment of the head frame to the table side rails at the thigh section. In this position, the patient's head could not be quickly lowered because it would require disengaging the skull clamp.

- Correct anatomic orientation to the midline structures of the posterior fossa or cervical spine
- Greater torsion or flexion of the neck for access to lateral structures (e.g., the cerebellopontine angle) without impairing venous drainage
- Elimination of the risk of eyeball compression because of the availability of secure head fixation using the three-pin head holder

The major disadvantage of the sitting position for the surgeon is the height of the surgical field. Arm and hand fatigue may develop unless the elbows of the surgeon are provided with support during lengthy procedures.

Advantages of the sitting position for the anesthesiologist include:

- Access to the anterior chest wall for resuscitation in the event of cardiovascular collapse
- Easier mechanical ventilation because of lower airway pressures and easier diaphragmatic excursions allowing hyperventilation when necessary
- Easier access to the endotracheal tube or airway
- Easier access to the anterior chest wall and extremities for monitoring
- An unobstructed view of the face when monitoring motor function of cranial nerves

Table 7–1

Surgical Structures in the Posterior Fossa

Pontomedullary cranial nerves (trigeminal–hypoglossal nerves)
Vertebral, posterior inferior, anterior inferior, and superior cerebellar arteries
Jugular foramen and internal auditory meatus
Cerebellopontine angle
Petrous pyramid and inferior tentorial surface

The major disadvantages of the sitting position are presented in the section on complications. In addition, patients at the extremes of age have an increased rate of complications.[3]

Despite its venerability, the sitting position presents complex challenges. It is difficult to establish, requires coordination of time and effort with intricate equipment, and needs abundant assistance from experienced operating room personnel for its creation to be smooth. Its mixture of physiologic assets and risks requires extreme vigilance by attending personnel if the patient is to be safe. Presently, there is considerable controversy concerning the use of the sitting position for posterior intracranial and cervical spine surgery. Some use it for most of these operations; some never use it; some may individualize the choice of position considering the specific requirements for surgical access, the medical condition of the patient, and the capabilities of the operating room team. However, the overall use of the sitting position has decreased over the past 15 years.[4, 5] In Great Britain, 20% of neurosurgical centers place patients in the sitting position for surgery on structures in the posterior fossa (a decrease from 53% in 1981) while only 7% of centers use the position for procedures involving the cervical spine.[5]

Many believe that use of the sitting position should be limited to busy neurosurgical practices where the number of cervical spine and posterior fossa procedures is sufficient to provide the operating room team experience with the techniques demanded by the posture. When the team is not sufficiently experienced, alternate positions should be used for access to the posterior fossa and cervical spine.

Physiologic Changes Occurring with the Sitting Position

Cardiovascular System

Gravity affects cardiovascular function significantly for the patient placed in the sitting position. General anesthesia exaggerates the normal physiologic changes that occur when humans are placed in an upright posture.[6, 7] Venous return decreases because of pooling of venous blood in the more dependent periphery, a situation that is exacerbated by the vasodilating and/or myocardial depressant effects of most general anesthetics.[8] This results in a decrease in stroke volume and cardiac output (-12%–20%) with a compensatory increase in pulmonary and systemic vascular resistance ($+50\%$–80%) (unless blocked by vasodilating anesthetics, which further exacerbates the reduced cardiac output). Heart rate will be unchanged or increased. Blood pressure may be unchanged or increased when an awake patient assumes the sitting position, but it usually decreases in anesthetized patients. Above the level of the heart venous return is aided by gravity and by the inspiratory subatmospheric pressure phase of spontaneous ventilation; it is obstructed by positive-pressure ventilation. Cerebral perfusion pressure decreases by about 15%. Local arterial pressure decreases by approximately 1 mm Hg for every 1.25 cm distance above the level of the heart. Lateral rotation of the head to 60 degrees begins to impede arterial flow through the contralateral vertebral artery; and at 80 degrees of rotation, flow is obstructed. With an intact circle of Willis that flow reduction would normally be compensated for by an increase in blood flow in the ipsilateral vertebral artery. However, in patients with diseased vessels or changes in the cervical spine, the compromised circulation with reduced compensatory mechanisms may cause cerebral ischemia.

The higher the surgical target lies above the level of the heart, the lower is the intravascular pressure within veins of the operating field. The resulting widening of the pressure differential between those veins and the right atrium promotes entrainment of air through incised venous channels. The structure of the dural sinuses maintains their sizes constant, neither expanding under increased pressure to store blood nor collapsing when venous pressure is low.[9] That characteristic makes them particularly vulnerable to the entrainment of air if they are incised when the head is above the heart during surgery.

Respiratory System

The sitting position permits caudad gravitation of abdominal contents, freeing diaphragmatic excursions and increasing ventilation of the lung bases. Vital capacity and functional residual capacity are increased in the sitting position when compared with the supine position. Positive-pressure ventilation requires less peak inspiratory pressure to expand the lungs of a sitting patient. Consequently, hyperventilation is easily achieved. If ventilation is not carefully monitored, excessive hypocarbia may occur, a vasoconstrictive decrease in cerebral blood flow may result, and cerebral ischemia may appear in patients with cerebrovascular disease. Because of gravity, the upper lung fields are less well perfused in the sitting position. Positive-pressure ventilation and any relative hypovolemia may further reduce perfusion to the upper lung zones, causing an increase in physiologic dead space. Increases in ventilation/perfusion mismatch may occur that could produce hypoxemia. With positive-pressure ventilation, the normally subatmospheric inspiratory phase becomes positive, producing an additional impedance to venous return and a further exacerbation of ventilation/perfusion mismatch. Medications that abolish hypoxic pulmonary vasoconstriction, such as sodium nitroprusside or high concentrations of volatile anesthetics, further exacerbate ventilation/perfusion mismatch. Their use in patients in the sitting position may require higher concentrations of inspired oxygen to prevent hypoxemia, as measured by pulse oximetry or arterial blood gas analyses.

Central Nervous System

In the head-elevated position, gravity produces a gradient in CSF pressure along the neuraxis with values in the lumbar region approximating 30 mm Hg whereas those in the vertex of the skull are subatmospheric (-5 mm Hg).[9] The decreased CSF pressure in the head lessens that component of intracranial pressure enough for a mass lesion to have a less detrimental effect on perfusion of the surrounding normal tissue. When the arachnoid membrane at the base of the elevated head is opened, CSF escapes from the subarachnoid space and ventricles, allowing air to enter the intracranial CSF pathway. As a result, the cerebral hemispheres are no longer supported by ventricular CSF, the brain does not float in subarachnoid CSF, and some degree of caudad displacement of the brain occurs. Whereas most patients tolerate these changes safely, exceptions are individuals

with severe hydrocephalus and thin, flexible cerebral mantles. In them, the caudad displacement of the surface of the brain from the overlying dura could avulse bridging veins or arterioles and produce a subdural hematoma.

Musculoskeletal System

When neuromuscular blocking agents are used, joints and extremities can be positioned beyond their normal ranges of motion. Overstretching and hyperextension of muscles, tendons, and joints may occur and nerves may be stretched or compressed. Care should be taken to assure that relaxed extremities do not have their ranges of motion passively exceeded by a chosen surgical position.

Temperature Control

Body temperature is not easily controlled in patients who are placed in the sitting position. Airway warming by means of air exchangers or heated humidification and the use of forced air convective heating blankets placed over the patient may prevent some of the thermal losses inherent in the position.

Monitoring

Routine monitors for the patients in the sitting position include a noninvasive blood pressure cuff, a pulse oximeter, an electrocardiogram, a temperature probe, an esophageal or a precordial stethoscope to detect breath sounds, an end-tidal carbon dioxide concentration ($PETCO_2$) sensor, and an inspired oxygen concentration detector. In addition, a 5-lead electrocardiogram should be attached to reveal arrhythmias (lead II) and myocardial ischemia (lead V_5). Intra-arterial blood pressure should be monitored continuously. Large-caliber intravenous lines should be placed to allow sufficient fluid volume replacement and blood replacement as necessary. A urethral catheter should be inserted to monitor urine output as an indication of volume status and should be cleared to drain freely.

Specific monitoring for the detection of venous air embolism is listed in Table 7–2 and includes Doppler ultrasonography with the probe placed over the precordium; a right atrial catheter for the measurement of central venous pressure as well as for the retrieval of intracardiac air; capnography or mass spectrometry for the measurement of $PETCO_2$;

Table 7–2

Monitors for the Detection of Venous Air Embolism

Technique	Yield
Transesophageal echocardiography	Shows air in heart chambers
Precordial Doppler ultrasonography	Sound shift if air in right side of heart
End-tidal CO_2	Decreases if dead space ventilation (nonspecific)
Pulmonary artery pressure	Increases if pulmonary embolism (nonspecific)
End-tidal N_2	Increases if vascular air enters alveoli
Right atrial catheter	Aspiration of air for diagnosis and treatment of venous air embolism
Arterial blood pressure	Decreases as cardiac output falls
Pulse oximetry	Hypoxemia indicative of decreased ventilation and/or cardiac output
Electrocardiogram	Dysrhythmias from myocardial ischemia
Esophageal stethoscope	"Millwheel" murmur of froth in right atrium
Gasp/cough	Reflex from stretch receptors in right atrium

mass spectrometry for the measurement of end-tidal nitrogen concentrations ($P_{ET}N_2$); an esophageal stethoscope for the detection of air-induced heart murmurs; and transesophageal echocardiography. The most sensitive of these monitors are transesophageal echocardiography and Doppler ultrasonography; less sensitive are $P_{ET}N_2$, $P_{ET}CO_2$, central venous pressure, and pulmonary artery pressure; the least sensitive is a millwheel murmur heard through the esophageal stethoscope.

Doppler Ultrasonography

With the probe placed over the precordium at the level of the right atrium, Doppler ultrasonography is advocated as the basic monitoring device for the detection of venous air embolism. This is the most sensitive device *commonly* available as an indicator of air in the right atrium. It is reasonable in price, noninvasive, and easy to use. The Doppler probe generates a 2.5-MHz continuous ultrasonic signal that is reflected by moving blood. An electronic converter changes the signal to audible sound. A frequency shift is produced by reflection of the signal by air rather than blood. A characteristic change in the audible sound (the noise made when shaking a thin metal sheet) is produced and can be heard by both the anesthesiologist and the surgeon. Volumes of air as small as 0.25 mL can be detected by the change in sound.[10] In the sitting patient the precordial Doppler probe covered with conductive jelly should be placed over the right atrium, usually just to the right of the sternum, in the fourth or fifth intercostal space where the maximum signal strength is detected. The position of the probe can be confirmed by injecting 5 to 10 mL of agitated

saline[11–13] or mannitol[14] through a catheter placed in the right atrium and listening for the sound change. Greater sensitivity in the detection of air embolism has been described with the use of *transesophageal* Doppler ultrasonography,[15] a technique that is more invasive but avoids difficulties with positioning the external probe on the chest wall.

Right Atrial Catheter

A catheter placed in the right atrium can be used for measurement of central venous pressure, can confirm the diagnosis of venous air embolism, and can be used to aspirate air from the atrium in the treatment of venous air embolism. Patient position influences the detection of air and its retrieval, a maneuver that is easiest with the patient in the sitting position. The aspiration of air has been therapeutic and has reversed hemodynamic compromise when larger quantities of intracardiac air (>50 mL) have been retrieved.[16, 17] The volume of air retrieved has been increased by the use of a large-bore multi-orificed catheter.[18] Whether the routine aspiration of smaller amounts of air can prevent the cardiopulmonary complications of venous air embolism or paradoxical air embolism is unknown. The right atrium may be catheterized by a variety of routes, which include the cephalic or basilic veins of the antecubital fossa (the right arm approach is easier for right atrial catheterization), the internal or external jugular veins, and the subclavian veins. A specialized Doppler ultrasound transducer can locate the jugular or subclavian veins before needle insertion.[19] When the catheter is placed in the neck, insertion sites should be sealed with bacteriostatic ointment under an occlusive dressing to prevent or minimize their becoming entrainment sites when the patient is placed in the sitting position.

Proper placement of the right atrial catheter in the high right atrium can increase its utility by situating its tip where the entrained air tends to collect (Fig. 7–2).[20, 21] The placement of a right atrial catheter for optimal air retrieval can be achieved by using radiography, pressure recordings, or intravascular electrocardiography.[22] The use of intravascular electrocardiography allows more precise placement than do the other methods (Fig. 7–3).

The technique for seating the tip of an intravenous catheter in the right atrium is as follows:

- In the solution line for the catheter, place a special electroconductive adapter that accepts attachment to the electrocardiographic monitor. The use of sodium bicarbonate solution to flush the catheter

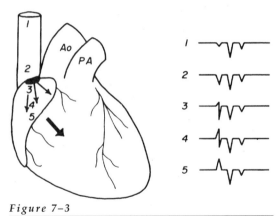

Figure 7–3

The intracardiac ECG lead from catheter position as it is placed in the right atrium. With a single-lumen catheter, the proper position is at 3. With a multi-orifice catheter the ECG tracing originates from the proximal orifice; the ECG tracing for proper positioning is at 2. (From Black S, Cucchiara RF: Tumor surgery. *In* Cucchiara RF, Michenfelder JD [eds.]: Clinical Neuroanesthesia. New York, Churchill Livingstone, 1990.)

rather than normal saline or lactated Ringer's solution improves the quality of the electrocardiographic tracing. Using a five-lead electrocardiographic monitoring system, set the ECG monitor for lead V and attach the V lead to the adapter. Observe the ECG tracing and advance the catheter.

- If the catheter has been placed from veins lying to the right of the midline, the P wave is initially negative (see Fig. 7–3, *1*). As its tip is advanced toward the sinoatrial node, the generator of the P wave, the negative P wave will become progressively larger (see Fig. 7–3, *2*). When the catheter tip is advanced just below the sinoatrial node, the P wave will become biphasic with a small initial upstroke and a larger downstroke (see Fig. 7–3, *3*).

- If the catheter has a single distal orifice, the small upstroke on the largely negative P wave is the optimal position for maximal air retrieval should it become necessary. However, with a multi-orificed catheter the electrocardiographic signal is believed to originate from the proximal orifice, usually 2 cm from the tip. Optimum placement of the multi-orificed catheter, therefore, is indicated when the P wave becomes most negative, just before the small upstroke develops. Placement is gained by advancing the catheter until the small upstroke appears and then

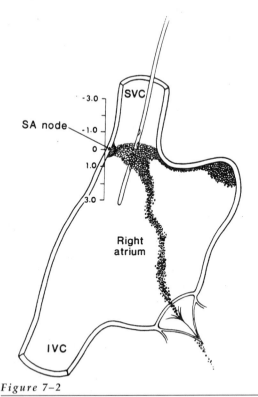

Figure 7–2

Localization of venous air emboli at the atrium–superior vena cava junction and in the upper portion of the right atrium in patients in the sitting position. The placement of a multi-orifice catheter as shown is most likely to aspirate air emboli. (From Black S, Cucchiara RF: Tumor surgery. *In* Cucchiara RF, Michenfelder JD [eds.]: Clinical Neuroanesthesia. New York, Churchill Livingstone, 1990.)

withdrawing it slightly until the upstroke has just disappeared and the P wave is all negative once again. That location places the proximal orifice of the catheter in the superior vena cava and allows the most distal part of its tip to float at the superior vena cava–atrium junction.

- When a catheter is introduced from veins to the left of the midline, the original P wave will be positive, an upstroke. It will become increasingly smaller and eventually negative as it approaches the sinoatrial node. Once the wave has become negative, the sequence of signals is similar to that just described for a right-sided approach.
- The correct positioning of the catheter tip by means of the intravascular electrocardiographic monitor should be reconfirmed with the patient in the final sitting position because changes in arm, neck, or head position may move the catheter tip.[23] When the location is satisfactory, the electrocardiographic lead is removed from the connection to the catheter to avoid any hazard of microshock during the subsequent surgical procedure. The conductive connector can either be removed from the line or insulated with a rubber cap or plug.
- At the end of the case the catheter should be withdrawn enough to relocate the tip from the right atrium into the superior vena cava to avoid atrial dysrhythmias or a perforation of an atrial wall.

Pulmonary Artery Catheter

Passage of air into the pulmonary circulation causes mechanical obstruction in the microcirculation and/or macrocirculation that may cause reflex vasoconstriction and hypoxemia. A catheter previously placed in the pulmonary artery indicates the event as an increase in pulmonary artery pressure.[24, 25] Return of pulmonary artery pressures toward normal indicates that the air in the circulation has cleared the pulmonary circuit by diffusion into the alveoli and exhalation through the lungs.[26] An increase in pulmonary artery pressure is more sensitive and specific than capnography in the detection of venous air embolism, but it occurs after a decrease in $PetCO_2$ is observed. However, the placement of a pulmonary artery catheter is invasive and retrieval of air through its lumen is difficult because of the small caliber and the slow speed of blood return.

Capnography

Measurement of $PetCO_2$ can be obtained by infrared analysis, mass spectroscopy, or Raman light-scattering analysis. Passage of air into the pulmonary circulation causes the aforementioned pulmonary vasoconstriction and increases dead space. Enlarged dead space decreases $PetCO_2$ and increases arterial concentrations of carbon dioxide ($PaCO_2$).[27] With the occurrence of an air embolism, decreases in $PetCO_2$ are evident after a sound change is heard by Doppler ultrasonography but before the onset of hemodynamic changes.[28] The magnitude of the decrease in $PetCO_2$ can be used to estimate the increase in dead space and may correlate with the amount of air that reaches the pulmonary circulation. However, the fall in $PetCO_2$ is not specific for venous air embolism alone. Other causes include increased minute ventilation, decreased cardiac output, decreased pulmonary perfusion, and obstructive lung disease. End-tidal CO_2 values will return to baseline after an episode of venous air embolism when the pulmonary intravascular air has diffused into alveoli and been exhaled, a process that usually requires 20 to 30 minutes after the cessation of air entrainment.

End-Tidal Nitrogen Concentration

Passage of air into the circulation results in the diffusion of nitrogen from bubbles in the blood into the alveoli and is detected through measurement of the end-tidal gases, including nitrogen.[29–31] Nitrogen can be detected by mass spectroscopy or by Raman light-scattering spectroscopy. Measurement of $PetN_2$ is more specific than capnography for the detection of an air embolism when the patient is breathing only O_2, nitrous oxide, and volatile anesthetic agents and can detect air emboli earlier than does a change in $PetCO_2$. The magnitude of the increase in $PetN_2$ is a measure of the amount of air entrained into the circulation.

Transesophageal Echocardiography

Visualization of all four chambers of the heart can be achieved with two-dimensional transesophageal echocardiography through a long-axis view of the heart at the level of the left atrium. This gives a view of the right atrium and right ventricle for venous air embolization as well as a view of the left atrium and left ventricle for visualization of paradoxical air emboli.[32, 33] Transesophageal echocardiography has been reported to be more sensitive than Doppler ultrasonography for detection of air emboli. It can consistently detect a bolus injection of 0.02 mL/kg air,[34] whereas consistent Doppler changes require a volume of 0.05 mL/kg. With continuous infusions of air (a model more indicative of the clinical situation) both Doppler ultrasonography and transesophageal echocardiography can detect air introduced at 0.05 mL/kg/min. Pulmonary artery pressure and PETCO_2 detect air at an infusion rate of 0.1 mL/kg/min.[34] Transesophageal echocardiography and Doppler ultrasound transducers can interfere with each other to the extent that monitoring transesophageal echocardiography is difficult when Doppler ultrasonography is in use. To circumvent the problem, routine continuous monitoring can be done with the Doppler probe. When air is detected by the Doppler device, it can be turned off and transesophageal echocardiography can be used to visualize the air in the right atrium for an estimation of the volume involved, to determine whether the entrainment is continuing, and to determine if air is passing across a septal defect into the left atrium.

Screening echocardiography has been advocated for the detection of a patent foramen ovale preoperatively in patients scheduled for surgery in the sitting position. Patent foramen ovale is the most common association with paradoxical air embolism, a potentially devastating complication that can result in myocardial and cerebral ischemia. Preoperative identification of patients with intracardiac defects has been proposed as a means of decreasing the risk of transseptal air.[35] Patients with a known patent foramen ovale can then be placed in an alternate position for the planned surgery. In the general population without cardiac disease, the incidence of patent foramen ovale at autopsy is 20% to 30%.[36] However, routine preoperative echocardiography detects an incidence of only 10% to 18%, a value much lower than expected.[37–41] Several techniques have been described for increasing the sensitivity and specificity of preoperative echocardiography as a screening method for the presence of patent foramen ovale. The combined use of phased-array two-dimensional transesophageal echocardi-

ography and the injection of agitated saline through a right atrial catheter while positive airway pressure is being applied has detected atrial transseptal fluid passage in 3 of 20 patients (15%).[42–44] The Valsalva maneuver has also been used as a provocative method of demonstrating right-to-left shunting for transesophageal echocardiography.[38, 42] Others have used a cough to achieve the same purpose.[37] However, even these maneuvers have failed to detect the incidence of patent foramen ovale that is expected in the normal population. More invasive use of transesophageal echocardiography has yielded a higher incidence of patent foramen ovale. Transesophageal echocardiography with the injection of contrast medium (normal saline and venous blood or, if patent foramen ovale was not detected, 3.5% oxypolygelatin and venous blood) produced an incidence of 25% patent foramen ovale as well as an incidence of 3.9% intrapulmonary shunting.[45] Transesophageal contrast echocardiography and color flow mapping have been reported to detect patent foramen ovale in 35% to 40% of patients.[46] The procedure is invasive, and proper interpretation of results requires sophisticated training.[47] The failure to detect patent foramen ovale preoperatively does not eliminate the possibility that the patient is at risk for developing paradoxical air embolism.[48] In one study in which all patients had preoperative transesophageal echocardiography and in which the detection rate for patent foramen ovale was 23%, intraoperative transesophageal echocardiography detected paradoxical air embolism in 12% of patients who did not appear to have patent foramen ovale on the screening examination.[41] Slightly consoling is the fact that the occurrence of paradoxical air embolism has been documented on intraoperative transesophageal echocardiography without neurologic sequelae.[49]

Transcranial Doppler Ultrasonography

Paradoxical air embolism in patients undergoing cardiopulmonary bypass has been diagnosed by the use of transcranial Doppler ultrasonography. Audio frequencies between 250 and 500 Hz are consistently dominant in the spectrum when air emboli occur.[50] The technique is noninvasive and may prove to be a useful monitor for paradoxical air embolism in patients having surgery in the sitting position.

Continuing vigilance and monitoring with

a precordial Doppler device, right atrial catheter, arterial catheter for pressure and sampling, capnography, and end-tidal nitrogen measurement remain absolute requirements for the early detection and treatment of venous air emboli.

Establishing the Sitting Position

Positioning a patient during general anesthesia has several criteria that should be met:

- Normal body alignment should be maintained without flexion or extension beyond the usual ranges of motion for that patient.
- No direct contact should exist between body parts and metal or hard surfaces that could lead to pressure necrosis or to burns if an electrocautery device is used.
- All body parts must be supported and all pressure points should be well padded to prevent pressure necrosis.
- Any areas where nerve compression might occur should be well padded to disperse pressure away from the nerve in question.

- Systemic circulation must be well maintained.
- Respiratory excursions should be maintained, and adequate room should be provided for chest and abdominal expansion.
- All monitoring lines should be accessible throughout the procedure.
- Positional changes should be accomplished slowly to allow maximum hemodynamic compensation (see also Chapters 2 and 3).

The specific technique for placing a patient in the sitting position is as follows (Fig. 7–4):

- The operating table should have a removable head section and separate controls for the leg section, back section, flexion, and head-down tilt.
- Significant padding and/or convoluted foam rubber padding should be placed over the operating table mattress to protect pressure points on the body of the patient.
- One or two large pillows should be placed upon the thigh section of the table. They serve to pad the gluteal area and protect the sciatic nerve. They should ele-

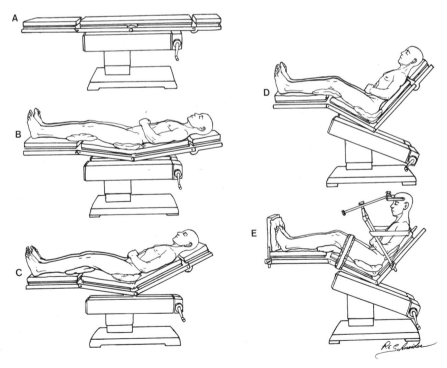

Figure 7–4

Table manipulation sequence for establishment of the traditional sitting position. *A.* Initially flat table. *B.* Top flexed and foot section lowered. *C.* Back section elevated. *D.* Table chassis is tipped down as back section is elevated farther. Foot section is adjusted to maintain legs at level of the heart. *E.* Head holder and frame in place; head section of table removed; thigh strap and footboard added.

vate the torso sufficiently for the upper end of the back section of the table to be at the level of the second or third thoracic vertebrae. In this manner the back section of the table top offers good support for the torso while allowing surgical access to the cervical spine if needed. In shorter adults or children, additional subgluteal padding may be needed to achieve the desired relationship between table edge and upper thoracic spine.

- While the patient is still supine a three-pin head holder is placed on the head with the pins positioned away from the intended surgical field. Using sterile technique, the scalp and periosteum of the skull at the pin sites should be infiltrated with local anesthetic (lidocaine 1% or bupivacaine 0.5%) to help prevent the hypertensive response to pin insertion into the outer table of the skull.[51] Antibiotic ointment should be applied around the pins to minimize the risk of bacterial contamination or air embolism. If the head holder needs to be repositioned using new pin sites, the old sites should be packed with antibiotic ointment to prevent air entrainment. In very young patients the skull must be firm enough to be immobilized in a pin head holder.

- The head holder is attached to a supporting arm that is affixed to a frame that is shaped like an inverted U. The limbs of the U insert into sockets that slide adjustably along the side rails of the *back section* of the operating table. Seating the U-frame in that manner allows the sitting patient to be lowered rapidly to a horizontal position in the event of hemodynamic compromise by simply lowering the elevated back section of the table. If the U-frame is attached to the thigh section of the table (see Fig. 7–1) the patient cannot be lowered to a horizontal position without a time-consuming process of removing the head from the holding system.

- Correct positioning of the head is crucial. Extreme neck flexion can (1) stretch the spinal cord with the potential for an ischemic transection at a cervical level and (2) obstruct venous drainage from the face and tongue sufficiently to produce edema that causes airway distress.[52, 53] Maintaining at least 2 to 3 cm (two fingerbreadths) space between the chin and the anterior chest wall should prevent excessive flexion. Extremes of head rotation

can alter flow in the vertebral artery system; in the presence of abnormal anastomoses in the circle of Willis brain perfusion can be threatened.

- Once all of the joints of the head clamp and its supporting frame are carefully tightened, the head is held in competent skeletal immobilization that gives surgical access to the dorsal field while providing access to the face and airway for the anesthesiologist.

Before the frame joints are fully tightened, the sitting position is achieved by elevating the back section of the table 60 to 90 degrees with the thighs flexed upon the trunk, the knees flexed, and the feet maintained at or near the level of the heart.

- Initially the table is flexed fully at the back-thigh hinge, then the foot section is lowered 30 to 45 degrees to flex the patient's knees. Any restraining straps across the thighs are loosened to free the motion of the table and prevent compression of the extremities.

- Next, the back section of the table is elevated into the desired sitting position. The maneuver should be performed slowly enough to allow the baroreceptor responses of the anesthetized patient to compensate for postural hypotension.

- Tilting the head end of the table chassis toward the floor further elevates the patient's legs while removing the projecting parts of the chassis from the area in which the surgeon needs to stand.

- The combination of back section elevation and chassis tilt is coordinated to further flex the thighs on the torso without significantly raising the patient's head and may require that the foot section be additionally adjusted to maintain the horizontal position of the lower legs at the level of the heart.

Alternatively the patient can be placed in the sitting position by flexing the table top, elevating its back section, and tilting the head end of the chassis upward, away from the floor (Fig. 7–5A). The U-frame can then be mounted on the side rails of the *thigh* section of the table. With this arrangement, should hemodynamic instability occur, the patient's head can be quickly lowered toward the horizontal by adjusting only the angle of the table chassis (Fig. 7–5B).

During these maneuvers the blood pressure

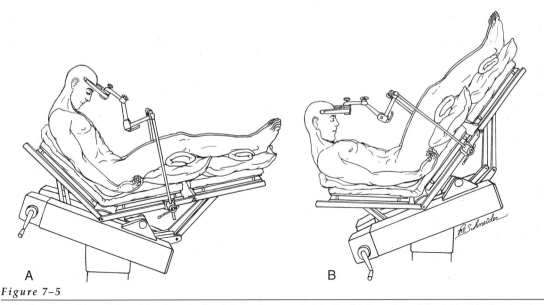

Figure 7–5

A. Correct position of the table when the head frame is connected to the thigh section of the table. The head end of the table chassis should be elevated when the patient is in the correct sitting position (note the differences with Fig. 7–1). *B.* The head can be quickly lowered to the level of the heart by rotating the elevated end of the chassis downward. (Redrawn from Miller RD [ed.]: Anesthesia, 3rd ed. New York, Churchill Livingstone, 1990.)

should be constantly monitored to detect any significant hypotension. Slow elevation of the head, together with the judicious use of fluids and/or vasopressors, is indicated to maintain blood pressure levels that provide adequate cerebral perfusion. General anesthesia should be adjusted to provide adequate sedation and analgesia, allow controlled ventilation, and minimize circulatory depression while posture is being altered.

All bony prominences should be well padded. The legs should be placed in thigh-high compressive stockings, although care should be taken during their application to avoid a tourniquet effect and subsequent ischemia to the leg. Sequential circumferential compression devices should be used to prevent pooling of blood in the leg veins and encourage forward blood flow. Arms should be well padded and flexed across the chest or abdomen to remain within the supporting bars of the U-shaped frame (see Fig. 7–4E). Crossing the hands in the lap permits access to intravascular lines for infusion and blood sampling. With large patients, placing the arms within the confines of the bars of the head frame may not be possible. Elbows and arms flexed around a padded frame should be supported with pillows or pads to prevent (1) downward traction on the shoulders and

stretch of the brachial plexus, (2) pressure on the ulnar nerve as it passes through the cubital tunnel on the dorsomedial aspect of the proximal forearm, (3) compression of the radial nerve above the elbow by the vertical bars of the U-shaped frame, and (4) contact with metal table parts that could permit grounding burns when electrocautery is in use. The legs should be free of pressure lateral to the knees where the common peroneal nerves course around the lateral portion of the fibula just distal to its head. Abdominal compression, lower extremity ischemia, and sciatic nerve injury may be avoided by preventing excessive flexion of the thighs on the torso.

When the patient is in the final sitting position, the arterial pressure transducer should be placed at the level of the operative site to measure the perfusion pressure there. The right atrial pressure transducer should be placed at the level of the heart. Each can easily be attached to a vertical mount on the operating table so that any adjustment made in the table height simultaneously adjusts the height of the transducers to preserve their relationships with sensing sites. The location of the right atrial catheter should be reconfirmed by electrocardiography. The Doppler probe should then be positioned.

COMPLICATIONS

Patient populations at increased risk for complications due to intraoperative positioning include the elderly; infants and children; those undergoing prolonged procedures; and those with pre-existing medical diseases such as obesity, malnutrition, debilitation, diabetes mellitus, cardiovascular disease, pulmonary disease, or hypothermia. The major pathophysiology among these conditions is decreased tissue perfusion and oxygenation resulting in ischemia.

Hypotension

Hypotension is the most frequent complication of the sitting position. Intravascular volume deficits, whether due to limited oral intake, therapeutic diuresis or that resulting from intravascular contrast substances used in diagnostic studies, preoperative bleeding, prolonged vomiting, or diarrhea, should be corrected before the induction of anesthesia because hypovolemia exacerbates hypotension. Blood pressure should be maintained within the patient's usual awake range or within a normal range if the patient presents with uncontrolled hypertension. Mean arterial pressure, measured at the level of the operative site, should be maintained above 50 mm Hg (the lower limit of the cerebral and spinal autoregulation curve) to assure that there is adequate cerebral blood flow in all regions of the brain. Most general anesthetics decrease cerebral metabolism such that this cerebral blood flow should be adequate to prevent ischemia. Any decreases in arterial pressure should be detected promptly and corrected rapidly. Hypotension occurring in patients in the sitting position may be especially detrimental in the presence of the following pre-existing diseases: hypertension, cardiovascular disease, cerebrovascular disease, previous carotid artery surgery that may be associated with altered limits of cerebral autoregulation and impaired cerebral perfusion, and abnormal baroreceptor function. It is exacerbated by general anesthesia. Volume infusion with either crystalloid or colloid before the induction of general anesthesia and the onset of positioning maneuvers may help prevent the occurrence of hypotension or minimize its severity and duration. When fluid resuscitation alone is not adequate to restore normal blood pressure, vasopressor medications should be used. Recommended are mixed alpha- and beta-agonists such as ephedrine; the pure alpha-agonist phenylephrine; or, when necessary, epinephrine. Fluid volume, myocardial function, cardiac rhythm, and depth of anesthesia must also be considered when treating hypotension.

Deliberate hypotension for patients in the sitting position is rarely used, even for patients undergoing high-risk surgical procedures.

Ventilation Difficulties

Endotracheal tube compression may occur with excessive flexion of the patient's head or by the patient biting on the tube. Whereas wire-reinforced endotracheal tubes usually do not kink when the head is flexed, they are easily compressed when bitten and may not return to their full caliber when the compressive force is removed. When they are used, some firm structure such as an oral airway or a bite block should be inserted between the teeth and taped in position to protect the tube against compression. Even with the endotracheal tube positioned correctly after intubation with the patient supine, its location will change to some degree as the head is moved during subsequent positioning. When the head is excessively flexed, the tube tip will migrate as much as 2 to 4 cm caudad, a distance that can result in its entry into the right mainstem bronchus. Even when a mainstem intubation has not occurred, the tip can be situated so that ventilation is preferentially aimed toward one lung, resulting in ventilation/perfusion mismatch. Listening to lung sounds *in the axilla* after positioning has been finalized should detect the presence of endobronchial intubation or preferential one-lung ventilation. Excessive lateral rotation or extension of the head can also move the tip of the endotracheal tube.

Venous Air Embolism

Venous air embolism is a common occurrence that is often undetected clinically. The reported incidence of venous air embolism depends on the method of detection being employed, varying between 1.6% and 6% with routine monitoring alone and 42% to 85% with Doppler ultrasonography.[54] The average incidence is 41% to 45% in patients undergoing posterior fossa craniotomy while in the sitting position and 11% to 24% in patients undergoing cervical spine surgery.[4, 55, 56] Venous air embolism occurs in 10% of neurosurgical cases done in the prone position.[57] Detection techniques have become more sensitive and now can diagnose venous air embolism before catastrophic hemodynamic events take place.[58] This allows the surgeon time to prevent further air entrainment and the anesthesiologist time to retrieve entrained air by aspirating the atrial catheter and to treat any hemodynamic changes. Significant morbidity and mortality of venous air embolism is now less than 1%.[4, 55]

Venous air embolism has widespread effects on the cardiopulmonary system, including increased pulmonary arterial pressure, decreased cardiac output, systemic hypotension, increased dead space ventilation, and shunting of blood in the pulmonary circulation with resultant hypoxemia, pulmonary edema, and systemic embolism. During slow continuous entrainment of air, the air is dissipated into the pulmonary circulation, producing sympathetic reflex vasoconstriction from mechanical obstruction of arterioles by small bubbles or from local hypoxemia.[59]

Together with the collapse of small airways,[60] this increases pulmonary artery pressure. Shunting of blood away from areas of air emboli can further exacerbate ventilation/perfusion mismatch and impair gas exchange; the result is hypoxemia and/or CO_2 retention with an increased $PaCO_2$ plus increased pulmonary dead space that decreases $PETCO_2$. Cardiac output may fall because of decreased venous return, right-sided heart failure due to the pulmonary hypertension, or more rarely from mechanical obstruction of the pulmonary outflow tract by a froth of bubbles. A rapid bolus injection of gas that exceeds the capacity of the pulmonary artery (5 mL/kg)[61] may produce an air lock within the right side of the heart. The right ventricular outflow tract is blocked by a compressible air bubble froth that obstructs venous return, impairs the effective pumping action of the ventricle, decreases cardiac output, causes acute right ventricular dilation and failure, and leads to pulmonary edema,[62] systemic hypotension,[63] and cardiac collapse. When the microvascular bubbles interface with blood and endothelial proteins, they activate the release of endothelial mediators. Complement is activated and cytokine released, causing neutrophil aggregation, more microvascular emboli, and the production of destructive oxygen free radicals that damage endothelium. Myocardial ischemia, dysrhythmias, and cerebral ischemia may result from severe hypoxemia, hypotension, or paradoxical air emboli.

Morbidity and mortality are directly related to the amount and rate of air entrainment. The symptomatic dose is unknown but is less than 50 mL. The lethal dose is greater than 300 mL.[64] Hemodynamically significant venous air embolism occurs in approximately 18% of patients experiencing venous air embolism. The incidence is decreased by careful surgical dissection, hemostasis, and the liberal use of bone wax to seal bone edges. Severe morbidity and mortality occur in about 1% of instances of venous air embolism.[55] Factors contributing to the incidence and severity of venous air embolism include the surgical site (cerebral venous channels are stented open by surrounding bone), the degree of head elevation, and the pressure differential between the surgical site and the right atrium that becomes greater in the presence of hypovolemia. Venous air embolism occurs more often with posterior fossa craniotomies than with cervical laminectomies.[4, 55, 56, 65] Children have greater hemodynamic derangements from venous air embolism than do adults.

VENOUS AIR EMBOLISM COMPLICATIONS: SITTING VERSUS HORIZONTAL PRONE

Several large retrospective studies have compared complication rates for patients in the sitting position with those occurring in the horizontal prone position. Most looked at the position and then at the associated complications.

- One study reported that the incidence of hypotension, perioperative myocardial infarction, and respiratory problems was the same in each group. However, increased bleeding requiring blood transfusion occurred in the prone position whereas increased cranial nerve preservation was present in the sitting position.[4]
- Another study reported that no intraoperative deaths had occurred from venous air embolism in patients in the sitting position although two patients suffered significant neurologic injury (0.05%). One death occurred in a patient in the three-fourths prone position.[58] Since that study, however, one postoperative death attributed to massive venous air embolism in a patient in the sitting position has occurred at that institution despite the use of the most sophisticated monitoring

equipment available and the retrieval of air (Weber J, personal communication, 1995).

- Another study compiled complications and then sought associated causal relationships. The authors concluded that the sitting position contributed to morbidity in 14 cases of supratentorial intracerebral hemorrhage.[64, 66]

Venous air embolus can and does occur during such diverse procedures as radical prostatectomies,[67] cesarean sections,[68] liver transplantation,[69] laparoscopic cholecystectomies, orthopedic surgery, and spine reconstructions.[70] Because many occurrences of venous air embolism have, undoubtedly, not been reported in the literature, its true incidence may be grossly underestimated.

PARADOXICAL AIR EMBOLUS

Any connection between the right and left sides of the heart can allow entrained air to appear in the arterial circulation, resulting in a paradoxical air embolism. If right atrial pressure is greater than left atrial pressure, intracardiac shunts through a patent foramen ovale or intrapulmonary arteriovenous shunts can lead to paradoxical air emboli. The migration of air can occur during the normal cardiac cycle[71] or as a result of venous air embolism causing increased pulmonary artery pressure, central venous pressure, and right-sided heart failure. The sitting position is contraindicated, therefore, in patients who have documented intracardiac defects or pulmonary arteriovenous malformations that could allow the occurrence of a paradoxical air embolus.

The most common association with paradoxical air embolism is the presence of a patent foramen ovale. A probe patent foramen ovale is present in 20% to 35% of the normal population at autopsy[36] and can be opened if pressure in the right atrium exceeds pressure in the left atrium. Venous air embolism, intermittent positive-pressure ventilation, and positive end-expiratory pressure (PEEP) can all elevate right atrial pressure. The sitting position is associated with acute reductions in left atrial pressure (as measured by pulmonary capillary occlusion pressure).[26] These factors combine to make sitting patients more at risk for paradoxical air embolism and its potential for myocardial, cerebral, or peripheral ischemia. Based on the incidence of patent foramen ovale (20%–35%), air embolus (40%), and elevated right atrial pressure (50%), the risk of paradoxical air embolism from intracardiac mechanisms can be calculated to be approximately 1 in 20 (5%).

Paradoxical air embolism can also occur through transpulmonary passage of air at doses exceeding 0.3 mL/kg/min[61] and has been detected clinically with the use of transesophageal echocardiography.[72] Whereas the lungs can usually inhibit transpulmonary air passage, there is a finite limit to this filtering ability.[61] Transesophageal echocardiography has been advocated as a means of detecting venous air embolism and paradoxical air embolism when the risk of air embolism is great (e.g., posterior fossa craniotomies done in the sitting position).

RESPONSE TO THE RECOGNITION OF VENOUS AIR EMBOLIZATION

Early detection of venous air embolism by the monitors just described has significantly reduced the complication rate of venous air embolism because its presence is now commonly identified before hemodynamic compromise has occurred. A team approach is needed to produce these results. The anesthesiologist makes the diagnosis and supports the cardiovascular system; the surgeon floods the surgical field with fluid (usually saline) to stop the entry of air and begins a meticulous examination to locate the portal of entry. Bone wax and sutures may be used to seal the vessel opening.

- Nitrous oxide should be discontinued and the patient ventilated with an FIO_2 of 1.0 to slow the increase in size of the entrained air bubbles (by the presence of nitrous oxide) and hasten their resorption.
- The application of jugular pressure at the anterior neck (without pressure over the carotid pulsation) can frequently raise the cerebral venous pressure in the wound sufficiently to identify the entrainment site by the presence of back-bleeding.[73] However, the maneuver is difficult to accomplish and prolonged jugular venous compression in the presence of a mass in the posterior fossa may significantly increase intracranial pressure.
- The right atrial catheter (or pulmonary artery catheter) should be aspirated at the earliest suspicion of air entrainment to

confirm the diagnosis and to remove the accumulating air.

- Vasopressors and fluid administration have been advocated to increase cardiac output and thereby aid in moving air through the heart and into the peripheral pulmonary circulation for absorption into the alveoli.
- A peak inspiratory hold (the Valsalva maneuver) has been reported to help prevent air entrainment and aid in the localization of the site of air entry.[74]
- The use of PEEP in the management of venous air embolism is controversial. Advocated by some as one more means of increasing central venous pressure to cause back-bleeding at the incision and help identify the site of air entry,[75–77] other studies have suggested that the levels of PEEP used can be ineffective in significantly raising central or intracranial venous pressure enough to affect the occurrence of venous air embolism.[78–80] PEEP has also been demonstrated to increase right atrial pressure to levels higher than left atrial pressure with the potential for causing paradoxical air embolism in the presence of a patent foramen ovale.[62, 71, 81]

When the measures described fail to identify the site of air entry, especially in the presence of hemodynamic compromise, the surgical site should be lowered below the level of the heart to reverse the hydrostatic gradient. An earlier recommendation, based on animal research, was to combine head-down tilt with the left lateral decubitus position as a means of trapping air in the apex of the right ventricle away from the pulmonary outflow tract. More recently, however, a study has demonstrated that body repositioning in that manner does not influence the effect of venous air embolism.[82] Increasing the rate of intravenous fluid administration may help maintain right-sided heart function in the presence of acute pulmonary hypertension, and the resulting increase in cardiac output may aid clearance of bubbles from the vena cava.[83]

Treatment of paradoxical air embolism consists of supportive therapy and continued mechanical ventilation with an FIO_2 of 1.0. In an animal study, this has been shown to increase the rate of removal of air from cerebral arteries.[84] Others have advocated the use of hyperbaric oxygenation.[85]

Because early detection and vigorous treatment of venous air embolism have signifi-

cantly reduced its morbidity, and because death ascribed to its effects is now very rare, the time and effort required to establish adequate surveillance of patients who are at risk is clearly justified.

Cardiac Dysrhythmias

The appearance of serious dysrhythmias (marked bradycardia, tachycardia, runs of premature ventricular contractions, or ventricular tachycardia) can herald surgical manipulation of the pons, medulla, or the roots of the fifth, ninth, or tenth cranial nerve and may indicate medullary or pontine ischemia.[86] Dysrhythmias may also indicate the presence of intracardiac air. Withdrawal of the surgical stimulus usually stops the dysrhythmia. However, if it does not stop, cerebral perfusion may be significantly compromised. Prompt use of medications to restore normal sinus rhythm and regain normal perfusion pressure is indicated, and aspiration of air from the atrial catheter should be attempted if venous air embolism is suspected. Other causes of dysrhythmias include hypercarbia, acidosis, and hyperkalemia or hypokalemia.

Nerve Injuries

The ulnar nerve, radial nerve, brachial plexus, sciatic nerve, and peroneal nerve are susceptible to injury in the sitting position.

- The most commonly injured nerve during anesthesia,[87] the ulnar nerve can be compressed between the medial epicondyle of the humerus and a sharp edge of the bed or head frame. Sustained pressure of the weight of the unpadded elbow upon the area of the cubital tunnel can also cause an ulnar neuropathy.
- The radial nerve may be damaged as the arm rests against the supportive bars of the frame that supports the head of a sitting patient. It is relatively superficial and vulnerable as it courses around the dorsolateral aspect of the humeral shaft about one handbreadth above the lateral epicondyle.
- Injury to the brachial plexus has been reported in patients with pre-existing disease of the cervical spine or a thoracic outlet syndrome.[88, 89]
- The sciatic nerve may be damaged in sitting patients when pressure on the ischial

tuberosities is prolonged in the presence of minimal padding from a reduced gluteal tissue mass or when too few artificial pads such as pillows or foam are used. The nerve can also be overstretched when the thighs are flexed on the torso while the lower leg is still extended or when the lower extremities are externally rotated.[90, 91]

- The peroneal nerve is the most commonly damaged nerve of the lower extremities.[87] Injury may occur if there is prolonged pressure in the popliteal fossa by pillows or if the legs are externally rotated so that there is pressure on the lateral surface of the head of the fibula. Footdrop can occur after either a sciatic or a common peroneal nerve injury. It is usually prevented by using a padded footboard on the table to prop the foot at an angle about 90 degrees with the long axis of the lower leg once the final sitting position is established. Heel pads should be applied to dissipate pressure on the Achilles tendon or the heels.

Pneumocephalus

A pneumocephalus denotes air within the CSF spaces of the skull, possibly including the ventricular system. It can occur after neurosurgical procedures involving patients in any position. Pneumocephalus occurs in 100% of sitting patients, in 72% of those in a park bench position, and in 57% of patients positioned prone. Rarely is it symptomatic, and it usually resolves spontaneously. Tension pneumocephalus occurs rarely but can produce neurologic deficits.[92–94] Delayed arousal from anesthesia after a craniotomy may suggest the presence of a symptomatic pneumocephalus. Radiologic evidence of air within the skull can confirm the diagnosis. Treatment consists of ventilation with an FIO_2 of 1.0. Rarely are burr holes or other techniques needed to aspirate the accumulated gas. The ability of nitrous oxide to expand an existing air mass and increase intracranial pressure makes its use hazardous if anesthesia must be administered to a patient who has recently had a craniotomy.

Injuries to the Cervical Vertebrae and Spinal Cord

Several reports of cervical spinal cord injuries, including quadriplegia, have involved patients whose surgery was done in the sitting position. Proposed causes were (1) excessive neck flexion stretching the spinal cord, (2) ischemic cord perfusion from loss of vascular autoregulation and intraoperative hypotension, and (3) excessive surgical retraction.[55, 56, 65, 95] Patients who have a spondylitic spine and cerebrovascular disease may be the most susceptible. Severe flexion and lateral rotation of the neck can severely traumatize an arthritic cervical spine. Head positioning should be done by slow, careful torsion and flexion that is never forced.

Edema of the Face, Tongue, and Neck

Swelling of the face, tongue, or neck can occur when patients are placed in the sitting position. When the head of an anesthetized, intubated patient with an oral airway in place is extremely flexed (the chin firmly on the chest), venous and lymphatic obstruction of the tongue can result in postoperative macroglossia.[53, 54]

Because of a higher-lying larynx and a relatively larger tongue, children may be particularly susceptible to this complication. Because the oral airway is a significant space-consuming object when used to protect an endotracheal tube, a bite block has been recommended for that purpose for patients in the sitting position whose neck will be flexed and head will be rotated.

Ischemia of the Lower Extremities

A very rare complication of the sitting position occurred in a patient on whom compression stockings had been placed. After prolonged surgery, deep venous thrombosis appeared in the legs. This complication should be obviated with the use of sequential circumferential compression devices.

Unilateral Blindness

Eye compression, from a horseshoe or other type of head frame on which the patient's face rests, may result in blindness from thrombosis of the retinal artery.[96] Prolonged ocular pressure, especially in the presence of hypotension, can be the cause. The use of the three-pin head frame for patients placed in the sitting position has virtually eliminated this complication, although it has still been reported to occur with prolonged use of the prone position.

Anesthetic Considerations

The use of nitrous oxide for patients in the sitting position continues to be controversial. Some avoid it because its high solubility (0.47 for nitrous oxide being 34 times that of 0.013 for nitrogen) increases the size of intravascular air bubbles if entrainment occurs. Others believe that the use of nitrous oxide allows earlier detection of venous air embolism as well as the measurement of residual intravascular air exhaled in the pulmonary gas after venous air embolism. Animal studies have reported a twofold reduction in the median lethal volume of venous air when 50% nitrous oxide is used and a threefold reduction with the use of 75% nitrous oxide.[97] However, the use of 50% nitrous oxide has no clinically detectable effect on the incidence or severity of venous air embolism in sitting patients if the nitrous oxide is discontinued when air is detected by Doppler ultrasonography.[98] The use of nitrous oxide may improve the sensitivity of $P_{ET}CO_2$ or pulmonary artery pressure measurements in detecting the presence of air emboli but does not improve the sensitivity of either Doppler ultrasonography or transesophageal echocardiography.[99] Purported advantages of the use of nitrous oxide are additional analgesia, rapid uptake and elimination of anesthetic gases providing more rapid emergence from anesthesia, and the earlier reliability of postoperative neurologic evaluations. However, one clinical study has reported that the use of nitrous oxide did not speed emergence from anesthesia when compared with isoflurane.[98]

Volatile anesthetics (primarily isoflurane) are the usual agents for patients in the sitting position. They provide smooth, easily controlled anesthetic depth that can be measured. Should the nitrous oxide need to be discontinued in the presence of venous air embolism, the main anesthetic will continue. Volatile anesthetics can also be used in the presence of motor function monitoring when neuromuscular blockers must be avoided. Short-acting narcotics (fentanyl, sufentanil, alfentanil) can be used to supplement volatile agents at the end of a procedure, allowing the presence of an endotracheal tube with minimal coughing while not interfering with awakening or with responses to commands necessitated by a neurologic examination.

The use of neuromuscular blocking agents to prevent coughing, straining, and movement allows the use of a lower concentration of volatile anesthetics. Relaxants with minimal cardiovascular effects (vecuronium, rocuronium, metocurine, and low-dose atracurium) should be chosen to avoid exacerbating the cardiovascular changes associated with the sitting position. However, pancuronium, with its vagolytic property, is often used to improve cardiac output.

Maintenance fluids should be administered at a rate of 2 to 4 mL/kg/h. Blood should be replaced to maintain a hemoglobin of 10 g/dL. That hemoglobin level provides the greatest oxygen-carrying capacity from hemoglobin saturation and lower viscosity of blood and promotes increased flow in tissues.

In the distant past the use of spontaneous ventilation was advocated so that a change in ventilatory pattern (sighing or gasping) could signal impingement on medullary respiratory structures, brain stem ischemia, or the presence of air emboli.[100, 101] However, spontaneous ventilation under general anesthesia is actually hypoventilation. Its subatmospheric inspiratory phase produces a lower pressure in the veins of the operative site than does controlled mechanical positive-pressure ventilation and may increase the risk of air entrainment and embolism. In addition, the gasp that occurs as a reflex response to massive venous air embolism can produce a large subatmospheric intrathoracic pressure and markedly increase the amount of air entrained.

THE LOW SITTING POSITIONS

The risks and benefits of these positions are similar to those of the classic sitting position with the exceptions that venous pooling of blood may be less, hypotension may be less, and the risk of venous air embolism may be reduced.[102] They are used for procedures about the shoulder, for dental operations, and for many procedures about the head and neck. Unless demanded by other aspects of the care of a high-risk patient, the intensive monitoring unique to the sitting position is rarely needed or used.

In most versions of the low sitting positions, the torso is placed in the midline of the operating table and the back section of the table top is elevated only about half the amount needed for the usual sitting position. However, the "reclining shoulder position" differs in that the surgical shoulder is shifted to lie somewhat beyond the lateral edge of the mattress and is raised off the supporting surface by padding. It is achieved by elevating the back section of the operating table surface only about 20 degrees, flexing the hips only enough to stabilize and support the buttocks, flexing the knees, and arranging the lower legs at about the level of the patient's heart. With the hips held firmly against undue lateral displacement, the torso is moved laterally until much of the shoulder to be operated on is off the edge of the table surface. Then a pad is placed under the target shoulder and moved toward the vertebral column. As a result, the shoulder is rotated and lifted off the table surface sufficiently to expose a significant area of its lateral surface for surgical preparation and access. In this position, the upper torso is rotated toward, but not as far as, the posture known as "semi-supine" (see Chapter 9). Other appropriate pads are arranged to relieve stress on the patient's head and neck. The head usually is retained in the sagittal plane of the torso to avoid adding rotary stress to the roots of the brachial plexus of the surgical site. The surgical arm and shoulder are prepped and draped as required, and the opposite arm is either retained at the side of the patient or placed in abduction of less than 90 degrees on a suitably padded armboard. The surgical team usually stands about the surgical field and the head of the patient, while anesthesia personnel and gear are arranged along the non-operative shoulder and hemithorax.

THE HEAD-ELEVATED PRONE POSITION

The head-elevated prone position is also known as the Concorde position (Fig. 7–6). It is becoming increasingly popular for surgery in the posterior fossa. To aid venous drainage from the surgical site, the head is usually elevated to some degree above the heart. Physiologic changes produced by this position include a slight cardiovascular challenge from venous pooling in the dependent periphery and an increased respiratory effort evidenced by the increased peak inspiratory pressures needed to mechanically ventilate the prone patient. Parallel ventral rolls should be used to allow better respiratory excursions and ventilation (see Chapter 10).

Because eye compression from a head rest may cause retinal artery thrombosis and blindness in a prone patient (see previous discussion), head support in this position is often provided by a three-pin head holder that frees the face and eyes from pressure. Conjunctival edema is seen frequently during and after the use of the prone position but is less likely to be present with the head elevated in the Concorde position. It resolves without sequelae.

Straps placed as seat rests at the caudal edge of the buttocks must be used to prevent the patient from sliding caudad, particularly if the three-pin head holder is not used to

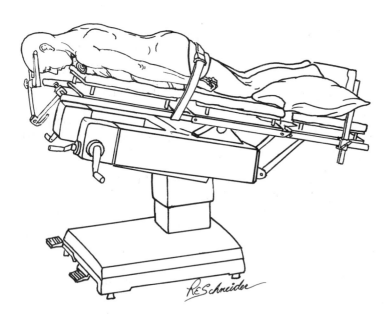

Figure 7–6

The head-elevated prone (Concorde) position. Head elevation is needed to aid venous drainage from the operative site. The restraining strap under the buttocks, anchored cephalad rather than directly downward onto the table frame, is necessary to maintain the torso in place on the ventral chest rolls.

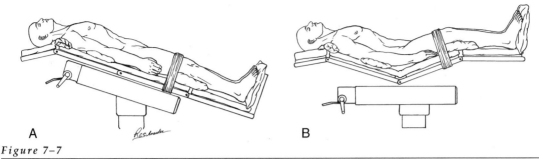

Figure 7–7

A. Head-elevated supine position, used for surgical exposure during thyroidectomy or laparoscopic cholecystectomy. The posture places the surgical field (thyroidectomy) above the level of the heart and promotes venous drainage away from the wound. A foot piece and thigh strap are needed to prevent hip and knee flexion and anchor the patient on the table. This position allows the abdominal contents to move caudad, providing better exposure of the gallbladder for the laparoscope. *B.* Alternative position for patient undergoing dental, neck, or ear, nose, and throat surgery. The hips and knees are flexed for lumbar comfort. The less-dependent lower extremities allow the posture to avoid most of the cardiovascular changes associated with the head-elevated supine position. To hyperextend the head for improved surgical access to the anterior neck (thyroidectomy) the head piece is angled floorward and an elevating roll is placed beneath the shoulders. The occiput must remain firmly supported by the head piece, however.

retain the head in position (see discussion of proper strap placement in Chapter 10). The knees should be flexed slightly by placing the lower legs on a pillow. The feet should be maintained at a 90-degree angle with the lower legs by placement of a padded foot rest. Arms are padded and retained at the patient's sides, making access to intravenous lines difficult.

Because the head is elevated to a lesser extent above the heart than is the case with the classic sitting position, the Concorde position offers a lower risk of air embolism. However, some risk is still present and is confounded by difficulty in monitoring for venous air embolism and by physical problems with resuscitation, should it become necessary. Doppler ultrasonography is not a good monitor for venous air embolism in this position and probably should be replaced by transesophageal echocardiography. Right atrial catheters are not usually placed in patients in this position so that retrieval of entrained air is impossible. Resuscitation would necessitate turning the patient supine.

THE HEAD-ELEVATED SUPINE POSITION

A variety of surgical procedures may be performed with the patient supine and the head tilted up to a variable degree (Fig. 7–7). These include eye, ear, nose, and throat procedures, dental operations, thyroidectomies, and laparoscopic procedures in the upper abdomen.

The posture has both hemodynamic and respiratory consequences.[103] Head-up tilt to greater than 20 degrees in anesthetized patients produces a 35% to 40% decrease in cardiac index. The direct myocardial depressant and vasodilatory effects of the anesthetic together with the loss of sympathetic tone cause the initial reduction in cardiac index. This decrease is exacerbated by the reduction in venous return inherent in the head-elevated posture.

In patients undergoing laparoscopic cholecystectomy, the cardiac index is further reduced to about 50% of normal by increased intra-abdominal pressure and neurohumeral effects caused by distending the abdomen with insufflated CO_2. The magnitude of the decrease in cardiac activity is directly related to the insufflation pressure in the abdomen. Although cardiac output partially recovers over time, the decrease in cardiac index can be avoided by maintenance of the supine position while the abdomen is insufflated. Slow insufflation to a maximum pressure of 10 mm Hg followed by a limited head-up tilt has been recommended.[103]

Venous return from the lower extremities is impeded in the head-elevated supine position by both the gravity effects of the posture and the compression of the inferior vena cava produced by a pneumoperitoneum. The resulting venous stasis increases the risk of deep venous thrombosis and pulmonary embolism. Head-up tilt benefits ventilation by caudad displacement of the diaphragm. However, the decreased cardiac index may offset any ventilatory improvement by worsening ventilation/perfusion mismatch.

The deleterious effects of positioning a patient in head-up tilt and then creating a tension pneumoperitoneum to facilitate a surgical procedure in the abdomen are well tolerated in healthy patients. However, when limited cardiopulmonary reserve is present, serious morbidity can result. In these patients the head-up tilt should be limited to 10 degrees.

An unanticipated consequence of abdominal insufflation in the presence of head-up tilt is the ability of the tension pneumoperitoneum to shift the tracheal carina cephalad in a manner similar to that seen with head-down tilt. Morimura and co-workers[104] confirmed the process by chest radiographs, and Iwami and associates[105] found that abdominal insufflation of carbon dioxide to 10 mm Hg shifted the carina cephalad by about 1 cm. Both groups emphasized the need to recognize the phenomenon in patients undergoing laparoscopic cholecystectomy.

PREANESTHETIC EVALUATION

In the preanesthetic interview for patients who are to be placed in a head-elevated position during the intended surgical procedure, important elements of the medical history include

- Previous operations. Patients with previous cerebrospinal shunting procedures may be at greater risk for subdural pneumocephalus in the sitting position.[104]
- Previous or existing cardiovascular or pulmonary disease
- The presence of intracardiac shunts

Key parts of the preanesthetic physical evaluation are

- The availability of vascular access for right atrial catheter placement. Patients in whom right atrial placement may be difficult include those who are obese (particularly those with short thick necks that obscure usual anatomic landmarks) and those with poor vasculature secondary to disease or chronic intravenous cannulation. These patients may need to be identified early so that adequate time is made available for catheter placement. The use of jugular or subclavian veins for right atrial catheterization has the added risk

of a pneumothorax and air entrainment in the sitting position.
- The presence of limitations of joint motion. Detecting joints with motion sufficiently limited to pose difficulties in establishing the sitting position dictates that an alternative posture be used for the procedure. When flexion of the neck and rotation of the head is intended for patients with cervical arthritis or a cervical disk, preoperative assessment of the mobility of the cervical spine should identify the limits of comfort and may prevent potentially incapacitating postoperative distress from head posture being forced beyond limits that could be tolerated awake.

CONCLUSIONS

The head-elevated positions pose continuing challenges for the anesthesiologist. When achieved during general anesthesia the posture produces significant changes in cardiopulmonary physiology and offers potential complications that require extreme vigilance in the care of the patient. In addition, the technical details of establishing the position and monitoring the progress of the patient require a coordinated effort of operating room personnel. Vital to success is the presence, adequacy, familiarity, and proven maintenance of the involved equipment. For the safety of the patient, the anesthesiologist *must* have significant experience in the techniques of establishing and monitoring the head-elevated positions and in the detection and treatment of their complications.

REFERENCES

1. deMartel T: Surgical treatment of cerebral tumors: Technical considerations. Surg Gynecol Obstet 52:281, 1931.
2. Stein BM: Supracerebellar-infratentorial approach to pineal tumors. Surg Neurol 11:331, 1979.
3. Frowein RA, Koening W, Loeschke GC: Age and other complication factors in neurosurgical operations in the sitting position. *In* Brock M (ed.): Modern Neurosurgery. New York, Springer-Verlag, 1982.
4. Black S, Ockert DB, Oliver WC, et al.: Outcome following posterior fossa craniotomy in patients in the sitting or horizontal positions. Anesthesiology 69:49, 1988.
5. Elton RJ, Howell RSC: The sitting position in neurosurgical anaesthesia: A survey of British practice in 1991. Br J Anaesth 73:247, 1994.

6. Coonan TJ, Hope CE: Cardiorespiratory effects of change in body position. Can Anaesth Soc J 30:424, 1983.

7. Spodick DH: Effect of upright tilt on the phases of the cardiac cycle in normal subjects. Cardiovasc Res 5:210, 1971.

8. Marshall WK, Bedford RF, Miller ED: Cardiovascular responses in the seated position: Impact of four anesthetic techniques. Anesth Analg 62:648, 1983.

9. Toole JF: Effects of change on head, limb, and body position on cephalic circulation. N Engl J Med 279:307, 1968.

10. Maroon JC, Goodman JK, Homer TG, et al.: Detection of minute venous air emboli with ultrasound. Surg Gynecol Obstet 127:1236, 1968.

11. Colley PS, Pavlin EG, Groepper J: Assessment of a saline injection test for location of a right atrial catheter. Anesthesiology 58:258, 1979.

12. Maroon JC, Albin MS: Air embolism diagnosed by Doppler ultrasound. Anesth Analg 53:399, 1974.

13. Tinker JH, Gronert GA, Messick JM, et al.: Detection of air embolism: A test for positioning of right atrial catheter and Doppler probe. Anesthesiology 43:104, 1975.

14. Losasso TJ, Muzzi DA, Cucchiara RF: Doppler detection of intravenous mannitol crystals mimics venous air embolism. Anesth Analg 71:568, 1990.

15. Muzzi DA, Losasso TJ, Black S, et al.: Comparison of a transesophageal and precordial ultrasonic Doppler sensor in the detection of venous air embolism. Anesth Analg 70:103, 1990.

16. Colley PS, Artru AA: Bunegin-Albin catheter improves air retrieval and resuscitation from lethal venous air embolism in upright dogs. Anesth Analg 68:298, 1989.

17. Michenfelder JD, Terry HR, Daw EF, et al.: Air embolism during neurosurgery: A new method of treatment. Anesth Analg 45:390, 1966.

18. Artru A: Modification of a new catheter for air retrieval and resuscitation from lethal venous air embolism: Effect of nitrous oxide on air retrieval. Anesth Analg 75:226, 1992.

19. Denys BG, Breishlatt WM, Reddy PS, et al.: An ultrasound method for safe and rapid central venous access. N Engl J Med 324:566, 1991.

20. Bunegin L, Albin M, Helsel P, et al.: Positioning of the right atrial catheter: A model for reappraisal. Anesthesiology 55:343, 1981.

21. Black S, Cucchiara RF: Tumor surgery. In Cucchiara RF, Michenfelder JD (eds.): Clinical Neuroanesthesia. New York, Churchill Livingstone, 1990.

22. Cucchiara RF, Messick JM, Gronert GA, et al.: Time required and success rate of percutaneous right atrial catheterization: Description of a technique. Can Anaesth Soc J 27:572, 1980.

23. Lee D, Kuhn J, Shaffer M, et al.: Migration of tips of central venous catheters in seated patients. Anesth Analg 69:949, 1984.

24. Marshall WK, Bedford RF: Use of pulmonary artery catheter for detection and treatment of venous air embolism: A prospective study in man. Anesthesiology 52:131, 1980.

25. Munson ES, Paul WC, Perry JC, et al.: Early detection of venous air embolism using a Swan-Ganz catheter. Anesthesiology 42:223, 1975.

26. Perkins-Pearson N, Marshall N, Bedford R: Atrial pressures in the seated position. Anesthesiology 57:493, 1982.

27. Smelt WL, de Lange JJ, Baerts WD, et al.: The capno-graph, a reliable noninvasive monitor for the detection of pulmonary embolism of various origins. Acta Anaesthesiol Belg 38:217, 1987.

28. Muley SS, Saini SS, Dash HH, et al.: End-tidal carbon dioxide monitoring for detection of venous air embolism. Indian J Med Res 92:362, 1990.

29. Drummond JC, Prutow RJ, Scheller MS: A comparison of the sensitivity of pulmonary artery pressure, end-tidal carbon dioxide, and end-tidal nitrogen in the detection of venous air embolism in the dog. Anesth Analg 64:688, 1985.

30. Matjasko J, Petrozza P, MacKenzie CF: Sensitivity of end-tidal nitrogen in venous air embolism detection in dogs. Anesthesiology 63:418, 1985.

31. Ozanne GM, Young WG, Mazzei WJ, et al.: Multipatient anaesthetic mass spectrometry: Rapid analysis of data stored in long catheters. Anesthesiology 55:62, 1981.

32. Glenski JA, Cucchiara RF, Michenfelder JD: Transesophageal echocardiography and transcutaneous O_2 and CO_2 monitoring for detection of venous air embolism. Anesthesiology 64:541, 1986.

33. Sato S, Toya S, Ohira T, et al.: Echocardiographic detection and treatment of intraoperative air embolism. J Neurosurg 64:440, 1986.

34. Furuya H, Suzuki T, Okumura F, et al.: Detection of air embolism by transesophageal echocardiography. Anesthesiology 58:124, 1983.

35. Fischler M, Vourc'h G, Dubourg O, et al.: Patent foramen ovale and sitting position. Anesthesiology 60:83, 1984.

36. Hagen PT, Scholtz DG, Edwards WD: Incidence and size of patent foramen ovale during the first 10 decades of life: An autopsy study of 965 normal hearts. Mayo Clin Proc 59:17, 1984.

37. Guggiari M, Lechat P, Garen-Colonne C, et al.: Early detection of patent foramen ovale by two-dimensional contrast echocardiography for prevention of paradoxical air embolism during sitting position. Anesth Analg 67:192, 1988.

38. Kronik G, Mosslacher H: Positive contrast echocardiography in patients with patent foramen ovale and normal right heart hemodynamics. Am J Cardiol 49:1806, 1982.

39. Lechat PH, Mas JL, Lascault G, et al.: Prevalence of patent foramen ovale in patients with stroke. N Engl J Med 318:1148, 1988.

40. Lynch JJ, Schuchard GH, Gross CM, et al.: Prevalence of right-to-left atrial shunting in the healthy population: Detection by Valsalva maneuver contrast echocardiography. Am J Cardiol 53:1478, 1984.

41. Papadopoulos G, Kuhly P, Brock M, et al.: Venous and paradoxical air embolism in the sitting position. A prospective study with transesophageal echocardiography. Acta Neurochir 126:140, 1994.

42. Black S, Muzzi DA, Nishimura RA, et al.: Preoperative and intraoperative echocardiography to detect right-to-left shunt in patients undergoing neurosurgical procedures in the sitting position. Anesthesiology 72:436, 1990.

43. Cucchiara RF, Nugent M, Seward JD, et al.: Air embolism in upright neurosurgical patients: Detection and localization by 2-dimensional transesophageal echocardiography. Anesthesiology 60:353, 1984.

44. Cucchiara RF, Seward JB, Nishimura RA, et al.: Identification of patent foramen ovale during sitting position craniotomy by transesophageal echocardiography with positive airway pressure. Anesthesiology 63:107, 1985.

45. Schwarz G, Fuchs G, Weihs W, et al.: Sitting position for neurosurgery: Experience with preoperative contrast echocardiography in 301 patients. J Neurosurg Anesth 6:83, 1994.
46. Nemec JJ, Marwick TH, Lorig RJ, et al.: Comparison of transcranial Doppler ultrasound and transesophageal contrast echocardiography in the detection of interatrial right-to-left shunts. Am J Cardiol 68:1498, 1991.
47. Petrozza PH: Preoperative echocardiography and the sitting position. J Neurosurg Anesth 6:71, 1994.
48. Losasso TJ, Muzzi DA, Weglinski MR: The risk of paradoxical air embolism (PAE) in sitting neurosurgical patients with and without a demonstrable right-to-left (R→L) shunt. Anesthesiology 77:A198, 1992.
49. Cucchiara RF, Nishimura RA, Black S: Failure of preoperative echo testing to prevent paradoxical air embolism: Report of two cases. Anesthesiology 71:604, 1989.
50. Bunegin L, Wahl D, Albin MS: Detection and volume estimation of embolic air in the middle cerebral artery using transcranial Doppler sonography. Stroke 25:593, 1994.
51. Colley PS, Dunn R: Prevention of blood pressure response to skull-pin head holder by local anesthesia. Anesth Analg 58:241, 1979.
52. Ellis SC, Bryan-Brown CW, Hyderally H: Massive swelling of the head and neck. Anesthesiology 42:102, 1975.
53. McAllister RG: Macroglossia: A positional complication. Anesthesiology 40:199, 1974.
54. Gildenberg PL, O'Brien RP, Britt WJ, Frost EA: The efficacy of Doppler monitoring for the detection of venous air embolism. J Neurosurg 54:75, 1981.
55. Matjasko J, Petrozza P, Cohen M, et al.: Anesthesia and surgery in the seated position: Analysis of 554 cases. Neurosurgery 17:695, 1985.
56. Young ML, Smith DS, Murtagh F, et al.: Comparison of surgical and anesthetic complications in neurosurgical patients experiencing venous air embolism in the sitting position. Neurosurgery 18:157, 1986.
57. Albin M, Carroll R, Maroon J: Clinical considerations concerning detection of venous air embolism. Neurosurgery 3:380, 1978.
58. Cucchiara RF: Safety of the sitting position. Anesthesiology 61:790, 1984.
59. Presson R, Kirk H, Haselby K, et al.: Fate of air emboli in the pulmonary circulation. J Appl Physiol 67:1898, 1989.
60. Lee BP, Chen HF, Hsu FC, et al.: Effect of pulmonary air embolism on discharge of slowly adapting stretch receptors. J Appl Physiol 76:97, 1994.
61. Butler BD, Hills BA: Transpulmonary passage of venous air emboli. J Appl Physiol 59:543, 1985.
62. Lam KK, Hutchinson RC, Gin T: Severe pulmonary oedema after venous air embolism. Can J Anaesth 40:964, 1993.
63. Aibiki M, Ogura S, Seki K, et al.: Role of vagal afferents in hypotension induced by venous air embolism. Am J Physiol 266:790, 1994.
64. Gottlieb JD, Ericsson JA, Sweet RB: Venous air embolism: A review. Anesth Analg 44:773, 1963.
65. Standefer M, Bay JW, Trusso R: The sitting position in neurosurgery: A retrospective analysis of 488 cases. Neurosurgery 14:649, 1984.
66. Bucciero A, Quaglietta P, Vizioli L: Supratentorial intracerebral hemorrhage after posterior fossa surgery. J Neurosurg Sci 35:221, 1991.
67. Albin MS, Ritter RR, Reinhart R, et al.: Venous air embolism during radical retropubic prostatectomy. Anesth Analg 74:151, 1992.
68. Karuparthy VR, Downing JW, Jusain F, et al.: Incidence of venous air embolism during cesarean section is unchanged by the use of a 5–10' head-up tilt. Anesth Analg 69:620, 1989.
69. Prager MC, Gregory GA, Ascher NL, et al.: Massive venous air embolism during orthotopic liver transplantation. Anesthesiology 72:198, 1990.
70. Albin MS, Ritter RR, Pruett CE, Kalff K: Venous air embolism during lumbar laminectomy in the prone position: Report of three cases. Anesth Analg 73:346, 1991.
71. Black S, Cucchiara RF, Nishimura RA, et al.: Parameters affecting occurrence of paradoxical air embolism. Anesthesiology 71:235, 1989.
72. Bedell EA, Berge KH, Losasso TJ: Paradoxical air embolism during venous air embolism: Transesophageal echocardiographic evidence of transpulmonary air passage. Anesthesiology 80:947, 1994.
73. Losasso TJ, Muzzi DA, Cucchiara RF: Jugular venous compression helps to identify the source of venous air embolism during craniectomy in patients in the sitting position. Anesthesiology 76:156, 1992.
74. Sharma K, Tripathi M: Detection of site of air entry in venous air embolism: Role of Valsalva maneuver. J Neurosurg Anesth 6:209, 1994.
75. Lee DS, Lechtmann MW, Weintraub HD: Effect of PEEP on air embolism during sitting neurosurgical procedures. Anesth Analg 60:262, 1981.
76. Muravchik S, DeLisser E, Welch F: The use of PEEP to identify source of cardiopulmonary air embolism. Anesthesiology 49:294, 1978.
77. Vorrhies RM, Fraser RAR, Poznak AV: Prevention of air embolism with positive end expiratory pressure. Neurosurgery 12:503, 1983.
78. Toung T, Ngeow YK, Long DL, et al.: Comparison of the effects of positive end-expiratory pressure and jugular venous compression on canine cerebral venous pressure. Anesthesiology 61:169, 1984.
79. Toung T, Miyabe M, McShane A, et al.: Effect of PEEP and jugular venous compression on canine cerebral blood flow and oxygen consumption in the seated position. Anesthesiology 68:53, 1988.
80. Zentner J, Albrecht T, Hassler W: Prevention of air embolism by moderate hypoventilation during surgery in the sitting position. Neurosurgery 28:705, 1991.
81. Perkins NAK, Bedford RF: Hemodynamic consequences of PEEP in seated neurological patients: Implications of paradoxical air embolism. Anesth Analg 63:429, 1984.
82. Mehlhorn U, Burke EJ, Butler BD, et al.: Body position does not affect hemodynamic response to venous air embolism in dogs. Anesth Analg 79:734, 1994.
83. Marco AP, Furman WR: Anesthetic problems: Venous air embolism, airway difficulties, and massive transfusion. Surg Clin North Am 73:213, 1993.
84. Annane D, Troche G, Delisle F, et al.: Effects of mechanical ventilation with normobaric oxygen therapy on the rate of air removal from cerebral arteries. Crit Care Med 22:851, 1994.
85. Bitterman H, Malamed Y: Delayed hyperbaric treatment of cerebral air embolism. Isr J Med Sci 29:22, 1993.
86. Millar RA: Neurosurgical anaesthesia in the sitting position. Br J Anaesth 44:495, 1972.

87. Kroll D, Caplan R, Posner K, et al.: Nerve injury associated with anesthesia. Anesthesiology 73:202, 1990.
88. Patel RI, Thein RMH, Epstein BS: Costoclavicular syndrome and the sitting position during anesthesia. Anesthesiology 53:341, 1980.
89. Saady A: Brachial plexus palsy after anaesthesia in the sitting position. Anaesthesiology 36:194, 1981.
90. Gozal Y, Pomeranz S: Sciatic nerve palsy as a complication after acoustic neuroma resection in the sitting position. J Neurosurg Anesth 6:40, 1994.
91. Keykhah MM, Rosenberg H: Bilateral footdrop after craniotomy in the sitting position. Anesthesiology 51:163, 1979.
92. Kishan A, Naidu MR, Muralidhar K: Tension pneumocephalus following posterior fossa surgery in sitting position: A report of 2 cases. Clin Neurol Neurosurg 92:245, 1990.
93. Kitahata LM, Katz JD: Tension pneumocephalus after posterior fossa craniotomy: A complication of the sitting position. Anesthesiology 44:448, 1985.
94. MacGillivray RG: Pneumocephalus as a complication of posterior fossa surgery in the sitting position. Anesthesiology 37:722, 1982.
95. Wilder BL: Hypothesis: The etiology of midcervical quadriplegia after operation with the patient in the sitting position. Neurosurgery 11:530, 1982.
96. Hollenhorst RW, Svien HJ, Benoit CF: Unilateral blindness occurring during anesthesia for neurosurgical operations. Arch Ophthalmol 52:819, 1954.
97. Munson ES, Merrick HC: Effects of nitrous-oxide on venous air embolism. Anesthesiology 27:783, 1966.
98. Losasso TJ, Muzzi DA, Dietz NM, et al.: Fifty percent nitrous oxide does not increase the risk of venous air embolism in neurosurgical patients operated upon in the sitting position. Anesthesiology 77:21, 1992.
99. Losasso TJ, Black S, Muzzi DA, et al.: Detection and hemodynamic consequences of venous air embolism: Does nitrous oxide make a difference? Anesthesiology 77:148, 1992.
100. Lall NG, Jain AP: Circulatory and respiratory disturbances during posterior fossa surgery. Br J Anaesth 41:447, 1969.
101. Warren JE, Tsueda K, Young B: Respiratory pattern changes during repair of posterior fossa arteriovenous malformation. Anesthesiology 45:690, 1976.
102. Von Gossein H, Samii M, Suhr D, et al.: The lounging position for posterior fossa surgery: Anesthesiological considerations regarding air embolism. Childs Nerv Syst 7:568, 1991.
103. Wahba RWM, Beique F, Kleiman SJ: Cardiopulmonary function and laparoscopic cholecystectomy. Can J Anaesth 42:51, 1994.
104. Morimura N, Inour K, Miwa T: Chest roentgenogram demonstrates cephalad movement of the carina during laparoscopic cholecystectomy: Correspondence. Anesthesiology 81:1301, 1994.
105. Iwami H, Nakane M, Aoki K, et al.: Abdominal insufflation pressure during laparoscopic cholecystectomy shifts the tracheal carina cephalad: Correspondence. Anesthesiology 84:491, 1996.
106. Toung TJK, McPherson RW, Ahn H, et al.: Pneumocephalus: Effects of patient position on the incidence and location of aerocele after posterior fossa and upper cervical cord surgery. Anesth Analg 65:65, 1986.

Chapter 8

Head-Down Tilt

John T. Martin

BACKGROUND

History

Tilting patients head down to facilitate surgical management of pelvic lesions has been practiced "since early times."[1] During the middle years of the 19th century, individual European surgeons, including Bardenhower of Cologne, had discovered that raising the hips of a laparotomized patient caused abdominal viscera to shift cephalad toward the concavity of the diaphragm, thereby improving suprapubic access to pathologic processes in the pelvis. Friedrich Trendelenburg, a renowned surgical pioneer, held professorial positions successively at medical universities in Rostock, Bonn, and Leipzig. Early in his career, Trendelenburg was influenced by Bardenhower, who apparently had publicized the posture,[2] and he began inclining patients' torsos 45 degrees head down to facilitate deep pelvic repairs of conditions such as vesicovaginal fistulas. Initially, he placed the bent knees of the supine patient over the shoulders of an attendant (Fig. 8–1), but table attachments were subsequently developed for the purpose (Fig. 8–2).

Visiting surgeons were impressed with Trendelenburg's successful techniques and emulated the master. Generalized use of the position resulted. Esmarch, in 1873, apparently created the Trendelenburg eponym for the posture.[2] Trendelenburg's pupil, New York surgeon Willie Meyer, published the earliest description of its use in 1885 and credited its discovery to his teacher.[3] Trendelenburg's own report of the posture appeared in 1890.[4] Widespread adoption of steep head-down tilt

for abdominopelvic operations followed on both sides of the Atlantic.

With few detractors, the popularity of Trendelenburg's position continued into the middle of the current century. In 1956, well-defined and lucid objections to its use were presented by Inglis, an anaesthetist in Birmingham, England, and Brooke, his surgical colleague.[5] They argued that the appearance of muscle relaxants had improved the ability of surgeons to pack viscera out of an abdominal wound, obviating the major reason for using the position. They also showed radiologically that steep head-down tilt moved the symphysis pubis into the surgeon's line of sight to the deep pelvis. Their extremely perceptive catalog of objections included respiratory embarrassment from viscera lying upon the diaphragm, masked hypovolemia, cardiopulmonary vascular overload, cerebral vascular congestion, gastric regurgitation during tilt, and nerve palsies in upper extremities. They concluded that the posture was obsolete. Nevertheless, its widespread use continued.

Resuscitative Value of Trendelenburg's Position

Early in the twentieth century, Walter B. Cannon, an eminent American physiologist, proposed that "shock" after trauma be treated by lowering the victim's head to promote the return of blood to the heart from the elevated lower extremities. Initially, he also believed that the maneuver also benefited cerebral circulation. The technique rapidly gained favor and was widely used during World War I.[6] However, Henderson and Haggard,[7] studying humans, reported that a head-down tilt of 45

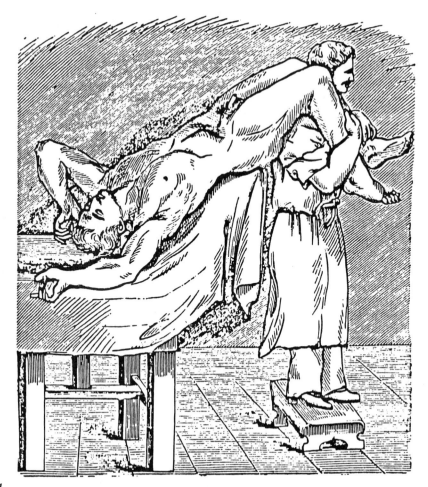

Figure 8–1

Pelvic elevation for urologic surgery advocated by Bardenhower and popularized by Trendelenburg. (From Meyer W: Uber die Nachbehandlung des hohen Steinschnittes sowie uber Verwendbarkeit desselben zur Operation von Blasenscheidenfisteln. Arch Klin Chir 31:494, 1885.)

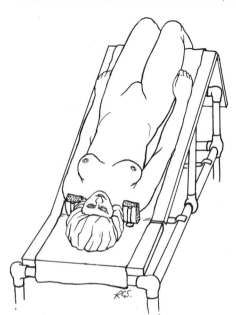

Figure 8–2

Early nonadjustable table modification using padded shoulder braces and legs bent at knees to stabilize Trendelenburg's position. (Redrawn from Bickham WS [ed.]: Operative Surgery. Philadelphia, WB Saunders, 1924.)

degrees resulted in no marked change in blood pressure. Subsequently, Cannon repudiated his original belief,[8] but its acceptance had become so deeply rooted in American medical folklore that head-down tilt remained a fixed part of the treatment of hypotension for more than three decades.

Starting in the 1950s with Cole,[9] continuing with the landmark studies of Weil[10, 11] in 1957 and 1965, Taylor and Weil[12] in 1967, and underscored by the report of Sibbald and associates[13] in 1979, critics of the resuscitative effectiveness of head-down tilt developed convincing evidence of its cardiovascular and intracranial dangers. A better understanding of the relationship between circulating volume and vascular capacitance evolved at about the same time. Consequently, the use of head-down tilt as a fundamental resuscitation technique fell into disrepute in most quarters.

Surgical Value of Head-Down Tilt

Surgeons attribute the following advantages to head-down tilt:

- Movement of the abdominal viscera cephalad to clear a lower abdominal or pelvic operating field
- Establishment of a vascular gradient from the wound to the subjacent heart that minimizes small artery bleeding at, and improves venous drainage from, the operative site
- Engorgement of vessels in the superior caval drainage system that assists with the placement of intravenous catheters

Surgical disadvantages include the following:

- Movement of the viscera into the wound when the chest is expanded and the diaphragm is shifted caudad during the inspiratory phase of intermittent positive-pressure ventilation
- Central venous engorgement masking blood loss from the wound until the patient is returned to the horizontal position[5]
- The potential for nerve, vessel, or muscle and bone injury to a very heavy patient who has been shifted against restraints by the forces of gravity
- The risk of air entry into patulous veins at the dissection site where the venous pressure is essentially subatmospheric because of the elevation of the surgical field above the level of the heart

The Anesthesiologist and Head-Down Tilt

From the standpoint of the anesthesiologist, placing a patient in a head-down position has real problems and few assets.[5]

- The amount of head-down tilt usually employed as an aid to catheterization of vessels in the neck has been shown to increase myocardial oxygen requirements in the awake patient with coronary artery disease.[14]
- Steep head-down tilt causes stasis in the congested vessels of the head and neck, often to the extent that superficial cyanosis is evident and worrisome. In florid individuals this effect becomes particularly disturbing. Obtaining blood gas data may be the only means of assessing the general status of the patient.
- Increased work of spontaneous ventilation occurs because of the weight of viscera that have shifted to lie against the diaphragm. The ventilatory effort is obviously worsened by obesity, requires ventilatory assistance for the anesthetized patient, and mandates the use of an endotracheal tube or other device to segregate the respiratory system from the gastrointestinal tract.
- Using vital signs to judge the extent of blood volume replacement may cause the significance of a volume deficit to be underestimated until poor perfusion becomes evident during blood redistribution caudad as the posture is terminated.[5]
- As a tool with which to treat "shock," tilting the patient head down has been in well-deserved disrepute for two decades.[11, 14]
- An asset of placing the patient head down, however, is the fact that vomitus can be drained out of the mouth and away from the trachea when sudden perianesthetic emesis is encountered.

Why, then, use head-down tilt at all? When visceral exposure can be improved, the operative procedure hastened, and the duration of anesthesia reduced, a case can be made for the use of the least necessary degree of head-down tilt. Countless thousands of surgical patients have survived the posture acceptably. However, when its use is capricious, in that it will neither speed surgery nor shorten the duration of the anesthetic, or when significant cardiopulmonary or intracranial pathology exists, employing any degree of head-down tilt is a physiologic transgression that is difficult to justify. As a "shock position," its value has been disproved.[13]

VARIETIES OF HEAD-DOWN TILT

The eponym "Trendelenburg" initially described a posture in which the surface that supports the supine patient (e.g., bed, operating table, transport cart) was tilted about 45 degrees head down. The subject's head was below heart level, while the abdomen, pelvis, and thighs were above it (see Figs. 8–1 and 8–2). Gradually, the eponym became carelessly used and any degree of head-down tilt was called "the Trendelenburg position," regardless of whether the patient was supine, prone, or lying on one side. Even more inappropriate has been the general application of the name "reverse Trendelenburg position" to any variety of head-up posture. Because the usefulness of the adjective "Trendelenburg" has been compromised by misapplication, the time has arrived to abandon the eponym and label tilts more precisely.[15]

Steep Head-Down Tilt

Draping the lower extremities of a supine, laparotomized patient over the shoulders of a diener, Trendelenburg's original maneuver, angulated the thighs and torso sufficiently to angulate the long axis of the abdomen about 45 degrees above the horizontal surface of the operating table (see Fig. 8–1). Later versions of head-down tilt varied between 30 and 45 degrees according to the capabilities of table

attachments or the desires of the practitioner. This range can be described as steep head-down tilt (SHDT).[15]

In most medical practices the use of SHDT almost completely disappeared during the middle years of this century. However, the recent development of laparoscopic abdominopelvic surgery in an abdomen that has been distended by peritoneal insufflation of a compressed gas has re-established the use of the posture for operations that may last a disturbing length of time.

Minimal Head-Down Tilt

During the early decades of the seventeenth century a German surgeon, Johan Schultes (1595–1645) known as "Scultetus" and for whom the bandage may have been named, apparently advocated a less drastic version of head-down tilt than the one later ascribed to Trendelenburg. It was referred to as the *scultetus position*.[16, 17] Although the eponym is no longer employed, surgical use of the posture can be presumed to have persisted in some quarters.

As reservations about the physical and physiologic safety of SHDT became more widespread, lesser degrees of tilt gained acceptance in operating rooms and on hospital wards. With early models of hospital beds, raising the foot of a bed enough to produce more than about a 20-degree tilt of the patient's long axis was often almost impossible. Possibly for that pragmatic reason, 10 to 20 degrees of head-down tilt became popular. That range can be referred to as minimal head-down tilt (MHDT) (Fig. 8–3).[15]

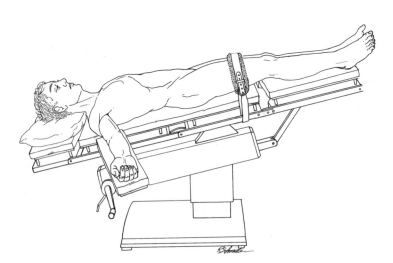

Figure 8–3

Minimal head-down tilt. Torso tilted approximately 15 degrees and held in place by friction with fixed mattress and restraining strap over distal thighs.

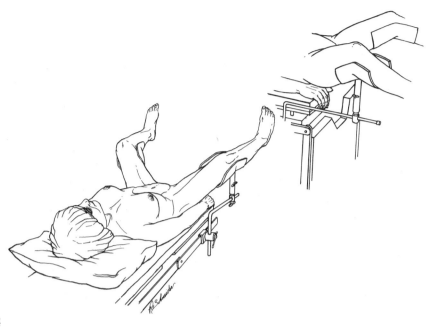

Figure 8–4

Minimal head-down tilt plus low lithotomy position. Leg support depicted has potential of compressing popliteal space and proximal calf because of unsupported weight of leg and foot. Compartmental damage to lower leg may result if use of position is lengthy (see Chapter 6). Note also the potential for damage to fingers when the depressed foot section of the table is returned to level (*inset*). (Modified from Barash PG, Cullen BF, Stoelting RK [eds.]: Clinical Anesthesia, 2nd ed. Philadelphia, JB Lippincott, 1992.)

MHDT is often requested in the operating room for surgical procedures in the lower abdomen, pelvis, and perineum. If SHDT was needed to move viscera cephalad and improve surgical access, the use of much lesser levels of tilt for that purpose seems open to serious question. In many situations, requests for MHDT appear to be more of a surgical habit pattern than a technical necessity. Physiologic stresses have been documented with MHDT (see later sections on the physiology of head-down tilt), a fact that seems not to have gained widespread surgical appreciation. Its routine use in the presence of cardiorespiratory or central nervous system disease deserves serious reconsideration.

Internationally, aerospace physiologists have studied awake volunteers placed for relatively long periods of time in only 6 degrees of head-down tilt. Their presumption is that the posture has a relationship to that assumed in the weightless state in space and that physiologic data acquired from it will enhance understanding of body system adaptations encountered during periods of weightlessness. Although their studies establish interesting data, extrapolation of their findings to an anesthetized patient is probably not justified.

Minimal Head-Down Tilt plus Low Lithotomy

When a lesion in the deep pelvis must be approached surgically through the lower abdomen as well as from the perineum, a position that will permit access to both regions simultaneously has proven desirable (Fig. 8–4).[18]

The patient is placed in the low lithotomy position with the lower extremities abducted in holders that flex the thighs on the trunk about 15 to 20 degrees and bend the knees sufficiently to maintain the lower legs roughly parallel to the long axis of the torso. Abduction is sufficient to move the extremities laterally out of the way of a surgical team member who is seated facing the patient's perineum. At the same time, flexion of the thigh on the trunk is not sufficient to interfere with team members standing at the flanks of the patient and working through an abdominal incision while needing occasionally to manipulate an instrument previously placed to protrude from the vagina. MHDT is then added to the arrangement.

The Hyperlordotic Position

To provide access to structures shielded by the symphysis pubis, two approaches have

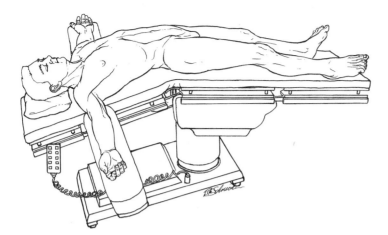

Figure 8–5

The hyperlordotic position for transabdominal access to the ventral pelvis and retropubic area.

been used. The exaggerated lithotomy position rotates the caudal edge of the pubis ventrad to improve perineal access to the prostate and related tissues (see Chapter 6 and Fig. 6–7). When accessing the area through an open abdomen, some surgeons prefer to tilt the pubis in the opposite direction by increasing the natural lordosis of the lumbar spine and rotating the pelvis to tip the abdominal edge of the pubis ventrad as the legs are lowered. To move viscera into the upper abdomen as much as practical without compromising transabdominal access to the pelvis, MHDT is added (Fig. 8–5). The result places the patient in a simultaneous head-down and foot-down position with markedly increased lordosis of the lumbar spine. The hyperlordotic position is similar to that of a diver in a swan dive with an 180-degree twist or of a patient who had been placed in a jackknife position (see Fig. 10–14) and then turned supine over the angulated table surface.

Mechanically, the hyperlordotic position is achieved in several ways. Supports in the form of pads, blankets, or large bags of irrigating fluid can be placed beneath the lumbar spine to produce the desired degree of lordosis. The elevatable transverse bar ("kidney rest") can be used as an adjustable support with or without additional padding. Depending on the preference of the surgical team, the table top can remain flat or can be angulated at the back-thigh hinge to lower its ends into a wide inverted "V" in a manner similar to that of the low jackknife position (see Fig. 10–14). Depressing the cephalad end of the table chassis further lowers the head of the patient without affecting the degree of lordosis. The patient's lower extremities are usually abducted sufficiently to place each

heel just at the edge of the table mattress to permit external access to the perineum and rectum should the need arise during the procedure.

A somewhat similar alternative used by some surgeons is to place the lower lumbar spine of the patient over the back-thigh hinge of the operating table and then to depress the back section of the table about 10 degrees. By adjusting the chassis so that the trunk is horizontal, the pelvis is tilted a modest amount without unduly stressing the lumbar spine.

Because of the slight amount of head-down tilt used in the hyperlordotic position and the fact that the lower extremities are also angulated downward, there is usually no reason to use wrist restraints or shoulder braces to retain the patient in position over the angulation point of the operating table. A strap over the lower legs may be used to retain the extremities apart and stabilize tactile access to the perineum if needed during the procedure. The arms of a patient usually extend beyond the point of angulation of the table surface if retained at the sides of the hyperlordotic torso. Consequently, the distal forearm, wrist, and hand can be unsupported and may be subject to injury after being covered by surgical drapes. A more prudent alternative is to retain each upper extremity on a well-padded armboard that is abducted to no more than 90 degrees from the long axis of the torso.

Despite its ability to improve transabdominal access to pelvic organs, several aspects of the hyperlordotic position have the potential of being major insults for the patient involved.

• Arching the lumbar spine excessively can

seriously stress the joints and ligaments of the angulated area. Postoperative backache can be anticipated, particularly in elderly patients with arthritic spines. Similar problems were encountered with the ancient, and now generally abandoned, technique of using the elevatable transverse bar of the operating table (then known as the "gallbladder rest") to arch a patient's thoracolumbar spine and improve access to the area of the gallbladder. The acute hyperlordotic surgical position is quite uncomfortable for an awake volunteer, and chronic hyperlordosis is a well-recognized cause of persistent back pain. MEDLINE offers more than 8000 references linked to the subject.

- The arched spine elongates and flattens the major vessels on its ventral surface, can reduce their caliber significantly, and may impede blood flow, particularly in the more thin-walled inferior vena cava. Consequent changes in pressure in collateral circulation may affect intraspinal perfusion, causing either congestion or ischemia of the contents of the spinal canal.

- The adverse effects of the head-down position on the contents of the cranial vault, on myocardial oxygen requirements, and on the pulmonary circulation are detailed elsewhere in this chapter.

- Placement of legs at levels lower than the atrium promotes venous stasis in distensible vessels of the dependent extremities and reduces volume return to the heart. Compressive dressings, whether intermittent or continuous, have been used to combat the vascular stasis.

An article by Amoiridis and co-workers[19] implicates the hyperlordotic posture in the production of an ischemic infarction of the spinal cord during a 10-hour intrapelvic operation in a 43-year-old man. Historically normotensive, the patient's systolic blood pressure had been 100 mm Hg or above for all but 15 minutes of the procedure. The patient had been in 17 degrees of head-down tilt and a similar amount of lower extremity depression (34 degrees total spinal angulation). These researchers offered detailed electrophysiologic and magnetic resonance imaging evidence to explain the pathophysiologic processes involved in the resultant paraplegia. Increased intraspinal pressure secondary to compression of the inferior vena cava by the hyperlordotic position was implicated, as was

a possible lumbar canal stenosis. In their patient, postoperative contrast studies identified focal areas of enhancement consistent with ischemic infarction of the lumbosacral spinal cord, adjacent meninges, and dorsal third of the bodies of the L2 and L3 vertebrae.

An epidural catheter had been placed preoperatively for subsequent pain control but had contributed only a minimal volume of morphine in normal saline to the epidural space before the onset of the neurologic deficit. Elsewhere, preliminary studies of intraoperative hyperlordosis place the apex of angulation variably in the body of the fourth lumbar vertebra or at the L4-5 interspace (well caudad to the termination of the spinal cord) rather than at L1 (Warner MA, personal communication, 1996). Clinical experience indicates that the T12-L2 vertebral segment has little ability to become hyperlordotic (Warner MA, personal communication, 1996). Although caution is indicated, further investigation is needed before indicting hyperlordosis per se as a cause of serious spinal cord pathology.

ESTABLISHING HEAD-DOWN TILT

Keeping the patient in position on the inclined operating table has been a recurring problem since the introduction of head-down tilt. For minimal amounts of tilt, less than about 20 degrees head low, the patient of average size can be retained in position by the presence of a padded strap placed across the thighs (see Fig. 8–3). Steeper tilt has been sustained by one of three methods: (1) wristlets affixed to the lateral rails of the table top (Fig. 8–6, *top left*); (2) shoulder braces on adjustable angle bars locked to the lateral rails of the table (see Fig. 8–6, *top right*); and (3) ankle straps affixed to the distal portion of the leg section of the table top plus flexion of the patients' knees (see Fig. 8–6, *bottom*). Specialized operating tables (Fig. 8–7) and mattresses (Fig. 8–8) have been adopted for the purpose.

Methods of Restraint
Wristlets or Shoulder Braces

Use of wristlets or shoulder braces to sustain head-down tilt threatens to pull (wristlets) or push (braces) the mobile shoulder mechanism caudad, closing the retroclavicular space by moving the clavicle onto the first rib (Fig.

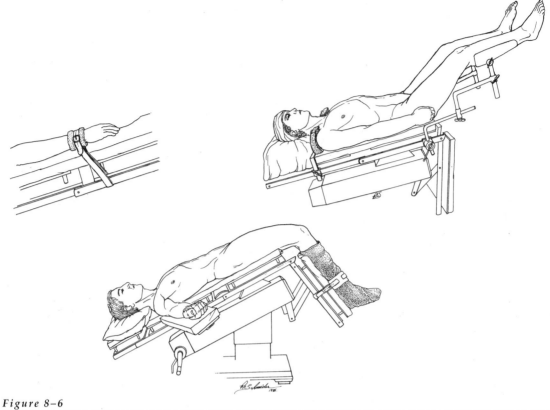

Figure 8–6

Restraints used to stabilize patient tilted head-down. *Top left.* Wristlets attached to table rail. *Top right.* Shoulder braces adjusted to lie against shoulder caps at the acromioclavicular joints. *Bottom.* Bent knees/anklets arrangement. (Additional padding not shown for clarity.)

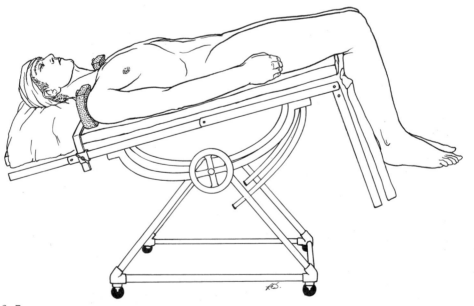

Figure 8–7

An early model surgical table that allowed adjustable head-down tilt. (Redrawn from Juilly GJ [ed.]: Practical Surgery of the Abdomen. Philadelphia, FA Davis, 1928.)

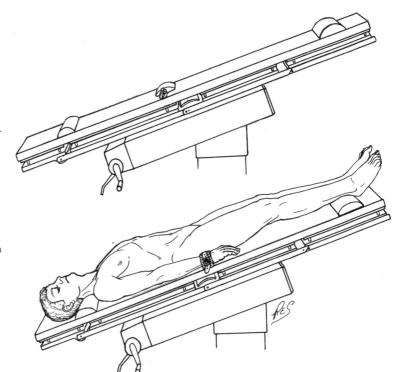

Figure 8–8

The Hewer mattress. Surface of corrugated rubber plus pads beneath the neck, lumbosacral spine, and ankles retains patient in head-down tilt without use of shoulder braces or restrictive straps. Wristlets were used only to retain arms at sides. (Redrawn from Hewer CL: Latest pattern of non-slip mattress. Anaesthesia 8:198, 1953.)

8–9). The retroclavicular neurovascular bundle of subclavian vessels and brachial plexus can be stretched (wristlets) and/or compressed (both wristlets and braces) by the closure. At risk is (1) perfusion of the extremity with the potential for a compartment syndrome and (2) abnormal neural function with dysesthesias or anesthesia of the extremity that may be permanent. Placing the shoulder braces medially against the root of the neck can directly compress vessels that emerge from the thoracic outlet as well as nerves that exit the cervical foramina and adjacent neck musculature. The traditional advice about the safest location for shoulder braces has been that they be situated laterally over the cap of the shoulder, but even there the risk of retroclavicular space closure remains (Fig. 8–

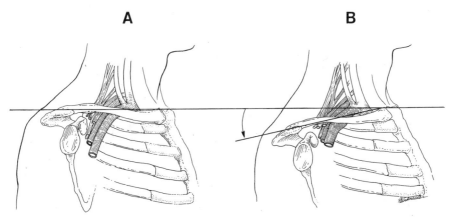

A   **B**

Figure 8–9

A. Normal relationships of structures in the retroclavicular space. *B.* Retroclavicular space closed by moving the shoulder mechanism caudad either by traction on the extremity (wristlets) or by pressure on the area of the acromioclavicular joint (padded shoulder braces). Note the approximation of the clavicle and first rib that threatens compression of the subclavian vessels and brachial plexus.

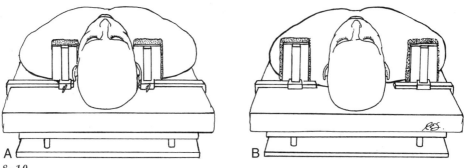

Figure 8–10

Shoulder brace placement problems. *A.* Braces placed tight against the root of the neck compress muscles, structures traversing the thoracic outlets, and nerves emerging from the lower cervical spine. *B.* Braces placed laterally over the shoulder cap avoid compression of the root of the neck but may still exert sufficient caudad pressure on the shoulder mechanism to depress the clavicle onto the first rib, closing the retroclavicular space and compressing the subclavian neurovascular bundle.

10). Heavier patients and steeper tilt accentuate the possibility of structural damage from wristlets and shoulder braces.

Bent-Knee/Anklet System

When SHDT is needed, a time-honored and successful technique has been to hold the patient in place by strapped anklets plus bent knees produced by the floorward angulation of the leg section of the table (see Fig. 8–6C). In this manner the flexed knee and lower leg become the restraining force rather than the upper extremity assuming that task by means of either wristlets or shoulder braces.

An issue of maximum importance in establishing the bent-knee/anklet method of torso restraint is the need to avoid severe compression of the upper calf muscles and vessels by the unyielding cephalad edge of the lowered foot section of the table. To accomplish this, the top of the patella is used as the guide for positioning the patient's knee relative to the hinge of the leg section of the table (Fig. 8–11). The patient is initially placed on the operating table so that the cephalad edge of the patella (index finger, upper hand, Fig. 8–11A) is caudad to the hinge connecting the leg and thigh sections of the table by a distance equal to the thickness of the mattress pad (and x-ray tunnel, if present) that supports the legs (see Fig. 8–11A, lower measuring hand). The patella becomes an important landmark because, as the leg lies extended, its cephalad margin is situated directly above the eventual point of angulation in the popliteal fossa when the knee is flexed. If an x-ray tunnel adds to the height of the table top, and if the

portion of it that is on the foot section of the table top will remain in place after that section is depressed, its thickness also must be added to the distance that the top of the patella will lie caudad to the hinge (see Fig. 8–11A).

The consideration of thickness is based on the fact that the metal leg section of the table top itself pivots as much as several inches beneath the surface on which the patient is lying. This places the intersection of the patient-contact surfaces of the thigh section and the depressed leg section caudad to its connecting hinge by a distance equal to the total thickness of whatever (mattress and radiolucent x-ray tunnel) rests on the surface of the leg section.

If the foregoing details are ignored, the cephalad edge of the depressed leg section of the table top can act as a transverse, compressive bar across the upper dorsal calf to obstruct venous return from the more distal lower extremity. When the details are observed as described, the posture is tolerable for the patient and serves as an effective restraint for the torso against the forces of gravity acting in the tilted position.

The mattress must be fixed to the table top with adhesive tape or Velcro-type fasteners, so that the weight of the patient cannot cause it to slide cephalad. Loose, footed leggings are used to minimize heat loss from the extremities, and the ankles are wrapped with suitable padding to protect pressure points. Padded straps, fastened securely to the distal portion of the foot section of the table top, are wrapped or buckled about the ankles of the awake patient. They must be snug but

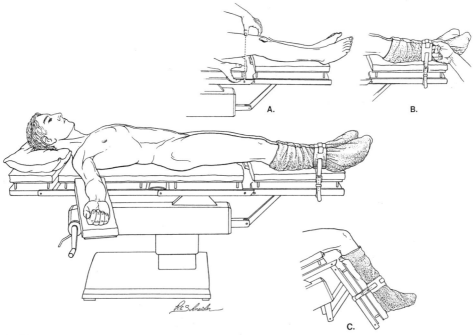

Figure 8–11

Arrangement of patient on operating table before instituting steep head-down tilt with bent knee/anklet restraining system. *A.* Right hand measuring thickness of table top and x-ray attachment at the hinge between the thigh and leg sections of the table top; left hand duplicating the measurement for proper placement of the proximal edge of the patella a similar distance caudad to that hinge. *B.* Padded anklets attached to distal table rail; finger tests snugness to preclude ischemia from tourniquet effect. *C.* Restraint mechanism in effect when foot section of table top is depressed as tilt of table surface is established, precluding need for shoulder braces or wristlets to stabilize patient. Armboard is abducted less than 90 degrees from the sagittal plane of the body to avoid stressing axillary neurovascular bundle. (Additional padding not shown for clarity.)

comfortable. As a check, an attendant should be able to insert a finger between the strap and the surface of the restrained ankle (see Fig. 8–11*B*). The maneuver is intended to detect straps that need to be loosened slightly to avoid pressure injuries to underlying structures and tourniquet-like ischemia of the foot after tilting.

Because the restraining force for the patient on the table is the flexed knee plus the continuity of the extremity across the joint (see Fig. 8–11*C*), this method does not require the use of straps or binders across legs or thighs that might interfere with the circulation sufficiently to increase the incidence of venous thrombosis and pulmonary embolism after surgery.[20]

Arm Arrangement

Intravenous cannulas are securely placed while the patient is supine. The patient's arms are restrained across the chest or placed alongside the torso and secured by a single wide draw sheet that encompasses the arm, elbow, forearm, and wrist and is tucked under either the patient's flank and hip or the mattress. Pressure points are padded about the elbow to protect the radial and ulnar nerves. Padded, metal toboggan-like (Wells Arm Protector, Mercury Enterprises, Inc., North Clearwater, FL) arm shields may be placed to protect the intravascular lines and blood pressure cuff from contact with the members of the surgical team (Fig. 8–12).

If one or both of the patient's arms are to be abducted and accessible throughout the operation, they should be placed on armboards that can be locked firmly in place. The arrangement should not allow an arm to be extended dorsally to elevate the shoulder on that side and force the head of the humerus against the axillary neurovascular bundle or stress the capsule of the shoulder joint. For similar reasons, the angle of abduction of the arm from the long axis of the body should be less than 90 degrees (see Fig. 8–11). Lesser amounts of abduction may be needed in the

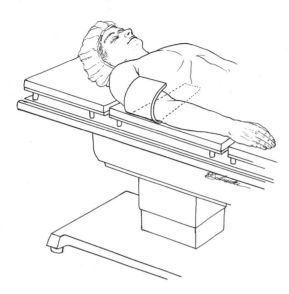

Figure 8–12

Wells arm protector, popularly referred to as a "toboggan." (Padding not shown for clarity.)

presence of gnarled skeletons or limited shoulder motion to keep the axillary musculature from being obviously stretched.

The position of the arm on the padded board, usually with the palm supinated, must assure that the weight of the elbow is placed on the olecranon process of the ulna to avoid undue pressure on the adjacent cubital tunnel and its ulnar nerve. Repeated attention must be directed to the position of the armboard during the operation, because it easily may be displaced, moved cephalad, or unintentionally rotated into unwanted abduction by the surgeon or an assistant who is preoccupied by events at the operative site.

After the patient is anesthetized, the trachea is intubated and control of ventilation is assured, the table is tilted to the desired plane. If the bent-knee/anklet arrangement is used, the leg section of the table top is angulated downward toward 90 degrees to flex the knees, and the restraining system is checked to assure that the proper relationship between the knees and the table hinge has been established.

The SHDT position warrants the use of an endotracheal tube for efficient ventilatory support even if neither the thorax nor the abdominal cavity will be entered. The position of the endotracheal tube should be reconfirmed once the patient has been tilted head down because the mediastinum and main carina frequently shift cephalad, possibly allowing the proximal portion of a main bronchus to slip over the previously "fixed" tube. The head should remain in a neutral position, if possible, tilted neither left nor right. As opposed to head rotation with spinal alignment maintained, lateral tilt of the head and neck may place additional stretch on the brachial plexus of the side with the obtuse angle between cervical and thoracic spine and compound the stretch/compression threat to the plexus if shoulder braces or wristlets are used for postural stabilization.[21] The occiput should be well padded to prevent pressure alopecia, particularly in a lengthy operation. An additional safeguard is occasionally rotating the head slightly to vary the point of occipital pressure on the mattress.

If the tilted low lithotomy position described by Lloyd-Davies[18] is used (see Fig. 8–4), the steps taken in its establishment are essentially the same as those already listed. The lower extremities, however, are placed in some form of leg holders before tilting the table (see also Chapter 5). Care must be taken to see that the angulation of the thighs on the trunk is not sharp enough to constrict vascular flow in the legs. For unobstructed perfusion of the extremities, the thighs should be flexed on the long axis of the torso considerably less than 90 degrees and usually are elevated only 30 to 45 degrees (see Fig. 8–4). Leg supports should be padded to prevent pressure on the peroneal nerve where it circles laterally around the fibula just beneath its proximal head.[22] Dry, soft padding over metal parts of the table and its attachments can protect bony prominences from pressure injury and also minimize the possibility of burns occurring when electrocautery is used.

McLachlin and colleagues[23] were concerned about the possibility of venous stasis in the lower extremities in the Lloyd-Davis combination of low lithotomy and head-down tilt. They studied patients in two comparable groups: the first had the lower legs (knees to ankles) placed parallel to and 15 degrees above the frontal plane of the body; the second had knees angulated to place the lower legs 15 degrees below the frontal plane. Venous dye clearance from the legs was compared in both positions and related to clearance in the horizontal supine position. Clearance was slowest supine and best in the group with 15-degree elevation, the posture now considered tilted low lithotomy (see Fig. 8–4 and Chapter 6). Schiller[24] considers this the basis for selection of the Lloyd-Davis posture for combined abdominopelvic procedures. By contrast, Warner advises that at the Mayo Clinic, after several generations of experience with SHDT stabilized by downward angulation of the anklet-retained lower legs, there has been no appreciable incidence of superficial or deep phlebitis attributable to the Clinic's version of steep tilt (Warner MA, personal communication, 1995).

Discontinuing Head-Down Tilt, With or Without Simultaneous Leg Elevation

When the head-low posture is no longer needed at the end of the surgical procedure, the patient should be returned to the horizontal position with great care. Vasocompensation being depressed by anesthesia, a sudden return to the horizontal supine position may unmask inadequate volume replacement and provoke hypotension by adding the vascular capacitance of the lower limbs to that of the more central circulation more rapidly than the body can accommodate. If leg holders had been used to elevate the lower extremities, the legs should be brought together, straightened slowly, and lowered simultaneously. Unilateral lowering of elevated extremities from tilted lithotomy positions should be avoided because of its potential for serious stress on lumbosacral articulations, particularly when protective muscle tone is relaxed by the influence of anesthesia or when lumbosacral arthritis is present.

PHYSIOLOGY OF HEAD-DOWN TILT

When an awake patient is maintained in head-down tilt, a rather stylized series of events commonly occurs, and with varying speed of onset. The individual becomes anxious and restless, often develops a pounding vascular headache, becomes dyspneic, may develop a stuffy nose, gradually becomes less cooperative, and often tries to sit up to escape the head-low posture (Fig. 8–13).

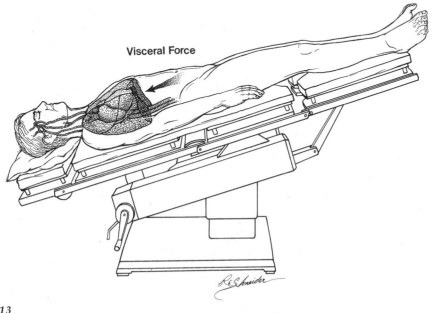

Visceral Force

Figure 8–13

Visceral pressure of head-down tilt. See text. (From Barash PG, Cullen BF, Stoelting RK [eds.]: Clinical Anesthesia, 2nd ed. Philadelphia, JB Lippincott, 1992.)

The sensorium of an obtunded patient can clear temporarily when tilted head down, but diminished awareness usually recurs and may advance to coma. Wilkins and associates[25] noted that jugular venous pressure was increased up to fourfold by head-down tilt. The sequence of events just described can be interpreted as a combination of impaired cerebral circulation; a vascular overload in the superior caval circuit; pulmonary vascular congestion, particularly in the apices; and disrupted ventilation due to interference with diaphragmatic excursions. The reasons for its occurrence are valid; and the steeper the tilt, or the more unhealthy the patient, the more rapid should be its onset.

The Circulatory System

As noted earlier, during World War I the eminent physiologist Walter Cannon advocated using Trendelenburg's position as a therapy for "shock," a nonspecific term used in that era to refer to any form of hypotension. He believed that head-down tilt increased the return of blood from the lower extremities and that cerebral blood flow improved.[6] Common desk chairs or wooden "shock blocks" became familiar devices with which to elevate the foot of a hospital bed, and several subsequent generations of physicians revered the head-down position as the obligatory first maneuver in the treatment of hypotension.

Serious reservations about the value of the "shock position" were expressed by Weil[10] in 1957 and later supported by Guntheroth and colleagues[26] and others. The mild rise in brachial artery blood pressure attainable in the head-down position was recognized as early as 1950 by Cole[9] as being due to the table tilt relocating the blood pressure cuff to a new level below the heart.

In 1965, Weil[11] anesthetized rats with pentobarbital sodium, bled them in a standard protocol, placed them in the supine, head-down, and head-up positions, and then compared them with anesthetized normotensive, normovolemic control rats that were similarly positioned. Of the rats that had been bled, 83.3% died when placed head down, while all rats that had been kept supine survived.

In the Shock Research Unit at the University of Southern California, Taylor and Weil placed seven hypotensive and six normotensive patients in 10 degrees of head-down tilt.[12] The normotensive patients had been admitted because of barbiturate intoxication (n = 2), hypocalcemia, stroke, septicemia, and adenocarcinoma of the colon (n = 1 each); those who were hypotensive were present because of barbiturate intoxication (n = 4), stroke, cirrhosis, and septicemia (n = 1 each). They encountered the following results:

- Hypotensive mentally obtunded patients became initially more alert after being tilted head down but then became anxious and uncomfortable.
- Similar but more severe distress was displayed by normotensive patients placed head down.
- The normotensive patients all tolerated the 10-degree tilt without changes in pressure.
- Of the seven hypotensive patients, all but one had further decreases in systolic, diastolic, and mean arterial blood pressures when tilted head down. A decreased cardiac index was measured in four of the seven patients.
- The values returned to previous levels, and cardiac output increased when the horizontal posture was restored.

Their findings constitute convincing evidence that the head-down position is not a reliable treatment for hypotension.

The change in arterial blood pressure seen just after a patient is tilted head down is caused primarily by baroreceptor activity.[27] The following events happen:

1. A rapid autotransfusion of up to 1000 mL of blood moves from the lower extremities into the central circulation.

2. The increased volume of blood is pumped from the heart as an initial increase in cardiac output, raising hydrostatic pressures in the arch of the aorta and in the carotid sinuses at the bifurcation of the carotid arteries.

3. Stimulation of baroreceptors on the great vessels reflexly causes a generalized vasodilation and a decreased stroke volume, leading to a reduced cardiac output and decreased perfusion of vital organs.[27]

4. The brain is especially vulnerable to decreased blood flow, because the head-down position increases cerebral venous pressure, which by itself congests the intracranial circulation and interferes with cerebral perfusion. A posturally induced migration of cerebrospinal fluid from the spine into the cranial vault raises the hydrostatic pressure of intracranial cerebrospinal fluid, additively impedes cere-

bral blood flow, and helps to cause stagnant cerebral hypoxia.[28, 29]

Decreased blood pressure of 5 to 10 mm Hg due to the head-down posture was encountered by Guntheroth[26] in mongrel dogs that were first bled to shock and then placed in a 30-degree head-down tilt, almost the original posture advocated by Trendelenburg. Subsequent studies with dogs that were placed in the head-down position after denervation of the carotid sinus and aortic arch showed that an increase in hydrostatic pressure in the baroreceptors was not then perceived as an increase in blood volume and did not cause the expected overall reduction in vasoconstriction or the secondary decreases in cardiac output and cerebral blood flow. These findings are strong evidence that cerebral blood flow is reflexly influenced by pressure in the great arteries.

Sibbald and associates[13] reported studies on 76 monitored intensive care unit patients who were either normotensive (n = 61) or hypotensive (n = 15), with sepsis (n = 30), acute cardiac dysfunction (n = 40), or miscellaneous acute conditions (n = 6). Each was placed in 15 to 20 degrees of head-down tilt. In normotensive patients, the preload of each ventricle was increased, cardiac output rose slightly, systemic vascular resistance fell, and mean arterial pressure was unaltered. The hypotensive patients did not exhibit increased preload, and their cardiac outputs decreased. These investigators concluded that the use of head-down tilt to treat shock was disadvantageous, because it caused an unpredictable further fall in mean arterial pressure in some of their hypotensive patients.

Gentili and colleagues[30] studied 22 elderly (mean age, 68.4 years) postoperative patients in an intensive care unit to determine the cardiopulmonary effects of 12 degrees of head-down tilt sustained for 15 minutes. They found no deterioration in any measured cardiac parameter, in PaO_2, $P\bar{v}O_2$, or venous admixture. Mean arterial pressure, cardiac index, and the stroke work of each ventricle increased significantly. Because of its uncertain effects on cerebral blood flow, they did not recommend the posture either for the treatment of hypotension or for use during cardiac resuscitation. However, they believed that it should be well tolerated by most patients during central venous access procedures.

Assessing various methods of improving the success rate of internal jugular vein cannulation, Armstrong's group made ultrasound measurements of the lateral diameter of the vessel in 35 volunteers.[31] No correlation was found between internal jugular vein size and the height, weight, age, or neck circumference of the subjects. Carotid artery palpation and full neck extension reduced the internal jugular vein diameter considerably. Vessel diameter increased as head-down tilt steepened. The most efficient methods of increasing internal jugular vein diameter were an abdominal binder and the Valsalva maneuver.

Kubal and co-workers[14] investigated the effects of MHDT on the cardiac function of patients with known coronary artery disease who were having invasive vascular monitoring established while awake before coronary artery bypass surgery. Significant increases in myocardial oxygen requirement and in central venous pressure were caused by 15 degrees of head-down tilt. One patient developed tilt-associated, ST segment changes on the electrocardiogram. Coronary artery disease patients are rarely able to supply myocardial oxygen requirements when demand is increased. Hence the appearance of myocardial ischemia on the electrocardiogram. Kubal indicated that after the study they had kept patients horizontal for catheter introduction and had encountered no difficulty with vascular access (Kubal K, personal communication, 1984).

Keusch's group[32] studied the electrocardiographic effects of introducing pulmonary artery catheters through the right internal jugular veins of 34 premedicated patients who were initially in sinus rhythm. Each patient was placed first in 5 to 10 degrees of head-down tilt and then in 5 degrees of head-up tilt plus right tilt. In each position, access to the pulmonary artery was equally facile and the overall incidence of dysrhythmias (85% head-down vs. 76% head-up-right tilt) was grossly similar. However, malignant dysrhythmias were twice as frequent in the head-down position (59% vs. 30%). When the posture was changed to head-up-right tilt, most of the malignant dysrhythmias became benign.

Commenting on Keusch and co-workers' report,[32] Baraka and associates[33] studied patients with coronary artery disease (n = 15) or needing valve replacement (n = 9) who were similarly anesthetized and were undergoing the introduction of flow-directed pulmonary artery catheters while in 20 degrees of head-down tilt. The incidence of arrhythmias was essentially similar in the two groups (14/15 who underwent coronary artery bypass grafting, 3/9 who received valves). Pulmonary artery catheter introductions were successful in all of the patients undergoing coronary artery bypass grafting, but in the valve replacement group three of the nine catheters could be introduced only after the patients were changed to 20 degrees of head-up tilt plus right lateral tilt. A fourth patient in the valve group, with tricuspid regurgitation and pulmonary hypertension, could not be catheterized in either position. The investigators concluded that head-up right lateral tilt may be superior to head-down tilt for pulmonary catheterization in both awake and anesthetized patients because it elevates the pulmonary outflow tract above the bulk of the right ventricle. They suggested that the whirlpool effect of tricuspid regurgitation into the right atrium denied entry of the flotation balloon into the ventricle of the patient who could not be successfully catheterized.

Reich and co-workers[34] examined the effects of either 20 degrees of head-down tilt or passive leg raising to 60 degrees in anesthetized patients with coronary artery disease who were undergoing myocardial revascularization while monitored with transesophageal echocardiography and a thermodilution pulmonary artery catheter. Minor hemodynamic improvement occurred with either maneuver, the only difference being that an increased cardiac index resulted from tilt but not from leg raising. However, both techniques resulted in right ventricular dilation, decreased right ventricular ejection fraction, and impaired oxygenation.

Sing and associates[35] studied the effect of head-down tilt on oxygen transport in eight hypovolemic postoperative adults in an intensive care unit. Initial pulmonary artery wedge pressures were 6 mm Hg or less in all subjects. Variables were measured with the patient supine and again 10 minutes after the institution of head-down tilt. Mean arterial pressure, pulmonary artery wedge pressure, and systemic vascular resistance all rose while cardiac index, oxygen delivery, oxygen consumption, and oxygen extraction ratios were each unchanged. They concluded that the increase in blood pressure produced by head-down tilt was not accompanied by an improvement in blood flow or tissue oxygenation.

The circulatory mechanics of a patient with heart disease can be sufficiently different from those of a healthy person to make added blood volume in the central circulation an affliction that is poorly tolerated and potentially decompensating. In the preanesthetic evaluation the effects of the desired degree of head-down tilt can be assessed. If the unanesthetized patient complains of dyspnea, or if the position results in a further decrease in blood pressure, an alternative posture should be sought for the operation. Several decades ago, Dripps strongly advised against placing an orthopneic patient either flat in bed or in head-down tilt after the induction of general anesthesia simply because he or she is asleep and cannot complain of dyspnea.[36]

SHDT, particularly in the patient with decreased cardiac reserve, is capable of increasing venous return and pulmonary blood flow enough to cause acute heart failure. This effect should also be kept in mind with regard to the patient with normal cardiac reserve in whom, during anesthesia and head-down tilt, pulmonary compliance progressively decreases or bronchospasm appears.[22]

Deklunder and colleagues[37] investigated the effects of brief (5 minutes) periods of SHDT (70 degrees) on 12 normal male subjects ages 19 to 24 using echocardiographic Doppler techniques. Tilt rapidly increased early passive filling of the left ventricle, transaortic flow velocity, and cardiac output. Blood pressure increased (7% systolic, 15% diastolic) and remained high throughout the tilt period despite peripheral vasodilation. These researchers believed that the cardiac responses to changes in posture in humans were related more to shifts of blood that passively filled the ventricles than to baroreflex regulation of arterial tone and that the reflexes mainly control vascular impedance.

Multiple cardiovascular variables were measured by Tomaselli and colleagues[38] in 12 male subjects in their fourth decades who were placed in 6 degrees of head-down tilt for 1 hour to simulate the onset of weightlessness. Whereas translocation of fluid from the lower extremities to the thorax began immediately with tilt, most cardiovascular measurements remained stable for the first 30 minutes of the procedure. In the second 30 minutes, leg fluid continued to translocate into the thorax but stroke volume, cardiac output, and mean stroke ejection rate were decreased while mean arterial pressure rose. Their data, from awake individuals in very slight head-down tilt, indicated that blood from the lower extremities was sequestered in the pulmonary circulation rather than being retained in the great veins.

The effect of posture on blood flow at the operative site can be stated in gross terms. Vascular pressures at a given tissue location will vary by 2.0 mm Hg for each 2.5 cm distance that the site is either above or below the zero reference point at the heart.[39] If the operative site is elevated above the level of the heart, venous blood and shed blood drain away from the tissues and structures in the operative site, and actual bleeding at the operative site may be reduced. Thus, the impression is obtained that blood loss from surgical wounds located caudad to the heart can be decreased significantly by placing the patient in head-down tilt.[40]

Calculations of the hemodynamics of head-down tilt, using the data of Enderby[39] mentioned earlier, indicate significant potential perfusion problems even with slight variations of tilt. The issue is detailed in the discussion of the tilted lithotomy position in Chapter 6 and depicted in Figures 6–8 and 6–9. With only 15 degrees of head-down tilt, a normotensive patient who is 6 feet tall and has an atrial mean arterial pressure (MAP) of 90 mm Hg can be expected to develop a MAP at the ankles of 66 mm Hg while that at the circle of Willis has risen to 104 mm Hg.[41] If the legs are elevated into one of the lithotomy positions, ankle MAPs may fall enough to threaten perfusion of the extremities. In the presence of intracranial pathology, that elevation of MAP at the circle of Willis is difficult to justify. Figure 6–9 indicates that steeper levels of tilt should produce greater degrees of MAP variance. As those MAPs become more abnormal and the operative procedures last longer, risk factors for the patient can be expected to increase even in the absence of disease. Significant cardiovascular, respiratory, or intracranial pathology can be worsened accordingly.

Laparoscopic surgery for problems in the lower abdomen is a relatively recent technique that appears to be increasing in popularity. Abdominal distention, produced by insufflation of carbon dioxide or an inert gas into the peritoneal cavity, is combined with some degree of head-down tilt to provide working room for the surgeon amid abdominopelvic viscera that are displaced cephalad to varying degrees. The intention is that the laparoscopic technique offers the patient less risk of wound healing and a shorter hospital stay than does the traditional abdominal incision for the same procedure. In some practices, however, the assumed reduction in patient risk has allowed potentially detrimental changes in protocols: the tilt has become as much as 45 degrees, the abdomen is significantly distended, the surgical times now last many hours, and intraoperative physiologic stresses can be assumed to have increased. Johannsen and associates[42] report a study of 16 women undergoing elective diagnostic laparoscopies with intra-abdominal insufflation pressures of 2 kPa (about 15 mm Hg), 30 degrees of head-down tilt, muscle relaxation, and controlled ventilation. One group was given halothane, the other was given a more balanced form of anesthesia. Multiple cardiac parameters were either measured or calculated. At the time of maximum hemodynamic stress, stroke index and cardiac index were reduced an average of 42% in each group while no significant changes occurred in either heart rate or mean arterial pressure. Total peripheral resistance increased by 50% in the halothane group and by 100% in the balanced group. Decreases in stroke index were related to changes in total respiratory compliance. Stroke index and cardiac index values remained abnormal until the patient was returned to the horizontal position and the abdomen was exsufflated. The authors deemed the changes produced by head-down tilt and abdominal insufflation to be much more important than the minor variation in values between the two types of anesthesia.[42]

The effects of head-down tilt on carotid blood flow and pulmonary gas exchange were investigated by Loeppky and co-workers.[43] Six subjects were studied supine, at serial intervals during 20 minutes of 30-degree head-down tilt, and after returning to the supine position. Common carotid artery blood flow was reduced 6% by tilt, briefly increased in the second minute, and rebounded to be 7% higher than control when the horizontal supine posture was restored. Tilt caused increases in oxygen uptake, carbon dioxide output, respiratory exchange ratios, and tidal volume in the first minute. About 200 mL of blood shifted within the circulation, providing a ventilatory stimulus. Finding that tilt can decrease blood and tissue oxygen stores and increase carbon dioxide stores by shifting blood volume toward and blood flow away from the dependent vascular compartment of the head, they speculated that an additional factor could have been ischemia of the elevated lower extremities. Periodic breathing accompanied the cerebral venous congestion produced by tilt. Reduced common carotid artery blood flow during tilt was only partially offset by decreased flow resistance in the carotid artery.

In the light of current evidence, the effects of head-down tilt on the cardiovascular system of a normovolemic patient are (1) increased central blood volume, (2) reflexly decreased cardiac output, and (3) reduced perfusion of vital organs. Surgical use of the position is intended to improve operative exposure, aid the drainage of shed blood away from the operative field, reduce bleeding in the wound, and minimize blood loss. In the presence of a normal cardiorespiratory function and an intact blood volume, and in the absence of intracranial pathology, the traditional Trendelenburg position should be, and historically has been, tolerated acceptably by the patient. However, on the basis of what is now known about the adverse effects of the posture on hypovolemic patients, the anesthesiologist must be particularly diligent in maintaining normal blood volume when this position is used during surgery.

The foregoing data, indicating that the SHDT of Trendelenburg's position is contraindicated in the treatment of shock, merit strong emphasis. There is, however, a posture that optimizes venous return in the presence of hypovolemia and hypotension: the *lawn chair position* gently elevates both the head and the slightly flexed lower extremities while keeping the torso level. (See discussion in Chapter 5 and also Figs. 5–3 and 5–4.) Cerebral congestion is minimized, cerebral venous drainage is aided, peripheral venous return is augmented, and the rise in central blood volume is unlikely to have the adverse reflexogenic intensity of the head-down position. Other measures of perfusion support should then be applied as needed.

The Respiratory System

During normal breathing the thorax expands in all directions except dorsally. In humans, the activity of the accessory muscles of respiration is abolished in deeper planes of anesthesia, and most of the work of breathing is done by the diaphragm. An SHDT position allows the abdominal contents to push cephalad against the diaphragm, so that its stretched musculature then not only must ventilate the lungs but also must lift the

weight of the abdominal contents. The result is a predisposition to atelectasis.[44]

In an important study, Fahy and associates[45] measured airway flow and esophageal pressures in 12 anesthetized, paralyzed, and intubated patients mechanically ventilated at rates of 10 to 30 per minute with tidal volumes of 250 to 800 mL during intra-abdominal insufflation of CO_2 for laparoscopic surgery. Measurements were made supine, in 10 degrees head-up tilt, and in 15 degrees of head-down tilt at intra-abdominal pressures of 0, 15, and 25 mm Hg. In five of the patients the additional effect of a lithotomy position was studied head down and head up. Calculations produced elastance and resistance values for the total respiratory system, lungs, and chest wall. Fahy and associates found that lung and chest wall impedances to inflation during mechanical ventilation increased with increasing intra-abdominal pressure, with head-down tilt, and with increasing body mass index. The increased lung impedance requires greater alveolar pressures for passive lung inflation and adds to the risk of pulmonary barotrauma. The increase in chest wall impedance increases intrathoracic pressure during positive-pressure lung inflation and has possible inhibitory effects on cardiac output. The researchers believed that the changes were the result of a decrease in lung volume and the development of microatelectasis.[46] They warned that these alterations might become clinically relevant in the presence of obesity and pulmonary disease and warned against the use of head-down tilt in those patients.

The work of breathing is increased by Trendelenburg's position. In 1966, Chiang and Lyons[47] studied 11 male volunteers in head-down tilts of 45 degrees and found that the position diminished pulmonary compliance, as demonstrated by a decreased lung volume at the same transpulmonary pressure and by an increased transpulmonary pressure while the same inflation volume was maintained. Increased pulmonary blood volume, as well as gravitational force on the mediastinal structures and diaphragm, were factors postulated to explain the decreased pulmonary compliance and the decreased functional residual capacity.

Obese patients are not good candidates for head-down tilt.[44] Whereas a heavy chest wall is difficult to lift as the chest expands, the added weight of the abdominal contents on the diaphragm decreases compliance and increases the risks of atelectasis and hypoxemia. Miller reported that Trendelenburg himself noted this intolerance of obese individuals for head-down tilt.[2]

SHDT reduces vital capacity. Studying the effects of various surgical positions on human lung volumes, Altschule[48] observed a 20% decrease associated with head-down tilt during operations. As early as 1946, Case and Stiles[49] measured vital capacity in 26 healthy awake adults, 22 to 78 years of age, first in the sitting position and then in a 20-degree head-down position; they found that the vital capacity of subjects placed head down averaged 14% less than when they were in the sitting position, with the greatest changes in older subjects.

In 1964, West and associates[50] performed a classic study of pulmonary perfusion and ventilation using normal dog lungs. They found that in the normal upright lung pulmonary arteriolar pressure at the apex is normally less than apical alveolar end-expiratory pressure, causing the capillaries of this portion of the lung to be collapsed. This area, defined by West and associates as zone 1, is ventilated but not perfused. The base of the lung is below the level of the heart, and the hydrostatic pressure in the venous end of the capillary is greater than both the left atrial pressure and the basilar alveolar end-expiratory pressure, causing these capillaries to be constantly opened. This functional region of the lung is known as zone 3. Between zones 1 and 3 is zone 2, an area in which the hydrostatic pressure of the pulmonary arteries is higher than the alveolar end-expiratory pressure but lower than the left atrial pressure. In zone 2 the capillaries are intermittently closed.

In an erect lung 30 cm long, the hydrostatic pressure of blood causes an apical to basal difference of 23 mm Hg in pulmonary artery pressures.[51] West pointed out that zone 1 does not occur in humans under normal conditions, because the pulmonary artery pressure is just sufficient to raise blood to the apex of the lung. If either or both pulmonary artery pressure and blood volume are reduced, or if alveolar pressure is raised, as with positive-pressure ventilation, then zone 1 does occur.

With the patient in the supine position, the anterior (ventral) part of the lung lies above the left atrium, and the plane from hilum to base lies at the level of the left atrium; these parts of the lung function as zone 2. The posterior (dorsal) part of the entire lung from apex to base becomes zone 3.[52] It may be

postulated, therefore, that with SHDT most of the lung becomes zone 3, because most of the entire lung then lies below the level of the left atrium.

According to Laver and co-workers, in zone 3 an excessive increase of left atrial pressure over alveolar pressure will enhance fluid transudation into the alveoli.[52] A prolonged head-low position, therefore, can contribute to pulmonary congestion and edema. Increased airway pressure during passive ventilation may help prevent this complication.

An evaluation of the usefulness of increased tidal volumes during head-down tilt was conducted by Tweed and associates[53] in 24 high-risk adult patients having lower abdominal surgery during head-down tilt. Steady-state measurements were made awake, after 30 minutes of conventional tidal volume ventilation (7.5 mL/kg) or high tidal volume ventilation (12.7 mL/kg) (the two conditions were introduced in random order), and after 5 minutes of manual hyperinflation of the lungs. Controlled ventilation used air/oxygen at FiO_2 0.5, and $FETCO_2$ was stabilized by the addition of dead space during high-volume ventilation. Significant deterioration of measured values occurred with conventional tidal volume ventilation; high tidal volume ventilation prevented the deterioration; and manual hyperinflation reversed it. It is reassuring to be shown that the use of head-down tilt does not compromise the value of large tidal volumes for passive ventilation of anesthetized patients, a practice widely applied to supine patients.

Healthy volunteers subjected to recumbency for 10 days had decreased physiologic dead space and decreased ratios of alveolar dead space to alveolar tidal volume.[54] The apex of the lung was better perfused. The enlarged alveolar capillary surface increased the diffusion capacity of the lungs. Early, the alveolar-arterial oxygen gradient decreased, but later the gradient increased. These recumbent patients were conscious and able to sigh. It might be expected that these changes would be exaggerated in the anesthetized patient who is tilted head down and that the resulting atelectasis might prevent any improvement in alveolar-arterial oxygen gradient.

Patients with chronically elevated left atrial pressures, such as those with mitral stenosis, increase their pulmonary blood volumes; and much of West's zone 2 in the lungs of normal upright patients may become zone 3 with elevated pulmonary capillary pressure. Such patients tolerate the supine position or the head-low position poorly, because the additional pulmonary blood volume that the postures produce may further increase pulmonary interstitial fluid, causing transudation of fluid into the alveoli. The result is atelectasis and hypoxemia.[52]

Because of the described hydrostatic pressure changes, the patient in SHDT can be considered similar to the patient with elevated left atrial pressure secondary to mitral valve disease. In these patients it may be beneficial to maintain constant airway pressure sufficient to produce alveolar pressure higher than the estimated left atrial pressure to simulate a relationship normal for zone 2. Values of 5 to 10 cm H_2O end expiratory pressure might be useful.

In 17 anesthetized, mechanically ventilated dogs, Loeppky and associates[55] examined the separate and combined effects of acute hypoxia, 30 degrees head-down tilt, and fluid loading on hemodynamics and pulmonary gas exchange. Tilt produced pulmonary vascular congestion and reduced total respiratory compliance during either normoxia or hypoxia. Compliance loss was doubled with fluid loading, the resultant pulmonary interstitial edema being confirmed by microscopy. Tilt added to hypoxia doubled the pulmonary vascular resistance increase attributable to hypoxia alone. They showed that increased blood volume and a shift in blood volume from systemic to pulmonary circulation contributed to the changes in pulmonary vascular resistance. A significant inverse relationship of pulmonary gas exchange efficiency to pulmonary driving pressure existed under these experimental circumstances.

The anesthetist must pay special attention to the position of the endotracheal tube after each change in the patient's posture, because a tube previously well positioned in the trachea can enter a bronchus after the patient is tilted into a steep head-down position. Heinonen and colleagues[56] reported that 20 of 49 patients (41%) who were subjected to 30 degrees of head-down tilt with an endotracheal tube in place had displacement of the "fixed" endotracheal tube to a site lower in the trachea. However, a study by Karpinos and co-workers,[57] measuring cephalad movement of the tracheal carina directly with patients in the supine, lithotomy (thighs flexed on trunk 80 to 140 degrees), and tilted lithotomy positions (head down 10 to 30 degrees) found that

relocation of the tip of the endotracheal tube in the trachea was a function of flexion of the neck rather than torso tilt. Nevertheless, with SHDT the potential remains for a cephalad shift of mediastinal contents to allow the tracheobronchial tree to move proximally along the endotracheal tube. If the tube tip is positioned close to the tracheal carina, a mainstem bronchus may slide over it. Because the orifice of the right upper lobe bronchus lies just beyond the carina in the right mainstem bronchus, a tube tip that has entered that bronchus has the potential of degrading ventilation of both lobes of the left lung plus the right upper lobe. In the presence of the ventilation/perfusion ratio alterations already present in SHDT, ventilating only two of five lobes threatens the rapid onset of severe respiratory embarrassment.

In spite of these changes in respiratory physiology, head-down tilt is a useful adjunct to the accomplishment of certain surgical procedures and need not be considered "all bad" by the anesthetist, as long as ventilation is controlled or assisted. The decreased functional residual capacity may allow more rapid changes in the uptake and blood level of inhalation anesthetic agents, although it also decreases pulmonary oxygen reserve. Tidal volume and ventilatory frequency adjustments should give a minute volume adequate for maintenance of good oxygenation and should prevent atelectasis without requiring diaphragmatic excursions so great as to interfere with the surgical operation. A small amount of constant positive pressure (5 to 8 cm H_2O) in the breathing circuit helps increase lung volume and decrease atelectasis.[58]

In the presence of specific lung disease, some degree of head-down tilt may be an asset when relative hypoxia is present despite artificial ventilation with 100% oxygen and positive end-expiratory pressure. Prokocimer and colleagues[59] reported a study that included two patients with bilateral lower lobe pneumonia whose marginal oxygenation was improved significantly by placing them in head-down tilt. The position was maintained until the pneumonia either had cleared or had advanced sufficiently to defeat any therapeutic advantage of the posture.

The Central Nervous System

In addition to its lack of usefulness as a "shock" position, no degree of head-down tilt should ever be inflicted on a patient with known or suspected intracranial pathology. The posture has a major potential for increasing intracranial fluid volume and further upsetting the perfusion dynamics within the brain. The brain includes three fluid compartments that contain cerebrospinal fluid, cerebral tissue water, and cerebral blood. A change in the pressure of one fluid compartment of the rigid cranial vault necessarily changes the pressure in the others unless the system can be decompressed through the foramina or foramen magnum.

The premise that the head-down position improves human cerebral circulation was disproved in studies done by Shenkin's group.[60] They tilted five awake, physiologically normal adults from the horizontal to a 20-degree head-up position and measured no change in cerebral blood flow; however, the mean carotid pressure decreased an average of 17%, and the intracranial cerebrospinal fluid pressure decreased from 133 mm H_2O to -9 mm H_2O. They then tilted four awake, physiologically normal adults 20 degrees head down and recorded a consistent 14% decrease in cerebral blood flow with a 10% increase in mean carotid blood pressure. Intracranial fluid pressure rose from 137 mm H_2O in the horizontal position to 290 mm H_2O in the head-down position. The constant cerebral flood flow, in spite of the decreased carotid artery pressure in the head-up position and the decreased cerebral blood flow with increased carotid pressure in the head-down position, is explained by altered cerebrovascular resistance as responses to changes in position. An increase in cerebrovascular resistance in the head-low position produces the decreased cerebral blood flow. Most surgical patients show some degree of conjunctival edema after being tilted head down for any length of time. Thus it is not surprising that a comparable degree of congestion in the cerebral circulation should result from gravity-induced increases in pressure in the jugular veins.

Measurements of cerebral blood flow in dogs anesthetized with thiopental and nitrous oxide, and given succinylcholine to permit controlled ventilation, showed increases in cerebral venous pressure up to 40 cm H_2O to be associated with moderate increases in cerebral blood flow.[61] This paradoxical increase in cerebral blood flow concomitant with an increase in outflow resistance is caused by an increased distention of venous channels and inhibition of the recurrent collapsibility of the thin-walled veins.

The intracranial pressure must rise to approximately 450 mm H_2O before cerebral circulation is impaired. Above this point Kety and co-workers, in 1948, demonstrated that the cerebral blood flow falls progressively, as autoregulation ceases to function normally.[62]

In mongrel dogs anesthetized with thiopental, nitrous oxide, and succinylcholine, Harper and Glass[63] found that an increase in the $Paco_2$ from 40 to 80 mm Hg increased cerebral blood flow 100%, whereas a decrease in the $Paco_2$ to 20 mm Hg decreased the cerebral blood flow 40%.

SHDT produces increased intrathoracic pressure, increased jugular pressure, and increased cerebral venous pressure. It also decreases cardiac output and reflexly lowers both carotid pressure and cerebral blood flow while simultaneously increasing cerebrospinal fluid pressure. One must be particularly careful, therefore, in ventilating the patient who is tipped head down. Overly aggressive use of positive pressure to expand the lung will further decrease cerebral blood flow and dangerously increase venous pressure, while insufficient ventilation will increase the $Paco_2$, and, with it, cerebral blood flow and intracranial pressure. In addition, respiratory alkalosis from too vigorous ventilation can so lower cerebral blood flow that the critical value for cerebral perfusion may be raised to a higher level,[64] compounding the deleterious effect of the positionally lowered cerebral blood flow.

A mean arterial pressure of 50 mm Hg or an average systolic blood pressure of 80 mm Hg is necessary for normal cerebral perfusion. Cerebral blood flow can be sharply decreased by pressures that are below 80 mm Hg systolic.[64] Taylor and Weil's work[12] showed decreased cardiac output in the hypotensive patient subjected to head-low tilt. We can hypothesize, therefore, that cerebral blood flow, normally decreased in the head-down position, must be even more impaired during hypovolemic, vasoconstrictive hypotension plus the head-low tilt. By contrast, when drug-induced vasodilative hypotension is present and the head is lowered, drug impairment of the reflex decreases in cerebral blood flow can be postulated to allow marked augmentation of intracranial blood volume and cause considerable rises in intracranial pressure.

Boyan, in 1953, reported on the effect of

hypotensive anesthesia for radical pelvic and abdominal surgery with patients in traditional SHDT.[65] Hypotensive anesthesia was permitted by the belief that as long as the systolic blood pressure was greater than the usual arterial capillary pressure (32 mm Hg), perfusion through the capillary bed would be normal and tissue metabolism would not suffer. No known complications from the head-down position were reported, and, because the patients did not show signs of anoxia, the posture was considered safe during radical surgery. The danger of hypotensive anesthesia combined with head down-tilt suggests, however, that the decreased blood pressure could combine with increased venous pressure to lessen local tissue flow to values that could be below the requirements of cerebral metabolism.[40] More sophisticated cardiovascular monitoring available in current practices, and unheard of at the time of the Boyan report, might resolve this controversy. Until then, the combination of deliberate hypotension and head-down tilt should be considered risky for the patient.

In normal adults the cerebrospinal fluid pressure and the pressure in the thin walled cerebral veins are identical. The cerebral venous sinuses, on the other hand, with their semirigid walls, do not respond directly to cerebrospinal fluid pressure. They depend on pressure in the right atrium transmitted to the internal jugular veins.[66]

The cerebral arterioles autoregulate to maintain constant flow despite changes of systemic pressure. The vessels dilate as pressure falls and constrict as pressure rises. When a sudden intracranial pressure rise lessens the gradient between intravascular and tissue pressures, an autoregulated vasodilative response occurs that attempts to preserve perfusion. Increased intrathoracic or intra-abdominal pressure elevates superior vena caval pressure, impairs cerebral venous drainage, and increases both cerebral blood volume and cerebrospinal fluid pressure.[66]

A progressive increase of intracranial pressure along with a decrease in vasomotor tone causes cerebral vasodilation and a further increase in intracranial pressure. If vasomotor activity leads to a situation in which arterial pressure equals intracranial pressure, brain swelling becomes severe and cerebral volume will vary directly with the blood pressure. Vasomotor paralysis, therefore, causes an increase in cerebral blood volume, and it is this increase in cerebral blood volume that is the primary cause of subsequent brain swelling.[67]

Any process that increases intrathoracic venous pressure also increases venous pressure within the skull and can result in cerebral edema. A rise in $PaCO_2$ causes venous engorgement that may provoke an acute onset of cerebral edema during surgery.

Cerebral perfusion pressure increases transiently while the patient is tilted head low, but if the carotid sinus reflex is functioning, the carotid blood pressure and flow will decrease rapidly.[68] Normal patients do not have appreciable changes in cerebral blood flow until the mean cerebral blood pressure is less than 50 mm Hg. Hypertensive and arteriosclerotic patients, however, may have a critical level that is considerably above 50 mm Hg. Elderly patients are more likely to have arteriosclerotic plaques in the carotid arteries and lose vessel elasticity. Also, some elderly patients have cervical osteoarthritis with buildups of calcium deposits, and turning the head to one side or the other can decrease flow in the opposite carotid artery by 10% to 27%.[69] This decreased flow is thought also to be due to compression of the carotid artery by the transverse process of the first cervical vertebra.[70] The combination of head-down tilt and head rotation may, therefore, be particularly threatening to the elderly or hypertensive patient.

The jugular veins act as a reservoir of blood at near-atmospheric pressure that is constantly filling and emptying. Positive-pressure lung inflation fills the reservoir, but its compliance is great enough to minimize transmission of pressure to the brain while the patient is supine. Head-down tilt, however, overfills the reservoir. Positive-pressure ventilation then may cause further overfilling of the jugular veins with transmission of greatly increased pressure directly to the cerebral veins.[71]

Satake and co-workers,[72] in Japan, using single photon emission computed tomography, measured regional cerebral blood flow during a brief head-down tilt of only 6 degrees in human male subjects. Significantly increased flows were observed in the basal ganglia and cerebellum. Trends toward increases in other regions did not reach statistical significance. This slight degree of head-down tilt is commonly reported in investigations of awake volunteers by space agency laboratories of various countries that study the simulated effects of weightlessness.

Other Physiologic Systems

Hayashi and associates[73] studied the effect of hypoglycemic stress on water and electrolyte metabolism during head-down tilt. Healthy male volunteers were subjected to postural changes (30 minutes standing, 120 minutes of head-down tilt, and 60 minutes standing) before and after the onset of insulin-induced hypoglycemia. After baseline studies as controls, tilt was found to decrease levels of antidiuretic hormone, cortisol, plasma renin activity, aldosterone, and catecholamines; atrial natriuretic polypeptide levels, urine flow (250%), and sodium excretion (150%) were increased. After insulin administration during tilt, antidiuretic hormone, cortisol, plasma renin activity, aldosterone, and catecholamine levels were increased; the response of atrial natriuretic polypeptide was exaggerated; and the increases in urine flow and sodium excretion were abolished. They concluded that head-down tilt alters endocrine homeostasis in awake volunteers and that stress during tilt further modifies endocrine function. How these data apply to a patient under anesthesia is uncertain.

Using sevoflurane anesthesia and 6 degrees of head-down tilt, Hirose and associates[74] compared the endocrine and renal functions of ten patients undergoing lower abdominal surgery to a similar group that was kept horizontal. Mean arterial pressures were maintained constant by adjustment of the inspired concentration of sevoflurane. Plasma catecholamine levels increased less during surgery in the tilted posture, but levels of plasma aldosterone, cortisol, and urinary sodium excretion were significantly increased by tilt. Plasma renin activity, antidiuretic hormone, and atrial natriuretic peptide levels, urine volume, creatinine levels, and water clearance showed no changes related to positioning. They concluded that MHDT reduces the rise in sympathetic activity and lessens renal tubular reabsorption of sodium during lower abdominal surgery under sevoflurane anesthesia. Other stress hormones increase more with tilt.

Linder and colleagues[75] investigated the effect of changing body position on intraocular pressure and visual function using two groups of 10 subjects who were visually normal with normal intraocular pressures. In the first group, measurements were made while posture was changed in steps from +90 degrees (upright) to −90 degrees (inverted).

The second group was maintained in 6 degrees of head-down tilt for 2 hours while similar measurements were made repeatedly. Steep tilt tripled intraocular pressure. Significant reductions in neurophysiologic function at both the retinal and the cortical levels were associated with head-down tilt, with maximum neural effect occurring after 20 minutes of 6-degree tilt.

COMPLICATIONS OF HEAD-DOWN TILT

As described in the previous section, most complications associated with tilting an anesthetized patient head down arise from aberrations in physiology caused by the position itself. Their severity is probably related directly to the degree of head-down tilt and the duration of its use. Other complications are technical and can be substantially avoided by careful attention to detail.

Hypotension

In the absence of surgical bleeding, hypotension is the product of vasodilation and decreased cardiac output resulting from reflexes induced by the head-down position. Cardiac dysrhythmias are sometimes associated. Blood pressure can be kept nearly normal by carefully replacing lost circulating volume and by decreasing either the concentration of anesthetic agents or the degree of head-down tilt. Very careful administration of vasoconstrictor drugs may sometimes be indicated.

Masked Blood Loss

During surgery, head-down tilt can mask the significance of blood loss. Unsuspected hypovolemia often appears as sudden hypotension when the patient is returned to the supine horizontal position. Blood volume deficits must be carefully estimated and replaced before the end of the procedure. Shifting from steep tilt to a horizontal position should be done slowly with repetitive checks of blood pressure to detect the onset of hypotension as the body adjusts to the newly enlarged circulatory capacitance. However, strict attention should be applied to avoiding excessive intraoperative volume replacement that may stress a weakened vasculature when tilt is terminated and reflex vasodilatation ceases.

Venous Air Embolus

In theory, air might be entrained into open pelvic or abdominal veins during use of SHDT, but this is a rare complication. Because air embolus may be more likely to occur if a hypotensive technique is also employed, previous placement of a right atrial catheter for air aspiration might be advisable if deliberate hypotension is intended.

Ocular Complications

Increased cerebral venous pressure is known to occur as a physiologic change with head-down tilt, and retinal detachment[76] or cerebral edema can result. In patients with normal intraocular pressure, head-down tilt produces little change; however, if glaucoma is present, increases in intraocular tension may be severe.[77, 78] The possibility of complications secondary to increased cerebral venous pressure may be minimized by using a less steep tilt and by decreasing the amount of pressure in the airway.[79]

Venous Thrombosis

Venous thrombosis has also been attributed to SHDT. Passive congestion of the cerebral vessels may predispose to formation of thrombi,[40] and thrombosis is also reported when occlusive braces, pads, or straps interfere with flow in the superficial veins.[80] Boyan,[81] however, reported the infrequent occurrence of venous thrombosis of the legs even during long operations for malignancy in which the legs were flexed at the knees. Nevertheless, if it is thought that a patient might be at higher risk for phlebothrombosis, a lesser degree of knee bend should be used, and care must be taken that braces and pads are not occlusive.

Endotracheal Tube Migration

Relocation of an endotracheal tube into a mainstem bronchus is possible after the patient is tilted head down. Cephalad displacement of the diaphragm and compression of the lung bases can shift the carina cephalad over the fixed tube. Abdominal insufflation may enhance this possibility. The position of the tracheal tube should be rechecked after each change in position, and the head should be kept in a neutral midline position to minimize the chance of the endotracheal tube's

pushing into a bronchus.[56] Recognition is always dependent on observation and superficial auscultation of the chest. Relying only on an esophageal stethoscope to verify bilateral equal ventilation may be misleading.

Atelectasis

Atelectasis may occur during SHDT as a result of either drug-induced hypoventilation or compression of the lung by the abdominal viscera during the anesthetic. Positive pressure on the airway to counteract the weight of the abdominal viscera against the diaphragm helps keep the lung bases expanded, and assisted or controlled ventilation should protect against hypoventilation. Positional pulmonary edema may occur secondary to the increased pulmonary blood volume.[82] Edema can be prevented only by less steep tilt, and treatment is removal from the position plus positive-pressure ventilation.

Neuropathy

The complication of head-down tilt most frequently reported is neuropathy, the most common being brachial plexus dysfunction[22, 83, 84] from one or more of the following causes:

- Stretching the nerves over the arch formed by the tendinous attachments of the pectoralis minor at the coracoid process
- Shoulder braces depressing the clavicles into the retroclavicular spaces and directly compressing the plexuses
- Tilting the patient's head to one side, further stretching the nerve roots on the contralateral side, the side of the obtuse angle
- The head of the humerus impinging upon the plexus if the arm is externally rotated, abducted, or hyperextended
- A cephalad shift of the torso after arms are restrained, wrist straps pulling the heads of the humeri caudad, or caudal displacement of the shoulder girdle by shoulder braces. This may, individually or in combination, stretch the plexus and its associated vascular structures between its fixed points in the neck and the shoulder or compressed between the clavicle and first rib. Dysesthesias and anesthesia in the upper extremities can result.

Prevention of neuropathies depends on careful positioning of the arms at the sides or across the chest without use of wrist straps or shoulder braces. If it is necessary to have the patient's arm or arms abducted during the operation, each armboard should be positioned so that the extremity is not hyperextended. Abduction should be less than 90 degrees, structures in the axilla should be relaxed, and good peripheral pulses in the extremity should be verified. Padding of shoulder braces does not eliminate the possibility of brachial plexus injury, but, on the rare occasion when a shoulder brace is necessary, it should be well padded and placed at the acromioclavicular junction rather than either against the root of the neck or over the clavicle.[85] If one arm must be extended on an armboard when shoulder rests are required, prudence may require the use of only a single rest placed over the cap of the shoulder of the nonextended arm. Muscle relaxants in conjunction with SHDT may increase the chance of incurring a peripheral neuropathy.[44] When such an affliction appears, it may resolve very slowly or be permanent.

Angulating the lumbar spine to establish the hyperlordotic position introduces the possibility of elongating and compressing the great vessels on the ventral aspect of the vertebral column. The consequent obstruction of blood flow in those vessels has been implicated as the cause for increased pressure in the collateral circulation distal to that blockade and altered perfusion of intraspinal vasculature. Infarcts of the spinal cord meninges and dorsal portions of adjacent vertebrae have been reported.[17]

Arthralgia

An occasional patient may complain of sore knees or hips after being tilted head down. Most frequently this occurs after the use of bent knees and ankle straps to retain the patient in steep tilt. Forces of gravity, acting on the tilted torso, possibly stretch the capsules of the knee and hip joints because the pain seems to be greater in those patients who have had muscle relaxants. The Hewer mattress[84] (see Fig. 8–8), used mainly in England, allegedly helps prevent such pain, as does decreasing both the amount of tilt and the dose of muscle relaxant. Symptoms rarely last longer than the first several postoperative days and, while the entity is a postural complication, its appearance does not imply abandoning bent knees and ankle restraints in favor of shoulder braces or wrist straps to secure the position.

Finger Injuries

When the low lithotomy position is combined with MHDT and the arms of the patient are retained alongside the torso, fingers may be at risk of curling down over the distal edge of the mattress and intruding into the space between the thigh and leg sections of the operating table (see Chapter 6, Fig. 6–15A). When the removed leg section is replaced as the posture is terminated, or is cranked up from its depressed position to be aligned with the long axis of the table surface, fingers may be trapped between the approximating edges of the table sections. The potential exists for crushing or amputation of one or more digits. Welborn[86] has recommended that the hand be formed into a fist and wrapped in a towel to prevent intrusion of fingers into the gap between the sections of the table top (Fig. 6–15B).

Regurgitation

Although head-down tilt is commonly used in the emergency treatment of vomiting during resuscitation, or during either anesthetic induction or emergence, concern has existed that tilt itself could provoke regurgitation.[5] Heijka's group[87] measured gastric, lower esophageal, and barrier pressures in the supine, moderate, and steep head-down positions in 10 healthy female subjects during balanced anesthesia. Except for a slight rise in intragastric pressure in steep tilt no significant changes in measurements were associated with changes in position. They concluded that SHDT should not predispose to regurgitation in healthy patients. Although these observations are reassuring, the possibility of occult regurgitation should be kept in mind when an anesthetized or obtunded patient is tilted steeply head down.

Pre-existing Hazards

Several pre-existing medical conditions are relative contraindications to the use of head-down tilt. These include the following:

- A ruptured viscus, where free pus may be present in the abdominal cavity
- A head injury or brain tumor that increases intracranial pressure
- Glaucoma
- Congestive heart failure
- A thoracic injury that compromises pulmonary physiology

- Entities that cause increased intra-abdominal pressure, such as extreme obesity, pregnancy in the last trimester, and ascites. Whereas compressed gas insufflation, used to distend the abdomen for laparoscopic procedures, seems to be reasonably well tolerated by most patients, the disturbing trend toward longer procedures, steeper tilt, and possibly higher intra-abdominal distention needs to be carefully monitored to determine its limiting factors.

PRACTICAL CONSIDERATIONS

1. Because it has proved ineffective and actually detrimental in the treatment of hypotension, no version of head-down tilt is useful as a "shock position."

2. The patient with coronary artery disease who is placed in MDHT for the insertion of catheters into central veins usually experiences an undesirable increase in myocardial oxygen demand. Electrocardiographic monitoring should be carefully regarded when patients with coronary artery disease require head-down tilt.

3. Most patients without pre-existing cardiac, respiratory, or cerebral disease may be operated on in head-down tilt without problems due to the posture itself.

4. Head-down tilt should be used only if it enhances surgical exposure and thereby shortens the operating time, or if it prevents blood loss.

5. The tilted patient should be secured in place on the operating table either by a special friction mattress (Hewer type,[84] see Fig 8–8) or by flexed knees plus ankle straps that are applied over adequate padding (see Fig. 8–11C).

6. The patient in SHDT who is restrained by anklets should be carefully positioned on the operating table (see Fig. 8–11) so that neither tension on the knee joints nor pressure on the calves of the legs is exaggerated when the foot section of the table is lowered.

7. Special care must be given to positioning the arms so that the brachial plexus is neither stretched nor compressed.

- Palms should be supinated if arms are extended on boards or should contact the lateral thighs if arms are placed alongside the torso. The intention is to avoid pressure on the ulnar nerve at the elbow as well as to avoid external rotation of the humeral heads that can threaten the axillary neurovascular bundle.
- Alternatively, the arms can be folded across the chest if pressure can be kept off of the cubital tunnel and its contained ulnar nerve.
- Even though not proven effective,[88] prudence suggests that pads should be applied about the elbow to minimize pressure on the ulnar nerve, particularly when an upper extremity is retained alongside the torso.

8. If an arm must be placed out to the side on an armboard, the long axis of the humerus should be abducted less than 90 degrees from the sagittal plane of the body and the weight of the elbow should be supported by the olecranon process of the ulna. Restraining straps should be used to prevent the arm from falling off the armboard or the palm from pronating to rest the elbow on the cubital tunnel. Even though known to be less than 100% effective in nerve protection, padding should be used to distribute pressure away from the cubital tunnel and the contained ulnar nerve.[88]

9. Shoulder braces should be avoided if at all possible. On the rare occasion when they must be used, they should be placed laterally so that their pressure is on the area of the acromioclavicular articulation and not directly on either the clavicle or the root of the neck.

10. The head should remain in the midline with padding under the occiput. Lateral flexion of the neck increases the chances of repositioning the endotracheal tube into a bronchus or stretching the contralateral brachial plexus. If minimal repositioning of the head is necessary as a precaution against occipital pressure alopecia during protracted surgery, the degree of rotation should not be extreme and axillary breath sounds should be rechecked to assure acceptable bilateral ventilation in the new position.

11. The trachea should be intubated during general anesthesia so that positive-pressure breathing may be given safely. Because the tube position may change as the patient is tilted, auscultation should be used to assure ventilation of all lung lobes whenever the position of the patient is changed.

12. Ventilation should be assisted or controlled in such a manner as to enhance gas exchange while minimizing interference with cerebral venous return.

13. Blood loss should be monitored carefully to prevent unrecognized hypovolemia and avoid hypotension as the patient is returned to the horizontal position.

14. SHDT, the Trendelenburg position, imposes physiologic stresses on the patient and has the potential for injury. Its use must be considered a special technique. It can be a safe adjunct to anesthesia and surgical treatment, but it obligates the surgeon to be quick and the anesthetist to be vigilant.

PREANESTHETIC EVALUATION

Patients scheduled for lengthy surgical procedures in head-down tilt should be screened in the preanesthetic visit for evidence of significant cardiac, respiratory, or intracranial pathologic processes. If a problem is found, either careful medical evaluation should be obtained to assure that the condition is stable and will not benefit from further preoperative therapy or an alternate position should be decided on. Pertinent information about potential problems with tilting the patient should be documented in the preanesthetic record so that others involved in management of the anesthetic may easily perceive the situation. In most instances, discussions of anesthetic risk should be held with the patient.

When leg holders are to be used for an extended period of time with the patient in tilted low lithotomy, a model should be selected that will stabilize the lower extremity without either compressing the calf or the popliteal fossa. Elective, controlled hypotension as a measure of minimizing loss of blood volume during prolonged periods of tilted low lithotomy is a technique that should be regarded as potentially dangerous and should be applied only when its absence constitutes a demonstrably greater risk.

REFERENCES

1. Editorial: Friedrich Trendelenburg (1844–1924). Trendelenburg's position. JAMA 207:1143, 1969.
2. Miller AH: Surgical posture with symbols for its record on the anesthetist's chart. Anesthesiology 1:241, 1940.
3. Meyer W: Uber die Nachbehandlund des hohen Steinschnittes sowie uber Verwenbarkeit desselben zur Operation von Blasenscheidenfisteln. Arch Klin Chir 31:494, 1885.
4. Trendelenburg F: Ueber Flasenscheidenfistel operationen und ueber Beckenhochlagerung bei Operationen in der Bauchhole. Sammlung Klinischer Vortrage 335:3373, 1890. Translated in Medical Classics 4:964, 1940.
5. Inglis JM, Brooke BN: Trendelenburg tilt: An obsolete position. BMJ 11:343, 1956.
6. Porter WT: Shock at the front. Boston Med Surg J 175:854, 1916.
7. Henderson Y, Haggard HW: The circulation in man in the head-down position and a method for measuring the venous return to the heart. J Pharmacol Exp Ther 11:189, 1918.
8. Cannon WB: Traumatic Shock. New York, Appleton & Co., 1923.
9. Cole F: Head lowering in the treatment of hypotension. JAMA 150:273, 1952.
10. Weil MH: Current concepts on the management of shock. Circulation 16:1097, 1957.
11. Weil MH: Whigham H: Head-down (Trendelenburg) position for treatment of irreversible hemorrhagic shock: Experimental study in rats. Ann Surg 162:905, 1965.
12. Taylor J, Weil MH: Failure of the Trendelenburg position to improve circulation during clinical shock. Surg Gynecol Obstet 124:1005, 1967.
13. Sibbald WJ, Patterson NAM, Holliday RL, et al.: The Trendelenburg position: Hemodynamic effects in hypotensive and normotensive patients. Crit Care Med 7:218, 1979.
14. Kubal K, Komatsu T, Sanchala V, et al.: Trendelenburg position used during venous cannulation increases myocardial oxygen demand. Anesth Analg 63:239, 1984 (abstract).
15. Martin JT: The Trendelenburg position: A review of current slants about head-down tilt. JAANA 63:29, 1995.
16. Collins VJ: Principles of Anesthesiology, p 163. Philadelphia, Lea & Febiger, 1976.
17. Dorland's Illustrated Medical Dictionary, 27th ed. Philadelphia, WB Saunders, 1988.
18. Lloyd-Davies OV: Lithotomy-Trendelenburg position for resection of rectum and lower pelvic colon. Lancet 2:74, 1939.
19. Amoiridis G, Wohrle JC, Langkafel M, et al.: Spinal cord infarction after surgery in a patient in the hyperlordotic position. Anesthesiology 84:228, 1996.
20. Robertson JD: Anaesthesia in abdominal surgery. In Evans FT, Gray TC (eds.): General Anaesthesia: Clinical Practice, 2nd ed. vol. 2. Washington, DC, Butterworth & Co., 1965.
21. Wood-Smith FG: Postoperative brachial plexus paralysis. BMJ 1:1115, 1952.
22. Stark DCC: Practical Points in Anesthesiology. Flushing, NY, Medical Examination Publishing Co., 1974.
23. McLachlin AD, Stavraky WK, Sweeney JP: Venous stasis in the lithotomy-Trendelenburg position. Can J Surg 10:414, 1967.
24. Schiller WR: The Trendelenburg position: Surgical aspects. In Martin JT (ed.): Positioning in Anesthesia and Surgery, 2nd ed. Philadelphia, WB Saunders, 1987.
25. Wilkins RW, Bradley SE, Friedland CK: The acute circulatory effects in the head-down position (negative G) in normal man, with a note on some measures designed to relieve cranial congestion in this position. J Clin Invest 29:940, 1950.
26. Guntheroth WG, Abel FL, Mullins GL: The effect of Trendelenburg's position on blood pressure and carotid flow. Surg Gynecol Obstet 119:345, 1964.
27. Dripps RD, Comroe JH Jr: Circulatory physiology: The adjustment to blood loss and postural changes. Surg Clin North Am 26:1368, 1946.

28. Little DM Jr: Posture and anesthesia. Can Anaesth Soc J 7:2, 1960.
29. Abel FL, Pierce JH, Guntheroth WG: Baroreceptor influence on postural changes in blood pressure and carotid blood flow. Am J Physiol 205:360, 1963.
30. Gentili DR, Benjamin E, Berger SR, Iberti TJ: Cardiopulmonary effects of the head-down tilt position in elderly postoperative patients: A prospective study. South Med J 81:1258, 1988.
31. Armstrong PJ, Sutherland R, Scott DH: The effect of position and different maneuvers on internal jugular vein diameter size. Acta Anesthesiol Scand 38:229, 1994.
32. Keusch DJ, Winters S, Thys DM: The patient's position influences the incidence of dysrhythmias during pulmonary artery catheterization. Anesthesiology 70:582, 1989.
33. Baraka A, Baroody M, Haroun S, et al.: Pulmonary artery catheterization in the anesthetized patient: Correspondence. Anesthesiology 72:390, 1990.
34. Reich DL, Konstadt SN, Raissi S, et al.: Trendelenburg position and passive leg raising do not significantly improve cardiopulmonary performance in the anesthetized patient with coronary artery disease. Crit Care Med 17:313, 1989.
35. Sing FR, O'Hara D, Sawyer MA, Marino PL: Trendelenburg position and oxygen transport in hypovolemic adults. Ann Emerg Med 23:564, 1994.
36. Dripps RD: Anesthesia. In Rhoads JE, Allen JG, Harkins HN, Moyer CA, (eds.): Surgery: Principles and Practice, 4th ed. Philadelphia, JB Lippincott, 1970.
37. Deklunder G, Lecroart JL, Chammas E, et al.: Intracardiac hemodynamics in man during short periods of head-down and head-up tilt. Aviat Space Environ Med 64:43, 1994.
38. Tomaselli CM, Kenney RA, Frey MA, Hoffler GW: Cardiovascular dynamics during the initial period of head-down tilt. Aviat Space Environ Med 58:3, 1987.
39. Enderby GEH: Postural ischaemia and blood pressure. Lancet 1:185, 1954.
40. Little DM Jr: Controlled hypotension. In Anesthesia and Surgery. Springfield, IL, Charles C Thomas, 1956.
41. Martin JT: Compartment syndromes: Concepts and Perspectives for the anesthesiologist. Anesth Analg 75:275, 1992.
42. Johannsen G, Andersen M, Juhl B: The effect of general anaesthesia on the haemodynamic events during laparoscopy with CO_2 insufflation. Acta Anaesthesiol Scand 33:132, 1989.
43. Loeppky JA, Hirshfield DW, Eldridge MW: The effects of head-down tilt on carotid blood flow and pulmonary gas exchange. Aviat Space Environ Med 58:637, 1987.
44. Slocum HC, Hoeflich EA, Allen CR: Circulatory and respiratory distress from extreme positions on the operating table. Surg Gynecol Obstet 84:1051, 1947.
45. Fahy BG, Barnas GM, Flowers JL, et al.: The effects of increased abdominal pressure on lung and chest wall mechanics during laparoscopic surgery. Anesth Analg 81:744, 1995.
46. Fahy B, Barnas G, Nagle S, et al.: Effect of Trendelenburg and reverse Trendelenburg posture on lung and chest wall mechanics. Anesthesiology 83:A1224, 1995 (abstract).
47. Chiang ST, Lyons HA: The effect of postural change on pulmonary compliance. Respir Physiol 1:99, 1966.
48. Altschulte MD: The significance of changes in the lung volume and its subdivisions during and after abdominal operations. Anesthesiology 4:385, 1943.
49. Case EH, Stiles JA: The effect of various surgical positions on vital capacity. Anesthesiology 7:29, 1946.
50. West JB, Dollery CT, Naimark A: Distribution of blood flow in isolated lung: Relations to vascular and alveolar pressures. J Appl Physiol 19:713, 1964.
51. West JB: Respiratory Physiology: The Essentials. Baltimore, Williams & Wilkins, 1974.
52. Laver MB, Hallowell P, Goldblatt A: Pulmonary dysfunction secondary to heart disease: Aspects relevant to anesthesia and surgery. Anesthesiology 33:161, 1970.
53. Tweed WA, Phua WT, Chong KY, et al.: Large tidal volume ventilation improves pulmonary gas exchange during lower abdominal surgery in Trendelenburg's position. Can J Anaesth 38:989, 1991.
54. Cardus D: O_2 alveolar-arterial tension difference after 10 days recumbency in man. J Appl Physiol 23:934, 1967.
55. Loeppky JA, Scotto P, Riedel C, et al.: Cardiopulmonary responses to acute hypoxia, head-down tilt and fluid loading in anesthetized dogs. Aviat Space Environ Med 62:1137, 1991.
56. Heinonen J, Takki S, Tammisto T: Effect of the Trendelenburg tilt and other procedures on the position of endotracheal tubes. Lancet 1:850, 1969.
57. Karpinos RD, Schaffer SL, Capan LM, Turndorf H: Tracheal length in lithotomy and Trendelenburg positions. Anesthesiology 83:A1219, 1995 (abstract).
58. Pender JW, Damron JC: General anesthesia. In Preston FW, Davis WC, (eds.): Lewis' Practice of Surgery. Vol. 1. General Surgery: Introduction; General Principles. Hagerstown, MD, Harper & Row, 1969.
59. Prokocimer P, Garbino J, Wolf M, Regnier B: Influence of posture on gas exchange in artificially ventilated patients with focal lung disease. Intensive Care Med 9:69, 1983.
60. Shenkin HA, Scheuerman WG, Spitz EB, et al.: Effect of change of position upon the cerebral circulation of man. J Appl Physiol 2:317, 1949.
61. Jacobson I, Harper AM, McDowall DG: Relationship between venous pressure and cortical blood flow. Nature 200:173, 1963.
62. Kety SS, Shenkin HA, Schmidt CF: The effects of increased intracranial pressure on cerebral circulatory functions in man. J Clin Invest 27:493, 1948.
63. Harper AM, Glass HI: Effect of alterations in the arterial carbon dioxide tension on the blood flow through the cerebral cortex at normal and low arterial blood pressures. J Neurol Neurosurg Psychiatry 28:449, 1965.
64. Shenkin HA, Bouzarth WF: Clinical methods of reducing intracranial pressure: Role of the cerebral circulation. N Engl J Med 282:1465, 1970.
65. Boyan CP: Hypotensive anesthesia for radical pelvic and abdominal surgery. Arch Surg 67:803, 1953.
66. McComish PB, Bodley PO: Anaesthesia for Neurological Surgery. Chicago, Year Book Medical Publishers, 1971.
67. Langfitt TW, Weinstein JD, Kassell NF: Cerebral vasomotor paralysis produced by intracranial hypertension. Neurology 15:622, 1965.
68. Youmans JR, Albrand OW: Cerebral blood flow in clinical problems. In Youmans JR (ed.): Neurological Surgery: A Comprehensive Reference Guide to the Diagnosis and Management of Neurological Problems, vol. 2. Philadelphia, WB Saunders, 1973.
69. Hardesty WH, Roberts B, Toole JF, et al.: Studies of carotid artery blood flow in man. N Engl J Med 263:944, 1960.

70. Boldrey E, Maass L, Miller E: The role of atlantoid compression in the etiology of internal carotid thrombosis. J Neurosurg 13:127, 1956.

71. Hunter AR: Discussion on the value of controlled respiration in neurosurgery. Proc R Soc Med 53:365, 1960.

72. Satake H, Konishi T, Kawashima T, et al.: Intracranial blood flow measured with single photon emission computer tomography (SPECT) during transient −6 degrees head-down tilt. Aviat Space Environ Med 65:117, 1994.

73. Hayashi Y, Murata Y, Seo H, et al.: Modification of water and electrolyte metabolism during head-down tilting by hypoglycemia in men. J Appl Physiol 73:1785, 1992.

74. Hirose M, Hashimoto S, Tanaka Y: Effect of head-down tilt position during lower abdominal surgery on endocrine and renal function response. Anesth Analg 76:40, 1993.

75. Linder BJ, Trick GL, Wolf ML: Altering body position affects intraocular pressure and visual function. Invest Ophthalmol Vis Sci 29:1492, 1988.

76. Daly A: Quoted in Hewer CL: The physiology and complications of the Trendelenburg position. Can Med Assoc J 74:185, 1956.

77. Gartner S, Beck W: Ocular tension in the Trendelenburg position. Am J Ophthalmol 59:1040, 1965.

78. Prasad VN, Narain B, Katara GS: Intraocular tension in Trendelenburg position. J All-India Ophthalmol Soc 16:125, 1968.

79. Wyke B: Neurological principles in anaesthesia. In Evans FT, Gray TC (eds.): General Anaesthesia: Basic Principles, 2nd ed., vol. 1. Washington, DC, Butterworth & Co., 1965.

80. Slocum HC, O'Neal KC, Allen CR: Neurovascular complications from malposition on the operating table. Surg Gynecol Obstet 86:729, 1948.

81. Boyan CP, Brunschwig A: Hypotensive anesthesia in radical pelvic and abdominal surgery. Surgery 31:829, 1952.

82. Laver MB, Austen WG: Lung function: Physiologic considerations applicable to surgery. In Sabiston DC Jr (ed.): Davis-Christopher Textbook of Surgery: The Biological Basis of Modern Surgical Practice, 10th ed. Philadelphia, WB Saunders, 1972.

83 Flagg PJ: The Art of Anaesthesia. Philadelphia, JB Lippincott, 1916.

84. Hewer CL: Maintenance of the Trendelenburg position by skin friction. Lancet 1:522, 1953.

85. Clausen EG: Postoperative ("anesthetic") paralysis of the brachial plexus: A review of the literature and report of nine cases. Surgery 12:933, 1942.

86. Welborn SG: The lithotomy position: Anesthesiologic considerations. In Martin JT (ed.): Positioning in Anesthesia and Surgery, 2nd ed. Philadelphia, WB Saunders, 1987.

87. Heijke SA, Smith G, Key A: The effect of the Trendelenburg position on lower oesophageal sphincter tone. Anaesthesia 46:185, 1991.

88. Kroll DA, Caplan RA, Posner K, et al.: Nerve injury associated with anesthesia. Anesthesiology 73:202, 1990.

Lateral Decubitus Positions

Chapter 9

Lateral Positions

Noel W. Lawson / D. Joseph Meyer, Jr.

BACKGROUND

Decubitus, derived from the Latin, means "a lying down." *Dorland's Illustrated Medical Dictionary* defines *decubitus position* as "the position of an individual lying on a horizontal surface, designated according to the portion of the body resting on the surface..."[1] The terms *lateral decubitus, lateral,* and *lateral recumbent* are synonymous, but general usage has favored *lateral decubitus* in describing surgical positions. The lateral decubitus position is conventionally referred to as right or left according to the side on which the patient has been placed. For example, a right lateral decubitus position is one in which the patient lies on the right side and is suitably arranged for surgery with the left side uppermost (Fig. 9–1).

A highly significant issue concerns the coupling of the adjectives *decubitus* and *lateral* when describing *any* lateral position. In the absence of that nomenclature, terming a posture as the *right chest position* allows indecision as to whether the patient should lie on the right chest or whether the surgeon intends to operate on the right lung, an impossible accomplishment if the *right chest position* is interpreted as having the right side down. But use of the proper descriptor, *right lateral decubitus position,* eliminates that type of confusion and protects both the patient and the care team from wrong-sided intervention. Nevertheless, the jargon can become unwieldy when applied to special circumstances, such as flexed lateral positions. Before the patient is positioned, all members of the care team must deliberately re-identify which bilateral organ is the surgical target and ensure its accessibility.

Figure 9–1

Standard right lateral decubitus position. *Top.* Lateral position without padding or head support. Neck angulation threatens perfusion of head and stresses brachial plexus. *Bottom.* Proper padding over bony prominences; chest pad protects down-side shoulder without compromising axilla. Note proper alignment of cervical spine. Flexed lower leg stabilizes torso against ventral tilt.

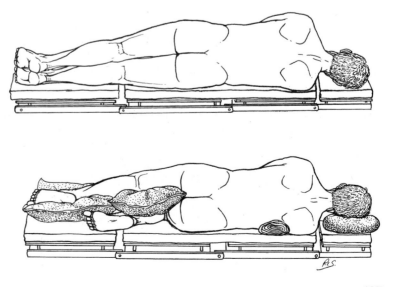

In the interests of clarity, the terms *up-side* and *down-side* are used in this chapter even though their repetition creates clumsy reading. They describe more clearly the side in question than do terms such as *dependent* and *superior*. *Dependent* is used to identify something that hangs down, such as the legs in the lateral jackknife position.

J. Marion Sims, a noted New York obstetrician and gynecologist of the middle nineteenth century, described the first extensive use of the lateral decubitus position for obstetric deliveries and surgical procedures (Fig. 9–2).[2] Thoracic surgery emerged almost a century after Sims' contribution. Its development paralleled that of anesthesia, which included the evolution of patient positioning to gain surgical access and the understanding of problems caused by an open pneumothorax. An extensive review of the history of thoracic anesthesia, though extremely interesting, is beyond the scope of this discussion and is covered in an earlier edition of this text.[3]

The lateral decubitus position has been associated most commonly with thoracotomies for cardiothoracic procedures but is often used to advantage for renal, obstetric, gynecologic, neurosurgical, and orthopedic operations. Orthopedists have used the lateral decubitus position extensively for total hip replacement as well as open reduction of hip fractures. Neurosurgeons may request the lateral decubitus position either for a craniotomy or for a laminectomy at any level of the vertebral column. The abdomen is freely mobile with the patient in the lateral decubitus position; thus, a laminectomy or craniotomy is less likely to be hampered by epidural or intracranial venous engorgement than might be the case in the prone position.[4] For surgeons who operate with the assistance of enlarging lenses, edema, caused by venous congestion, increases light reflection and distorts vision. As surgery is performed more frequently with the aid of a microscope or magnifiers, the issue increases in importance. The lateral position can also obviate the need for the sometimes bizarre prone positions that

have been proposed to minimize peridural venous pressure.[5, 6] Thus, there are many variations of the lateral decubitus position, each being selected according to purpose and each presenting peculiarities and advantages.[7]

THE LATERAL DECUBITUS POSITION AND ITS MODIFICATIONS

The Classic Lateral Decubitus Position

Patient positioning in the early days of lung surgery was dictated more by the necessity to control the direction of spillage of pulmonary secretions than by the need to provide the best access to the operative site.[8] However, development of endobronchial blockers and double-lumen endotracheal tubes has obviated these spillage concerns, allowing postural choices that more easily facilitate the surgery.[9] The standard lateral decubitus position has been widely accepted (see Fig. 9–1).

The lateral decubitus position optimizes surgical conditions for most thoracic operations. Most often a 90-degree angle is established between the patient's back and the surface of the surgical table (see Fig. 9–1).[3] This position is standard for most lung operations such as pneumonectomy, lobectomy, bronchoplasty, and decortication. It is also used for a variety of cardiovascular procedures, including division of a patent ductus arteriosus, resection of an aortic coarctation, and a mitral valve commissurotomy. The lateral decubitus position permits the most complete access to one hemithorax through an intercostal incision. The level of the intercostal incision may be varied from high in the axilla to resect the first rib in a thoracic outlet syndrome to a location that is more caudad on the chest wall for esophageal or diaphragmatic procedures. There are three standard variations of the intercostal incision that provide additional access to thoracic structures at any level when combined with positioning.

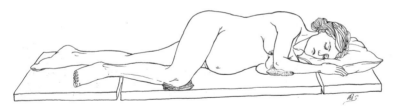

Figure 9–2

The lateral Sims position. Flexed upper leg affords access to the perineum while stabilizing the torso.

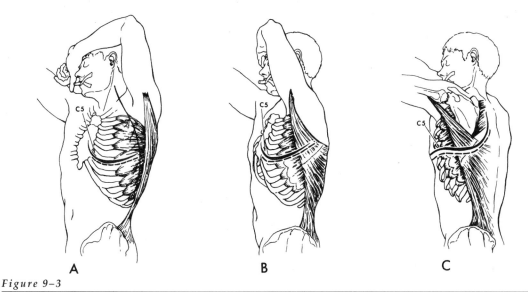

Figure 9–3

Standard thoracic incisions. *A.* Anterior. *B.* Lateral. *C.* Posterolateral. Figures indicate need to position ipsilateral upper extremity out of the surgical field without injuring the axillary neurovascular bundle. (From Alley RD: Thoracic surgical incisions and postoperative drainage. *In* Cooper P [ed.]: The Craft of Surgery. © 1964. Published by Little, Brown and Company.)

These are the anterior (anterolateral), lateral, and posterolateral approaches (Fig. 9–3).[3]

The anterior incision preserves the long thoracic nerve and latissimus dorsi muscle; the lateral incision divides these structures. The posterolateral incision, or "scapular displacing" incision, requires division of the rhomboid and trapezius muscle.[10] Standard intercostal incisions may be combined with, or extended to, other incisions in the neck, abdomen, or groin. Thoracoabdominal incisions offer access for major liver trauma, thoracoabdominal aortic aneurysms, or gastroesophageal disease.

Tilting of the operating table, or changing the obliquity of the back to the table through 45 and 135 degrees can provide additional access to the ipsilateral mediastinum, pericardium, hilum of the lung, or gastroesophageal junction (see Fig. 9–3). The lateral decubitus position is the base from which special oblique positions are developed to provide access for both neck and chest or thorax and abdomen. For example, if the thoracic aorta must be cross clamped, the thorax may be positioned at 90 degrees, but the pelvis may be tilted dorsad to less than 90 degrees to facilitate cannulation of femoral vessels. This technique has proven useful for aortofemoral shunting as might be required for repair of a descending thoracic aortic aneurysm, dissection of the aorta, or traumatic aortic disruption.[3]

Flexed Lateral Positions

With the patient in the classic lateral decubitus position, the table top and its attachments can be adjusted to produce two versions of lateral flexion.

The lateral jackknife position: With the patient in the classic lateral decubitus position the back-thigh hinge of the table top is bent to form an acute angle, opening floorward, with its apex located under the iliac crest. After restraining tapes are placed to stabilize the patient, the table chassis is tilted sufficiently to return the long axis of the torso to a level (horizontal) position and increase the dependency of the lower extremities (see Fig. 9–5).

The kidney position: In this version of lateral flexion, the angulation of the table surface is identical to that of the lateral jackknife position but the transverse elevating bar of the table (commonly referred to as the "kidney rest") is raised under the downside iliac crest to increase the acuteness of the patient's lateral bend. Leveling of the long axis of the torso may or may not occur.

The Lateral Jackknife Position

Some thoracic surgeons prefer this position (Fig. 9–4) as a means of increasing the distance between the up-side iliac crest and the adjacent costal margin, stretching the flank

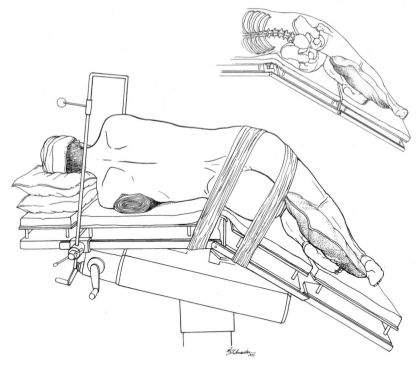

Figure 9–4

The lateral jackknife position. With the torso level, the lowered legs are intended to pull open the up-side intercostal spaces. The flexion point of the table top is shown properly located at the down-side iliac crest to allow rotation of the pelvic brim away from the rib cage, as the legs are lowered. Hip straps are anchored to thrust cephalad, as depicted, to prevent caudad slippage of the iliac crest, consequent compression of the flank at the flexion point (see text for discussion), and potential caval compromise due to angulation of the lumbar spine (*inset*).

muscles, and causing the intercostal spaces of the up-side hemithorax to be pulled open farther than is the case in the classic (non-flexed) lateral decubitus position.

However, the physiologic costs of the position can easily be very high. Furthermore, once the intercostal space is incised and held open by retractors, most of the postural help with exposure is ended. Closure of the incision usually requires that the lateral flexion be terminated.

An immediate reduction in pulmonary compliance will become evident to the experienced team member whose hand is on the breathing bag when the up-side flank is drawn taut by lateral flexion of the trunk. The result is a reduction in functional residual capacity beyond that inherent in the standard lateral decubitus position (see Physiology of the Lateral Decubitus Position).

The dependent extremities immediately pool approximately 1 unit of blood in an adult.[11] Lateral flexion may obstruct venous return by postural compression or occlusion of the inferior vena cava at the "break point"

of the table. This phenomenon is more frequent when the patient is placed in the right lateral decubitus position rather than in the left, apparently due to the proximity of the inferior vena cava to the right flank.[12] The combination of caval obstruction and venous pooling can produce a precipitous fall in blood pressure.

Hydrostatic forces of the dependent extremities can cause a surreptitious volume deficit as lower extremity edema ("third spacing") develops during a lengthy surgical procedure. As a result, additional infusion volume may be required to support the circulation during the operation. Once the supine position is resumed postoperatively, this volume will mobilize and the resultant hypervolemia can then become detrimental to the patient with cardiovascular compromise.

Because of these significant problems, the lateral jackknife position has fallen into general disuse, although it still may be requested for special cases. It can be employed safely by the wary, but routine or casual use is fraught with hazards.

The Flexed Lateral (Kidney) Position

Urologists usually employ a modified lateral decubitus position for renal surgery. Colloquially referred to as the "kidney position" or the "nephrectomy position," it is another flexed version of the lateral decubitus position. The additional lateral angulation caused by elevating the kidney rest until the up-side flank is taut imposes such severe skeletal stresses and ventilatory restrictions that most unanesthetized individuals cannot achieve the posture at all. Hence, musculoskeletal complaints are not unexpected after use of the kidney position. They may be attributed erroneously to the anesthetic technique rather than to the stresses of the position.

The surgeon intends to avoid entering either the pleural or peritoneal cavities during renal surgery. The most frequent surgical route to the kidney is from its lateral aspect (Fig. 9–5). The lateral approach necessitates (1) dividing the great muscles of the flank, (2) avoiding intercostal nerves and vessels, (3) avoiding both the pleura posteriorly and the peritoneum anteriorly, and (4) vigorously using retractors to enlarge the space between the twelfth rib and the iliac crest. Despite all these efforts, the resulting exposure is frequently adequate only for the lower pole of the kidney.[13]

The lateral approach includes the classic

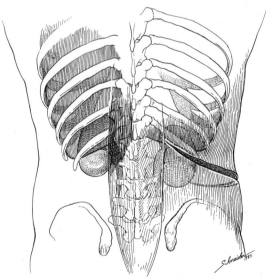

Figure 9–5

The attachments of the diaphragm in relation to the twelfth rib. Note the potential for a pneumothorax because the pleural cavity can be entered through the diaphragm at the dorsal end of the flank incision.

subcostal twelfth rib resection, an eleventh intercostal space incision, a dorsolumbar flap, and various combined thoracoabdominal incisions (see Fig. 9–5). All of these approaches validate the need for the patient to be placed on the operating table in the flexed version of the lateral decubitus position.

The patient is placed in the chosen lateral decubitus position, and the table is flexed at the level of iliac crest instead of under the flank or lower ribs, as is frequently the case with the lateral jackknife position (Fig. 9–6). Usually the surgeon requests that the kidney rest be elevated as well. In contrast to the minimal advantages of the lateral jackknife position, these maneuvers achieve the purpose of significantly separating the iliac crest from the lateral costal margin. Improved kidney exposure can be obtained with minimal danger of violating either the pleural or peritoneal cavities. Fear of entering the pleural and peritoneal cavities is probably unwarranted. Although complications are rarely seen, the anesthesiologist must always consider pneumothorax in the event that cardiovascular or respiratory compromise develops. Smith and co-workers[14] demonstrated that opening the peritoneal cavity is associated with no more morbidity than not opening the cavity.

The debate regarding the best placement of the patient over the kidney rest is mostly of historical interest. Flocks and Culp[15] advocated a posture that allowed the kidney rest to strike just above the iliac crest (see Fig. 9–6A). Smith and co-workers[14] recommended positioning the twelfth rib over the kidney rest (see Fig. 9–6B). Finally, Grayhack and Graham[16] recommend that the kidney rest be placed directly under the iliac crest (see Fig. 9–6C). All variations of the lateral decubitus position have been shown to decrease vital capacity.[17] Elevation of the kidney rest into the soft tissues cephalad to the down-side iliac crest compresses the flank and restricts descent of the ipsilateral hemidiaphragm. This flank encroachment in the right lateral decubitus position might directly compress the vena cava and impede venous return in a manner similar to that of the right lateral jackknife position. Extreme left lateral deflection could stretch and narrow the vena cava and decrease venous return. A decreased cardiac output is the result of either malposition. Most anesthesiologists today recognize that placing the kidney rest directly beneath the down-side iliac crest offers the least interfer-

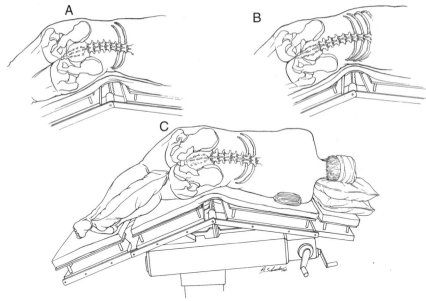

Figure 9–6

Flexed lateral decubitus (kidney) position. *A.* The point of flexion (kidney rest) is placed in the down-side flank cephalad to the iliac crest, restricting the descent of the down-side hemidiaphragm. *B.* Placement of kidney rest beneath the down-side eleventh and twelfth ribs, adding compression of the lower thorax to the diaphragmatic obstruction of *A. C.* The kidney rest properly placed beneath the down-side iliac crest, offering the least interference with the functions of the down-side lung and diaphragm.

ence with the functions of the down-side lung and diaphragm.[13]

Renal surgery in the pediatric population presents many of the same problems and hazards that are seen in adults. However, the child does not seem to require as extreme a degree of flexion as does the adult, nor does the posture create as many physiologic stresses.[13] (Further information about pediatric positioning can be found in Chapter 15.)

The Semiprone Position

A modification of the lateral decubitus position is referred to variously as the *semiprone, left lateral prone,* or *post-tonsillectomy* position (Fig. 9–7; see also Fig. 20–1). It is indistinguishable from that prescribed by Sims in 1857 (see Fig. 9–2).[2] While the semiprone position is occasionally required for a surgical procedure, its most common use is to aid in maintaining a clear airway in the awakening patient.

The Sims Position

Sims used the position that he described during successful repair of vesicovaginal fistulae (see Fig. 9–2). It was adapted to general obstetric procedures and remained popular for many years. In the recent past its popularity has waned markedly.

The classic Sims position is established by placing the patient in the left lateral decubitus position with the lower leg extended and slightly flexed at the knee (see Fig. 9–2). The upper leg is flexed at the hip and the knee, imparting a measure of stability to the patient. The torso is allowed to rotate forward to further stabilize the position. A significant difference between the Sims position and the standard lateral decubitus position is the arrangement of the legs. The down-side lower extremity is flexed in the standard lateral decubitus position for increased stability, whereas the up-side lower extremity is flexed in the Sims position to help stabilize ventral tilt and facilitate perineal exposure (compare Fig. 9–2 with Fig. 9–1).

The advantage of the Sims position in obstetrics is that the perineum is in full view and more accessible than is the case with either the currently popular lithotomy position or birthing chairs.[18] The Sims position is also more comfortable for vaginal delivery in women who have pelvic joint pathology. Most of these women relate that this position was their preferred posture for intercourse. Its additional advantages include avoidance

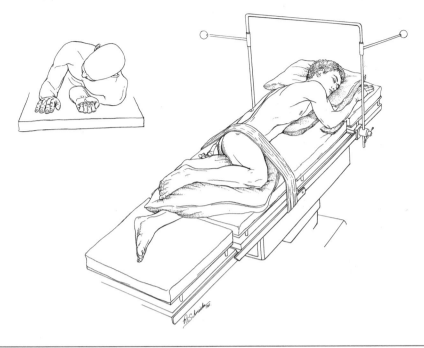

Figure 9–7

The semiprone position. Usual placement for the down-side arm is behind the torso. Axillary compression is risked in the posture of the down-side arm (*inset*). Flexed upper leg stabilizes the semiprone torso (compare with legs in Fig. 9-1).

of the supine hypotensive syndrome and diminished danger of maternal aspiration.

The Sims position has been found to be effective in performing proctosigmoidoscopy and rectovaginal examination as well as vaginal delivery.[19] Perhaps a lack of suitable recent descriptions and experienced personnel has impeded the rediscovery of this position. Furthermore, the advent of regional anesthesia for labor and delivery has precluded its use. Spinal or epidural anesthesia is a relative contraindication for delivery or examination in this position because the patient must be in control of her lower extremities to maintain this inherently unstable position. In addition, currently the Sims position is not deemed suitable for complicated deliveries.

Willis[20] notes that a modified Sims position is a curled lateral decubitus position with the knees together and the vertebral column flexed to permit widening of the interlaminar spaces (Fig. 9–8). Although not employed as a surgical posture, it is useful to the anesthesiologist for establishment of epidural and spinal anesthesia.

The Semisupine Position

Historically, mitral commissurotomy was most often performed with the patient in a modified lateral decubitus position called the semisupine position. The thorax was allowed to roll dorsally about 40 to 50 degrees into a semisupine position (Fig. 9–9) and carefully stabilized.

The up-side arm, raised over the head to rotate the scapula out of the thoracotomy field, was fixed to an appropriate support in a manner that protected the brachial neurovascular structures from stretch or occlusion.

Combined Lateral Decubitus and Supine Position

Repair of intracardiac and aortic defects during the same surgical procedure may require multiple changes of the patient's position. A median sternotomy is necessary for the cardiac repair and access to the aortic root, whereas a left thoracotomy is required to approach the descending aorta.

Changing the position of the patient is both time consuming and detrimental to maintaining a sterile field. Iwa and co-workers[21] have described a method by which the patient is placed in a right lateral decubitus position and then adjusted to a 45-degree semisupine position (Fig. 9–10). Stability is achieved by straps and Vacu-Pacs (Olympic

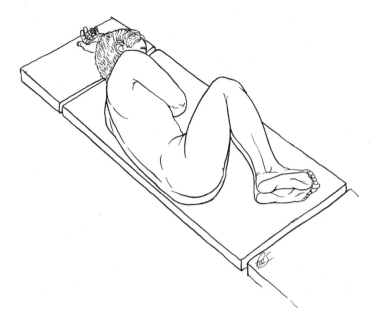

Figure 9-8

The modified Sims position is often referred to as the curled lateral decubitus position and is useful in establishment of subarachnoid and epidural anesthesia. (Full padding deleted for clarity.)

Medical, Seattle, WA) or "bean bags" (see Stability, Supports, Restraints, and Precautions). The fully supine position for sternotomy is attained by rotating the table top 45 degrees to the left. Conveniently changing the patient to a 60-degree semisupine lateral decubitus position simply requires that the table be leveled and then rotated to the right an additional 15 degrees. This multipostural arrangement has been employed by these investigators for (1) the Rastelli operation for pseudotruncus, with communication from the descending aorta; (2) radical surgery for the tetralogy of Fallot, with giant bronchial arteries; (3) coarctation of the aorta, with a ventricular septal defect; (4) corrective surgery for aortic arch aneurysms; and (5) dissecting aneurysms.

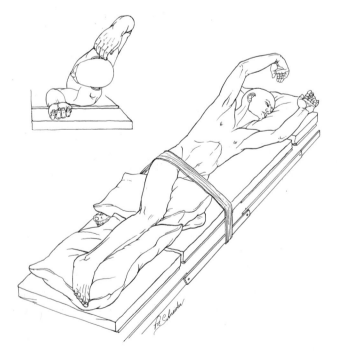

Figure 9-9

The semisupine position. The up-side arm is shown in a classic thoracotomy position, which rotates the scapula out of the surgical field. (Appropriate support mechanism is deleted; full padding deleted for clarity.) It may also be placed on the pillow next to the face. An equally effective position for the up-side arm during thoracotomy is shown in Figure 9-13.

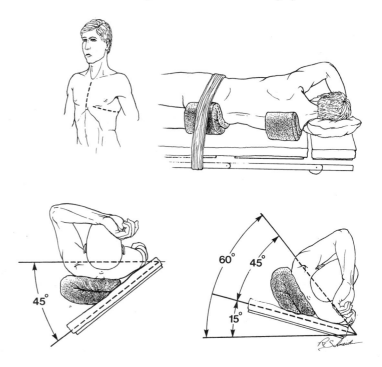

Figure 9–10

Operations requiring both a median sternotomy (in the supine position) and a left thoracotomy (in the right lateral decubitus position) can be facilitated by adjusting the table rather than moving the patient. The patient is stabilized firmly in the right lateral semisupine position on a level table. Tilting the table top to either side can alternately expose the sternal and lateral thoracic surgical fields with minimal risk to sterile conditions. (Redrawn from Iwa T, Nagai A, Yoshida C: Positioning for simultaneous intracardiac repair and/or ascending aorta and descending aorta surgery. Jpn J Surg 2:385, 1981.)

ESTABLISHING THE LATERAL DECUBITUS POSITION

General Considerations

All of the preceding variations of the lateral decubitus position must begin with the basic position. Because the lateral decubitus position is inherently unstable, it places the relaxed anesthetized patient at considerable risk for pressure and stretch damage. Therefore, careful attention to detail is crucial in establishing the position.

The side of the surgery must be specified on the consent document and in the record of the preanesthetic evaluation; it should be confirmed by the patient whenever practical. A person who is involved in the administration of the anesthetic must discuss the desired position with a knowledgeable member of the surgical team before induction.

The patient is transferred from the transporting stretcher to the operating table and remains supine until venous access, induction of anesthesia, endotracheal intubation, and appropriate monitoring are established.

Many methods have been proposed for placing patients in the lateral decubitus position. However, the manner in which it is accomplished is often more dictated by the circumstances rather than rote methodology. If several general principles are followed, the posture can be attained with little risk of sequelae.

- The first general principle identifies the anesthesiologist as the most appropriate person to coordinate the move. This choice relates to the need to control the airway; manage the intravenous infusion and monitoring devices; and protect the relaxed head, neck, and extremities during the turn. The possibility of injury to the relaxed neck is sufficient justification alone to assign the management of the move to the anesthesiologist. Once the posture is established, refinements can be directed by the surgeon.
- The second important principle is that the shoulders and pelvis of the paralyzed anesthetized patients must be maintained in the same plane during the turn to avoid torsional stress on the spine. Simultaneously, the anesthesiologist protects the head and neck.
- The third principle requires two team members plus the anesthesiologist as a minimum number of persons needed for a safe turn. Specific problems such as obesity, fracture, and serious joint disease necessitate additional help.

To turn a patient from supine into the left lateral decubitus position, two assistants, excluding the anesthesiologist, may place them-

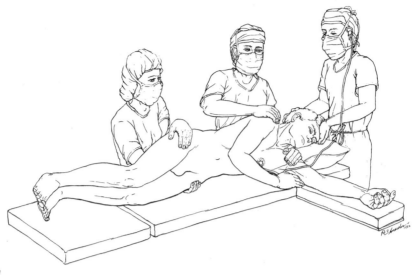

Figure 9–11

The stations of the assistants and the arrangements of their hands are demonstrated at the conclusion of the turning of a patient into the left lateral decubitus position. Note control of the head by the anesthesiologist.

selves beside the patient in one of several configurations. One may stand on each side of the table or they may stand together at the same side of the patient. The latter is less confining in coordinating the move and, for clarity, the turn is described with both positioning assistants at the right side of the supine patient.

The Turning Technique

The turn starts by abducting the patient's arm that will eventually be on the down side to avoid its being trapped under the trunk after completing the turn. A left lateral decubitus position would start with the left arm abducted. One assistant is responsible for the patient's hips (the hip assistant), the other for the shoulders (the shoulder assistant).

If both assistants are on the right side of the patient, the shoulder assistant places his or her left hand under the patient's neck and grasps the opposite (left) shoulder (Fig 9–11). That assistant's right hand is placed on the patient's right shoulder. Placement of the hand across the neck to the left shoulder is not acceptable, because this encroaches on the airway during movement. The hip assistant, meanwhile, passes his or her right hand under the patient's hips to grasp the pelvis in the area of the left anterior iliac crest. The assistant's left hand is placed on the right anterior iliac crest. This allows the hip assistant to face the other positioning team member and remain in visual contact with the patient during the move (see Fig. 9–11). This visual contact would not be possible if hand placement were reversed.

The anesthesiologist may rotate the patient's head toward the direction of the turn, to the left in this example, before moving the torso; this maintains the stability of the airway. However, if a cervical spine pathologic process is present, the head should be kept in the sagittal plane and moved simultaneously with the torso.

After the assistants indicate that they are ready, the anesthesiologist identifies the signal for starting the turn (e.g., "turn on the count of three"). At that signal, the move into the lateral decubitus position is achieved by simultaneously pulling on the patient's down-side or left hip and shoulder and pushing on the up-side or right hip and shoulder. Once in the lateral decubitus position, stability can be maintained by the hand of a team member being placed on the patient's up-side hip or shoulder while the extremities are satisfactorily rearranged. Then this basic position is further refined to suit the requirements of the particular procedure.

The left lateral decubitus position can also be achieved with both assistants on the left side of the supine patient. On the "turn" signal, the shoulder and hip assistants push on the down-side shoulder and hip and pull on the corresponding up-side parts.

A third approach is for the shoulder assistant to stand on the side toward which the turn will be made. The hip assistant is on the opposite side of the table. This technique is a combination of the two previous methods. However, it has the advantage of placing an assistant on each side of the patient with one controlling the arms and the other controlling the legs. It is especially applicable when the patient is obese, and additional assistants are required. Conflicts regarding space are avoided, and the possibility of the patient's falling from the table in either direction is minimized.

Stability, Supports, Restraints, and Precautions

Stability of the pelvis can be enhanced by flexing the lower leg at the hip and knee while the upper leg is straightened (see Fig. 9–1). This positioning can be done by the hip assistant while the shoulder assistant stabilizes the patient. Additional stability can be achieved by carefully placing broad strips of nonelastic adhesive tape, Velcro-type bands, or quick-release belts across the hips and fixing them securely to the sides of the table (Fig. 9–12). These strips, bands, or belts are particularly necessary for the semiprone (see Fig. 9–7) and semisupine (see Fig. 9–9) variations of the lateral decubitus position. If a strap is used to stabilize the torso, it should be placed just caudad to the axilla (see Fig. 9–12). Placement further cephalad increases the risk of brachial plexus injury while more caudal placement (across the lower ribs) impairs ventilation. Many clinicians prefer the use of padded rests in front or back, or both, of the pelvis and sternum. These devices may be used in addition to the straps; however, they must not be allowed to interfere either with respiration or with circulation to the extremities.

Other methods must be used if the flexed lateral decubitus position is used for total hip replacement because the straps or tape would interfere with access to the surgical site. The evolution of modern plastics has led to the development of the "bean bag" for retaining patients in inherently unstable surgical positions, such as the lateral decubitus position, obviating the need for straps or tape at the surgical site.

The bean bag (Vacu-Pac) is an impervious pliant pillow, valved to the atmosphere and filled with tiny plastic beads. It is placed on the table, and the patient is arranged as de-

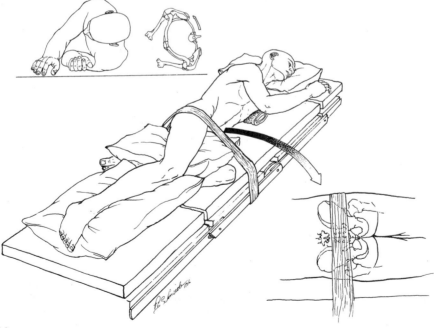

Figure 9–12

Proper placement of padding restraints and chest roll. *Upper inset.* Flexion and extension of the up-side arm will rotate the scapula (arrow) out of the thoracotomy field in a manner similar to that achieved by suspension of the arm. *Lower inset.* Stabilizing hip straps placed to avoid compression of the up-side femoral head and potential avascular necrosis.

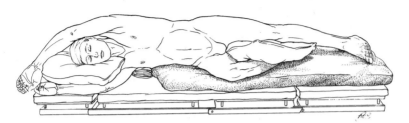

Figure 9–13

Right lateral decubitus position with upper arm flexed and extended to pull scapula away from standard thoracotomy site. Note that chest roll is caudad to the axilla. A "bean bag" that is shaped using a vacuum is beneath the patient as a molded support (see text for details). (Up-side arm support not shown for clarity.)

sired upon it (Fig. 9–13). At the conclusion of positioning it is molded carefully to the body contours, and wall suction is temporarily attached to its valve. As the air is removed, the beads are forced together and, in effect, the pillow becomes a solid mass. The valve can then be closed and the vacuum line detached. The pillow will keep its exact molded shape, similar to a plaster cast, as long as air is excluded; it returns to its original soft air-filled condition when the valve is opened.

Bean bags reduce the danger of pressure points for the patient because the body weight is evenly distributed with an effect equivalent to being supported by a buoyant fluid. The bean bags are radiolucent, nonconductive, and easily cleaned; they impart a measure of stability to the lateral decubitus position not previously obtained with other methods. The use of padded rests, as previously described, is obviated; however, any straps still required can be excluded from the operative site. Accidental puncture of the pillow may destroy all body support unless the alert anesthesiologist quickly reattaches the vacuum line. Unless the puncture is large or the vacuum line is weak, continuous suction to the "bean bag" under these circumstances maintains the firmness of the support until the conclusion of the case. A minor disadvantage of the plastic bead pillow is that additional assistants are often required to hold the patient in position while the pillow is molded and the vacuum applied. For surgical procedures that require repetitive and significant manipulation (e.g., hip arthroplasties) bean bags may also not offer sufficient stabilization. Additional padded pelvic fixation devices may be needed instead.

Positioning of the upper extremities adds somewhat to the postural stability of the lateral decubitus position. The down-side arm may be flexed and tucked under the pillow that supports the head (see Fig. 9–13), but prolonged flexion greater than 90 degrees is not advocated because it may tighten the arcuate ligament over the cubital tunnel and increase pressure on the ulnar nerve. The up-side arm placement usually adds little to stability, but the arm must be positioned according to surgical needs. Standard thoracotomy incisions require that the upper arm be extended and flexed to pull the scapula away from the site of the operation (see Fig. 9–13).[8] Managing the upper extremities for nonthoracic operations performed in the lateral decubitus position offers more options.

Two-level ("airplane") armboards, supporting one arm on each board, may be used to stabilize the upper extremities in the lateral decubitus position. However, the use of a two-level armboard may increase the susceptibility of the upper extremities to nerve stretch or compression. "Fixed" extremities allows undue stretch or stress on the brachial plexus when imperceptible shifts in the torso occur during surgery (see Complications of the Lateral Decubitus Position).

Suspension of the upper arm to the anesthesia screen is likewise discouraged. If the need to remove the upper arm from a high thoracic incision dictates its being loosely bound to a well-padded screen or drape support, care should be taken to avoid abduction of the humerus to more than 90 degrees. Periodic palpation of the axilla may be warranted to ensure its contents are not distorted by the humeral head. Perfusion of the extremity may be monitored by palpation of the radial artery and/or assessment of capillary refill. Whereas the arm may be against the anesthesia screen, it should never be used as a stabilizing force because traction on the neurovascular bundle is likely to occur, and a plexus injury or perfusion deficit can easily result (see Complications of the Lateral Decubitus Position).

Padding and pillows are required at bony prominences and between extremities to facilitate venous drainage as well as to prevent either nerve compression or the development of painful cutaneous pressure points. Flexion of the down-side leg at the knee and hip and extension of the up-side leg in the lateral decubitus position not only provides stability but ensures that the bony prominences of the lower extremities rest not against each other but against soft tissues (see Fig. 9–1). Pillows are then placed between the knees to avoid pressure from the weight of the uppermost extremity. Pillows or foam rubber pads are placed between the arms and under the elbows for the same reason. A sufficient amount of padding under the head (see Fig. 9–1) is needed to prevent lateral flexion of the neck that can stretch the brachial plexus, particularly if the arms are in a fixed position. Isolated palsy of the long thoracic nerve has been blamed on extreme lateral flexion of the neck.[22] Disposable foam rubber "donuts" are suitable head supports because they can be built up to align the cervical and thoracic spine. Furthermore, sections can be cut from the donuts to avoid prolonged pressure on the down-side eye, ear, and facial nerve. However, cost constraints may force some institutions to prefer a stack of wrinkle-free blankets rather than a stack of foam rings as support for the head in the lateral position.

A small pad or roll should be placed under the down-side thorax just caudad to, but not in, the axilla (see Figs. 9–1, 9–4, 9–12, and 9–13).

- This supportive device is often referred to as an *axillary roll*, but the term implies an improper and potentially dangerous location. Also, the term *roll* can be interpreted as implying length but little width when the device needs to be wide enough to spread its lifting pressure over the area of several contiguous ribs. More usefully termed a *chest pad*, it is correctly positioned just caudad to the axilla, supporting the shouldermost portion of the down-side rib cage.
- The purpose of the pad is to take pressure off the head of the down-side humerus and to avoid compression of the axillary neurovascular bundle.
- Improperly located in the axilla, the chest pad can cause vascular obstruction and compromise intravenous infusions or intra-arterial monitors if cannulae are present in the down-side arm.

Proper use of the chest pad may produce a secondary benefit. The vital capacity and tidal volume of conscious subjects placed in the lateral decubitus position is reduced by 10%.[9] These disturbances are of little concern today and are easily corrected in the anesthetized patient by the use of an endotracheal tube and controlled ventilation. Nevertheless, use of a chest pad improves compliance of the otherwise restricted down-side hemithorax. The freer excursion of the down-side thorax can reduce peak inflation pressure and avoid possible compromise of cardiac output and arterial oxygenation often seen when high inspiratory pressure is required. This issue becomes a major one during one-lung anesthesia.

Establishing the Kidney Position

The kidney position is established by first placing the patient in a basic lateral decubitus position on the appropriate nonoperative side (see Achieving the Lateral Decubitus Position).

- The flexion point between the trunk and thigh sections of the table should be located and the crest of the patient's down-side ilium placed over this point (see Fig. 9–6). The flank or lower ribs are thus avoided (see Fig. 9–6A and B). This minimizes the risk of vena caval obstruction and prevents undue compression of the down-side rib cage when the table is flexed. It also ensures optimum separation of the up-side costal margin and iliac crest during surgery.
- The table is flexed (or "broken") so that the muscles of the up-side flank become taut.
- Positioning of the patient on the table is extremely important. Care should be taken to see that the iliac crest does not slip off of the table break.
- The final step may be taken in establishing the kidney position by raising the kidney rest (also called the "kidney bar" or "elevator") underneath the iliac crest. The end point is the height at which lateral flexion has caused the up-side flank to become tight.

Lateral flexion for infants and small children in the kidney position may be obtained by placing an appropriately sized towel or rolled sheet at the flexion point. Flexion of the table is often unnecessary for these patients.

Hypotension can be countered by wrapping the dependent legs with compressive (but nonocclusive) elastic bandages to minimize venous stasis, by slow lateral flexion of the trunk, and by carefully raising the kidney rest. Frequent blood pressure determinations should be taken during this active process to detect early obstructive angulation of the inferior vena cava as it occurs. The acute onset of hypotension usually signals caval obstruction as opposed to the more gradual onset noted with orthostatic venous stasis.

Occasionally some urologists add a variable degree of head-up tilt to the flexed lateral decubitus position. They find it useful when performing a heminephrectomy for tumors of the upper pole of the kidney. Tolerable head elevation is added to the established kidney position slowly with careful vascular monitoring to detect the onset of hypotension that would limit tilt (Warner MA, personal communication, 1995).

MANAGEMENT OF MONITORS, INFUSIONS, AND THE AIRWAY

Nothing is unique to the lateral decubitus position per se that dictates specific monitors. Choices are indicated by the disease processes of the patient. Placing the patient in the lateral decubitus position imposes some unique problem with monitors, infusions, and the airway. The "finger on the pulse" method of monitoring, deemed antiquated by some, remains a useful adjunct to the modern machine.

Electrocardiographic Leads

The use of multiple lead electrocardiographic (ECG) monitoring, particularly lead V_5, is now recommended for all patients presenting for surgery with evidence of coronary artery disease.[23, 24] All leads are recorded for future reference. Two leads (II and V_5) should be displayed simultaneously. Recording devices should be available to make accurate measurements of ST segment changes, interpret difficult dysrhythmias, and confirm artifacts.

Many patients who present for thoracic surgery have concomitant cardiac disease. Placement of the ECG leads may present significant problems.

- The V_5 lead may be effective in its usual location on patients who will be placed

in the left lateral decubitus position for a right thoracotomy. The V_5 lead should be covered with an impermeable adhesive sheet (e.g., a Steri-drape), to prevent it from being dislodged during positioning and to protect it from surgical cleansing solutions that would upset contact.

- For a left thoracotomy, performed with the patient placed in the right lateral decubitus position, the V_5 electrode patch is in the surgical field. Several alternatives have been proposed as follows to overcome this obstacle: (1) It may be omitted in patients younger than 40 years of age who have no symptoms of coronary artery disease.[25] (2) A sterile needle electrode may be inserted in a substitute V_4 position after skin preparation. (3) To avoid loss of critical ECG data in the treacherous early period of anesthesia and positioning, Noback[24] advocates that a standard disposable electrode pad be placed in the V_5 position before anesthesia, removed before skin preparation, and replaced by a sterile needle electrode in the V_4 location before draping.

Blood Pressure Measurement

Whereas either indirect or direct methods of measuring blood pressure are applicable for a patient placed in the lateral decubitus position, direct intra-arterial pressure monitoring remains the standard against which all indirect methods are evaluated. Automatic oscillometric devices offer distinct advantages over manual auscultatory techniques. Subjectivity is reduced and repeatability is enhanced. Further, oscillometric units often function in situations where auscultatory techniques fail, such as in obese patients and children.[26] In general, when the chest is not entered, indirect blood pressure measurements are used for surgical procedures in the lateral decubitus position. If the chest is entered, an intra-arterial line is usually placed for rapid, beat-to-beat blood pressure monitoring and frequent arterial blood sampling.

Monitoring blood pressure in the lateral decubitus position presents unique problems related to the type and placement of the sensors. The hydrostatic forces produced by gravity on the vertical distance between the arms in the lateral decubitus position are significant. Gravity alters the pressure reading by 2 mm Hg per inch (or 0.8 mm Hg/cm) that the sensor is above or below the heart.[27]

The vertical distance between the arms of the average adult male in the lateral decubitus position is approximately 16 inches (40 cm). Thus, the discrepancy in blood pressure between the up-side and down-side arm could be as much as 32 mm Hg. Blood pressure measured in the upper arm would be approximately 16 mm Hg lower than the true pressure in the heart and brain.[28] When using direct arterial pressure measurements, the influence of hydrostatic pressured is easily negated by raising or lowering the calibrated transducer to the level of the heart. The effects of gravity on the fluids in the transducer extension tubing provide the countering force.

Discrepancies of 5 to 20 mm Hg have been found to occur between direct and indirect pressure measurements within the same patient and on the same arm. Direct readings are usually higher.[29, 30] The greatest variabilities are found in patients who are hypertensive, obese, hypothermic, or in shock.

Noback[24] recommends that cuff blood pressure measured in the lateral decubitus position should be taken in the up-side arm to avoid alterations induced by compression of the down-side axillary artery. The cuff and peripheral pulses are more readily accessible in the up-side arm. Blood pressure is more likely to be underestimated in the up-side arm, minimizing the risk of unrecognized hypotension, which may cause more problems than would an error in the assessment of hypertension. The down-side arm may be used equally as well provided that the axillary artery is not compressed and vertical differences in pressure between the arms are remembered.

Several factors must be considered when deciding to use the up-side or down-side arm for placement of the radial arterial cannula. The right radial artery is the artery of choice when the operative procedure is resection of an aneurysm of the descending thoracic aorta because the left subclavian artery may require occlusion by the surgeon during the resection. In most other instances, either artery can be used during surgery in the lateral decubitus position. We prefer to use the down-side arm when feasible, because the radial artery is on the accessible volar surface of the wrist, and the arm lies in a more stable, protected, and visible position than does the up-side arm during the procedure. In addition, shorter transducer extension lines can be used to avoid artifacts due to resonance in long tubing. Accurate pressures can be obtained from the down-side arm as long as body weight and bony structures are not allowed to compress its axillary artery.

Placement of the radial arterial cannula in the uppermost arm does not prevent damping or obliteration of the arterial trace if the rules of proper positioning are transgressed. Hyperabduction of the upper extremity, as might occur when the arm is suspended from an anesthesia screen, has been reported to obliterate the radial pulse in greater than 80% of young patients.[11]

Intravenous Catheters

Other than the availability of veins, no major indications exist for or against the use of the down-side or up-side arm as the site of peripheral intravenous infusion. Compression of the down-side neurovascular bundle, either by a misplaced chest pad or by a malpositioned humeral head, can obstruct the flow of an infusion. Accumulated solutions elevate pressure in the recipient vessel and may force extravasation from the puncture site, particularly if the infusion is pressurized.

The right internal jugular vein is the best choice for cannulation of the superior vena cava or right atrium regardless of which lateral decubitus position will be used. Subclavian insertions have fallen into disfavor because of a high incidence of complications,[25] including pneumothoraces and direct trauma to the brachial plexus and vessels, events that are indistinguishable from injuries associated with improper lateral decubitus positioning (see Complications of the Lateral Decubitus Position).

Direct monitoring of central venous pressure requires placement of the pressure transducer at the level of the cardiac atria. In the supine patient, the phlebostatic axis provides a reliable external reference point. It is defined as the junction of the fourth intercostal space and the midpoint of the anteroposterior diameter of the thorax. Central venous blood pressure monitoring in the laterally positioned patient is complicated by the inability to accurately and systematically define a phlebostatic axis.[31, 32] Thus, the baseline value of central venous pressure will always be in question. Nevertheless, if transducers and patient positions are maintained, trends in central venous pressure may be accurately recorded.

Pulmonary Artery Catheters

Whereas pulmonary artery catheters are especially useful in patients with cardiac disease undergoing pulmonary resections,[24] most catheters will float into the right middle or lower lobe of the lung and cause data collected from a patient who is in the lateral decubitus position to be questionable. Fluoroscopy may be required to place the pulmonary artery catheter into the left pulmonary artery if a right pneumonectomy is to be performed. Kopman and Sandza[33] report a highly successful technique of ensuring selective catheter placement in which the balloon is floated into the pulmonary artery trunk, the patient is turned in to the lateral decubitus position, and the resultant increase in blood flow through the down-side lung will carry the balloon and catheter tip to that lung. Radiographic confirmation of the final position is still required, but the need for fluoroscopy is obviated when successful.

A sudden onset of "idiopathic" ventricular dysrhythmias during and after changes of posture with central venous lines in place should suggest the possibility of catheter-induced endocardial irritability, especially if the disorder does not respond to standard therapy.[34, 35] Monitoring pressure waveforms differentiates among venous, atrial, or ventricular displacement of the catheter and facilitates repositioning.

Body Temperature

Large surface areas are exposed to ambient temperatures during thoracotomies and mandate thermometry. The posterior nasopharynx is the site of choice for measuring temperature[36] because esophageal temperature tends to be spuriously low when the chest is open or to fluctuate with the temperatures of irrigation solutions. An accurate representation of the brain temperature can be measured when a thermistor probe is inserted through the nares at a length equivalent to the distance from the tip of the nose to the earlobe. In those cases in which Foley catheters are indicated, Foley catheter thermometers accurately track core temperatures. Infrared tympanic membrane thermometers have gained recent popularity as a rapid, safe, and accurate means for monitoring core temperature.[37]

Pulse Oximetry and Capnography

Both monitors have become standards of care. Extensive reviews of capnography and ox-

imetry[38] can be found in the literature. In general, pulse oximeters are easy to use and provide early warning of impending hypoxemia, thereby giving the anesthesiologist ample lead time to correct the cause. We prefer to measure pulse oximetry at the ear, nose, or lip of a patient in the lateral decubitus position. The patient's position may interfere with flow to the extremities, adversely affecting oximeter performance. Intraoperative hypothermia, hypovolemia, hypotension or use of vasoconstrictor drugs may further compromise extremity perfusion and oximetric accuracy.[38] However, the plethysmographic capability of the oximeter has been proposed as a means to ascertain that the position has not interfered with blood flow to the arm or leg. In general, studies supporting such usage have been uncontrolled or anecdotal and should be interpreted with caution.[38]

The waveform of the capnograph can be helpful in diagnosing airway obstruction, relaxation, and malposition of double-lumen tubes.[39] There is usually a gradient between the capnograph CO_2 concentration and arterial P_{CO_2}, with the latter normally being higher. The size of the gradient may vary during the course of the operation,[40] making blood gas determinations necessary when tight control of acid-base status is critical.

The Airway and the Lateral Decubitus Position

A variety of endotracheal tubes and techniques have been developed to provide special conditions for patients being operated on in the lateral decubitus position. Double-lumen tubes and bronchial blockers are commonly used when one-lung anesthesia is intended.

Several studies confirm that flexion and extension of the adult neck after initial placement of the endotracheal tube will move its tip more than an inch within the trachea.[41, 42] By changing the distance between the teeth and the vocal cords, neck flexion moves the tube tip toward the carina, risking endobronchial intubation if the tube tip was originally positioned near the carina. Neck extension risks extubation if the tube tip is barely past the larynx. Proper location of endotracheal or endobronchial tubes must be determined immediately after the lateral decubitus position has been established, and any necessary corrections must be made before proceeding with an operation. Failure to do this results in a high incidence of tube nonperformance on initiating one-lung ventilation.[43] If possible, tube position should be verified by direct visualization through a fiberoptic bronchoscope.

In general, it is advisable to place an endobronchial tube in the down-side (nonoperative) lung. Bronchial intubation of the operative side may result in displacement during surgical manipulation. The possibility of bronchial rupture can be minimized by deflating bronchial balloons before the patient is turned into the lateral decubitus position. Proper function must be determined again after the balloons are reinflated.

PHYSIOLOGY OF THE LATERAL DECUBITUS POSITION

The functions of most organ systems appear to be little affected when the patient has been carefully positioned in the lateral decubitus position. Exceptions occur when postural extremes are used,[44] such as in the lateral jackknife or flexed lateral positions. Alterations in the mechanics and distribution of ventilation and circulation are primary considerations.

Cardiovascular System

Cardiovascular collapse is possible when the anesthetized patient is turned from the supine to the lateral decubitus position, especially after lateral flexion. Sudden postural changes are tolerated poorly in the anesthetized patient. Slow, gentle, deliberate repositioning of the anesthetized subject is required with constant checking of the blood pressure. General anesthesia depresses the carotid and aortic baroreceptors so that they can no longer effectively compensate for cardiovascular instability produced by altered body posture. Changes in body position should be made in the lightest possible plane of anesthesia because the homeostatic compensatory mechanisms of the circulation are depressed in direct proportion to the concentration of the anesthetic agent in use. In addition, the lateral decubitus position shifts the mediastinum toward the down side and rotates the heart on its axis. Such changes can interfere with venous return and cardiac output. Hypotension due to positional change can be rapidly detected and changes in position made. In the event that positional changes may not be per-

formed, the anesthesiologist is left with two principal options for treatment of cardiac output: volume expansion or vasoactive drug therapy. Both options should be exercised with caution. The transfusion of excessive fluid as the primary measure to combat hypotension in this situation may lead to cardiac decompensation when the patient is returned to the supine posture at the end of the case. Replacement of insidious third space fluid in the dependent extremities of the patient in the lateral jackknife or flexed lateral position can lead the unsuspecting anesthesiologist into creating an eventual overload when these fluids are mobilized postoperatively. Two instances of unilateral pulmonary edema due to volume overload have been reported after urologic surgery.[45, 46] Vasopressors may be used judiciously in an attempt to reduce venous capacitance and increase preload. Nevertheless, the experienced anesthesiologist is well aware of the risks of increased afterload and impaired peripheral perfusion with the use of these agents.

Eggers and associates[47] demonstrated that marked reductions in arterial pressures occurred with almost all lateral positions during anesthesia compared with the supine position. The lowest mean arterial blood pressure was noted in those patients placed in the right lateral decubitus and right lateral decubitus jackknife positions. The left lateral decubitus position produced little change in blood pressure compared with the supine. Cardiac output remained remarkably stable in any lateral position compared with the supine. Studies have concurred with Eggers findings.[48, 49] Werner and colleagues[49] report that neither opening the pleura nor subsequent pulmonary surgery (both lungs ventilated) causes any clinically significant derangements in systemic hemodynamics.

Impairment of venous return is not usually a problem except in exaggerated lateral positions, such as the jackknife or kidney position with the patient's legs placed in a markedly dependent position.[44] Kidney rests, mistakenly compressing the patient's flank rather than elevating the down-side iliac crest, are another source of vena caval occlusion. The right lateral decubitus position appears to place the patient at greater risk for vena caval constriction with kidney rests than does the left, possibly because of the proximity of the vessel to the right (down-side) flank. Application of positive end-expiratory pressure may cause inferior venal caval constriction in patients in the left lateral decubitus position.[50] Large intra-abdominal masses are reported to have caused obstruction of the vena cava and hypotension when the patient was placed in the lateral decubitus position for surgery.[12]

Respiratory System

Mechanics

Computed tomography has demonstrated that dense lung areas form immediately on induction of anesthesia.[51] The densities are located in the dependent regions of both lungs in the spontaneously breathing supine patient. Their studies suggest that these densities are atelectasis and that their formation is presumably due to a loss of forces that normally keep the lung expanded. Atelectasis formation in each lung may also be affected by moving the anesthetized patient from the supine to the lateral decubitus position. Although the total atelectatic area remains essentially unchanged in the lateral decubitus position, the atelectatic regions in the down-side lung increased from 50% of the total area to 90% of the total atelectatic area. This change may be obliterated with the use of selective positive end-expiratory pressure.

The single most important effect of posture on ventilation is simple mechanical interference with chest movement limiting expansion of the lungs.[52] Movement of the diaphragm is the dominant inspiratory force, contributing from 60% to 100% of the change in intrathoracic volume. The upward and lateral movement of the ribs contribute less to lung expansion than does the diaphragm, but both components can be restricted by positioning. Vital capacity of normal conscious subjects in the lateral decubitus position is reduced by 10%, a decrease comparable to that noted after changing from the sitting to the supine position.[53] The kidney position can produce up to a 15% reduction in vital capacity. Reduction of vital capacity is thought to be due to restriction of the thoracic cage in all directions, but lateral and anterior movement of the down-side ribs and impairment of movement of the ipsilateral diaphragm produces the greatest reduction.[54] The tidal volume in anesthetized individuals also decreases between 10% to 14% when they are placed in the lateral or kidney position, respectively.[55, 56] The same degree of reduction could be expected during spinal anesthesia with any additional increase being the result of intercostal muscle paralysis.

Ventilation/Perfusion Ratio in the Awake Patient

The functional residual capacity of an awake adult declines by 0.8 L after changing from the upright to the supine position.[57] Subsequent to the induction of anesthesia in the supine position, the functional residual capacity diminishes an additional 0.4 L.[58, 59, 60] This reduction occurs mainly in the dependent lung regions.[61, 62] Thus, turning the patient from supine to lateral decubitus reduces the volume of the down-side lung, whereas that of the upper lung is maintained or even increased.

Gravity causes a vertical gradient in the distribution of pulmonary blood flow in the lateral decubitus position, such that blood flow to the down-side lung is significantly greater than to the up-side lung. In the awake patient, ventilation is relatively increased in the down-side lung so that the overall ventilation/perfusion relationship of the lungs is not greatly altered from that of the supine position.[17, 39, 63] Preferential ventilation of the down-side lung reflects the fact that the lateral decubitus position in the awake patient forces the dome of the down-side diaphragm more cephalad into the thorax while the upper dome is flattened. The result is twofold: further reduction of functional residual capacity in the down-side lung yet better ventilation than the up-side lung.[9, 39, 62] The explanation offered is that, with a reduced volume and functional residual capacity of the lower lung, the diaphragm on the down-side lies higher in the chest and is more stretched. This effect gives that hemidiaphragm better mechanical efficiency for contraction than the hemidiaphragm of the up-side lung.

Ventilation/Perfusion Ratio in the Anesthetized Patient

General anesthesia, whether with spontaneous or controlled ventilation, causes major alterations in the distribution of ventilation and perfusion from that described in the awake subject in the lateral decubitus position.[9, 39] These variables differ even further with open pleura, paralysis, and the presence of pathologic processes in the up-side lung.[49, 64]

The degree of overperfusion or underventilation of alveoli is expressed as a shift in the ventilation/perfusion ratio. The lateral decubitus position in the awake patient allows gravity to produce a vertical downward gradient increase of ventilation and blood flow that favors the down-side lung. Induction of anesthesia does not cause any appreciable change in the distribution of the pulmonary blood flow from that of the lateral distribution while awake. However, general anesthesia does alter the distribution of ventilation in the anesthetized, spontaneously ventilating subject. The greater portion of the tidal volume is now distributed to the up-side lung.[9, 39, 62, 65] This distribution is related to the decreased functional residual capacity of the down-side lung. The lower lung is less compliant while the upper lung is more compliant. Muscle relaxants and positive-pressure ventilation also remove any mechanical advantage of the lower diaphragm noted in the awake state. The anesthetized patient in the lateral decubitus position with a closed chest exhibits an increased mismatch of ventilation and perfusion. The up-side lung is well ventilated but poorly perfused. This finding occurs regardless of the use of muscle relaxants.

Opening the chest wall and pleura does not alter pulmonary blood flow distribution from that of the closed thorax in the lateral decubitus position. However, further ventilation/perfusion mismatch occurs for three reasons: (1) positive-pressure ventilation is now required; (2) the upper lung, no longer restricted by the chest wall, becomes even more compliant and receives additional ventilation, according to the law of Laplace; and (3) positive atmospheric pressure on the up-side lung causes a downward displacement of the mediastinum into the dependent hemithorax. The exposed up-side lung tends to collapse because of unopposed elastic recoil. Mediastinal shift can cause decreased venous return to the heart and sympathetic activation, presenting a clinical picture of shock. Positive-pressure ventilation in the anesthetized, paralyzed, patient with an open thoracotomy in the lateral decubitus position can rectify the problems of mediastinal shift and paradoxic respiration. The application of positive end-expiratory pressure to both lungs redirects the majority of ventilation to the down-side lung. However, ventilation of the up-side lung is impractical from the surgeon's standpoint and has led to further refinements of one-lung anesthesia employing the double-lumen endotracheal tubes. The ability to differentially ventilate the down-side lung with or without positive end-expiratory pressure has greatly facilitated the safety of anesthesia for thoracic surgery. Furthermore, other mechanisms, such as surgical interference with blood flow of the up-side lung and hypoxic pulmonary vasoconstriction, also direct blood flow away from the surgically collapsed lung into the ventilated lung. The ventilation/perfusion ratio approaches normal. An extensive review of techniques for anesthesia for thoracic surgery is beyond the scope of this chapter; however, several other texts are recommended.[9, 39]

Alterations of the ventilation/perfusion ratio in the lateral decubitus position have practical value in giving anesthesia for thoracic surgery or in managing the patient in the intensive care unit.[64, 66] The effects of the lateral decubitus position on gas exchange in patients with extensive lung disease have been examined in several studies.[48, 67–69] The best oxygenation in unilateral lung disease (i.e., pneumonia) occurs consistently when the unaffected lung is down side and the patient is breathing spontaneously with or without low levels of continuous positive airway pressure.[64] Improvement in oxygenation has been demonstrated in mechanically ventilated patients with unilateral pneumonia on rotation from supine to the lateral position with the diseased lung uppermost.[70]

The effect of the lateral decubitus position on oxygenation in patients with bilateral lung disease is not clear.[67] Neither right or left lateral decubitus position is distinctly advantageous in improving oxygenation, although Zach and colleagues report a slight advantage in the right lateral decubitus position in awake patients.[71] No changes in oxygenation are reported in normal individuals with either side down compared with normal individuals supine.[64, 72]

COMPLICATIONS OF THE LATERAL DECUBITUS POSITION

The potential complications of surgical positioning hold much in common. Their etiology is usually attributed to abnormal pressure or stretch, or both.[73–75] In the past, many were believed to be preventable, although a cause was not always discernible. The role of the anesthesiologist is to modify the potentialities for harm as much as possible without interfering with the requirements of the surgeon.

Anesthetized patients are often placed in postures that they could not tolerate if awake. Anesthesia abolishes recognition of protective muscular and vascular reflexes, which ordinarily evoke complaints of pain. Legal precedents have placed the onus of responsibility for safe positioning on anesthesiologists.[53] Having produced a state of painlessness, we become the patient's fiduciary. In essence, a fiduciary is a person (or institution) who holds something of value for another in trust.

Cutaneous and Musculoskeletal Systems

Pressure injuries to the skin, soft tissues, and ligaments are probably the most common positional injuries that the lateral decubitus position shares with others.[76] Temporary baldness of the occipital scalp after long operations complicated by hypotension has been reported.[53] Lawson[77] reported permanent alopecia in 60 patients after open heart surgery. Moving the patient's head at frequent intervals eliminates the occurrence of alopecia. Scalp biopsy specimens disclosed "obliterative vasculitis" in the deep cutis; these represent "decubitus" ulcers in the purest sense.

Postoperative backache after anesthesia and surgery has been reported to occur in 2% to 20% of all patients[53] Backache is related to surgical position and duration of the procedure but not to the type of anesthesia. Brown and Elman,[78] in a small series, noted a 12% incidence of backache for the lateral decubitus position. Backache is a common complaint for patients who have had surgery in the lateral decubitus position in our experience as well. The incidence is much lower than that observed for the prone, lithotomy, or supine position, but the etiology still may be related to stretched lumbosacral ligaments.[79]

Whiplash injury to the cervical spine is a reported complication of positioning.[44] Undue tension on the cervical ligaments can be guarded against by controlling the head during the turn from supine to the operative position and by preventing sudden changes in position. Avoidance of markedly abnormal head positions (e.g., torsion, lateral flexion, and extension) lowers the incidence of whiplash injury. Jaffe[80] reported a patient affected with Horner's syndrome that persisted for 3 days postoperatively. He related this syndrome to lateral flexion of the head in the lateral decubitus position and stretch of the cervical sympathetic chain.

Two cases of acute postoperative parotitis after surgery with the patient in the left lateral decubitus position have been reported.[81, 82] The mechanism of these occurrences is believed to be either subluxation of the temporomandibular joint during a placement of a nasogastric tube or direct compression secondary to patient position. The swelling resolved within 1 to 2 weeks without sequelae.

Neurologic Complications

The Brachial Plexus

The brachial plexus is anchored in the neck at the transverse processes of cervical vertebrae and in the upper arm by the axillary fascia. That fixation, plus the proximity of mobile bony structures, places the components of the plexus at risk for stretch and compression injuries during anesthesia.[73] Ischemia of the intraneural vasa nervosa is the principal cause of positional nerve injuries. These injuries result primarily from stretching the nerve and secondarily from compression of a nerve already susceptible to damage by stretch. Stretch, rather than compression, is the major cause of damage to the brachial plexus in most surgical positions.[44, 73] In the lateral decubitus position, however, compression is the leading cause of brachial plexus injury.

- Compression of the plexus may occur when the lower shoulder and arm are allowed to remain directly under the rib cage after turning the patient into the lateral position (see Fig. 9–9, *inset*).
- Depression of the clavicle into the retroclavicular space compresses the brachial plexus between the clavicle and the first rib.
- The presence of a cervical rib should be sought in the preoperative chest radiograph, because an unsuspected cervical rib would increase the vulnerability of the brachial plexus to compression injury.
- A properly placed chest pad reduces the chances for a compression injury to the brachial plexus (see Fig. 9–1). However, the chest roll may become a compressive force itself if it is misplaced into the axilla. (An axillary compartment syndrome has been described, resulting from a change in position of the patient from lateral decubitus to semiprone.[83] The chest roll was not of sufficient bulk to support the chest

wall in the semiprone position, and compression of the down-side shoulder ensued.)

- In the absence of a chest pad, the entire humerus, including the humeral head, must be positioned ventrad to the rib cage to free the plexus from the weight of the trunk.

Stretch becomes a factor in producing brachial plexus injury in several situations:

- Excessive dorsal extension or lateral flexion of the neck widens the angle between the head and the shoulder tip and stretches the plexus between its fixed points at the traverse processes and the axillary fascia.
- Suspension of the up-side arm from an anesthesia screen stretches the brachial plexus around the clavicle and tendon of the pectorals minor if the arm is hyperabducted.
- Postural instability that allows dorsal semisupine positioning of a patient who was initially placed in the lateral decubitus position will stretch the brachial plexus if the up-side arm has been tightly fixed to an anesthesia screen to stabilize the torso.
- Common clinical practice permits maximum abduction of the arm to 90 degrees, but injuries have occurred with as little as 60 degrees of abduction when accompanied by forearm rotation.[7, 8]
- Brachial plexus stretch is accentuated by

dorsal extension or lateral flexion of the head.

The Suprascapular Nerve

An entrapment neuropathy of the suprascapular nerve is an infrequent, and easily overlooked, source of pain after a surgical procedure in which the patient was in the lateral decubitus position (Schweiss JF, personal communication, 1986). Derived from the fifth and sixth cervical roots through the upper trunk of the brachial plexus, the nerve traverses the neck and shoulder to reach the upper border of the scapula where it passes through the suprascapular notch and is fixed by the foramen. Stretch of the nerve (Fig. 9–14) apparently may occur by circumduction of the upper extremity across the chest or by marked lateral tilt of the head toward the contralateral shoulder.[85]

If the laterally positioned patient shifts ventrad (semiprone) during surgery, the down-side arm is forced ventromedially and may move the scapula sufficiently to stretch the nerve (see Fig. 9–14). If the laterally positioned patient shifts dorsad (semisupine) with the up-side arm fixed tightly to an anesthesia screen, circumduction of that arm across the chest can occur with the potential for a suprascapular stretch injury (see Fig. 9–14).

Pain derived from the suprascapular nerve is deep, poorly circumscribed, and roughly

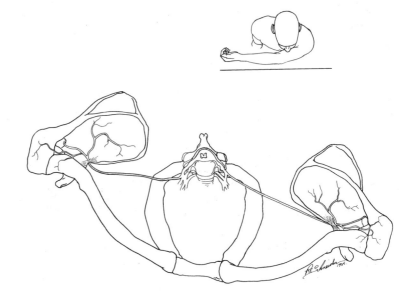

Figure 9–14

Circumduction of the arm across the chest can occur in the lateral position, injuriously stretching the suprascapular nerve. Rotating the torso to the semisupine position with the up-side arm fixed or to the semiprone position with the down-side arm immobilized (see Figs. 9-4 and 9-12) may produce enough scapular displacement to stretch the nerve.

localized to the posterior and lateral aspects of the shoulder.[84]

Peripheral Branches of the Brachial Plexus

The nerves of the brachial plexus may be injured after their exit from the axilla. The median and ulnar nerves can be damaged if the arm is allowed to hang over the edge of the operating table. The radial nerve is particularly susceptible to damage in the lateral decubitus position if the extended downside arm is pushed cephalad against the vertical bar of the anesthesia screen, compressing the nerve between the humerus and the bar.

The Long Thoracic Nerve

Long thoracic nerve injury is a rare and potentially disabling curiosity after anesthesia and surgery. The long thoracic nerve arises from spinal roots (anterior branches of C5, C6, and C7) that form the brachial plexus. It is a long nerve that serves only as the motor innervation of the serratus anterior muscle. It has no sensory component. Injury to it produces a "winged" scapula. The lateral decubitus position has been associated with serratus anterior palsy. The etiology is uncertain, but the long thoracic nerve may be stretched by lateral angulation of the neck and head away from the up-side shoulder. This association may be coincidental, having been noted in other surgical positions as well. Martin[22] reviewed a series of isolated long thoracic nerve injuries and could identify only 11% associated with a surgical procedure. The etiology in nearly all cases was contentious and poorly understood. For undetermined reasons, the palsy nearly always involved the right side. In the Martin study, an independent neuropathy could not be ruled out in many cases and appeared to be coincidental with otherwise uneventful perioperative periods. Recovery may occur within 6 to 24 months.

Because many factors may be involved during the perioperative period, complete prevention of brachial plexus injury due to operative position may not be attainable. However, awareness of its susceptibility to stress and the institution of obvious precautions may reduce the risk of it being traumatized.

Nerves of the Lower Extremity

Compression of the common peroneal nerve, the most frequent nerve injury in the lower extremity for patients placed in a lateral decubitus position, occurs less frequently than does injury to the brachial plexus, but it is not rare.[53] Damage occurs if the patient lies on a poorly padded operating table, and the nerve is compressed as it courses around the lateral aspect of the proximal fibula.[73, 74]

The sciatic nerve may be injured in an emaciated patient who is placed in a lateral position for repair of a fractured hip.[11] When the pelvis is rotated into a semisupine posture to expose the operative site, the dependent side rests obliquely down against the table and can compress the sciatic nerve between the table surface and the ischiopubic ramus. Supporting hip straps for the lateral decubitus position can also be a source of sciatic damage to the up-side hip if the straps are pulled too tight. Strap buckles should not be placed over the infragluteal region of emaciated patients for the same reason. Traditionally, we have believed that straps should not be placed over the femoral head because of the possibility of aseptic necrosis from a compression of the vessels that cross the hip joint from the pelvis to supply the head (Fig. 9–15). The obese patient placed in the lateral decubitus position is at risk for a gluteal muscle crush injury that can produce rhabdomyolysis, compartment syndromes, and a consequent sciatic nerve palsy.[85]

The possibility of nerve injury within the spinal canal from positioning has been reported by Schweiss (personal communication, 1986). A permanent cauda equina syndrome was noted in an elderly patient after a hip replacement. Both lower extremities were noted to be weak, but this finding was attributed to his previously immobile state related to his arthritic pain. His surgery was performed under an easily accomplished, uncomplicated spinal anesthetic. He was positioned in a sharply flexed lateral decubitus position. Numbness of his left toes and foot were noted in the postanesthesia care unit. The condition progressed over a 3-day period to become a cauda equina syndrome. A computed tomographic scan noted a severe spinal stenosis at the L3-4 level that was the same level at which the anesthetic was given. A decompression laminectomy was performed but without recovery of function. No hematoma was found. One could easily ascribe the lesion to the spinal anesthetic, which has been the historic norm. However, one cannot rule out the effect of a prolonged flexed lateral position over a pre-existing spinal stenosis

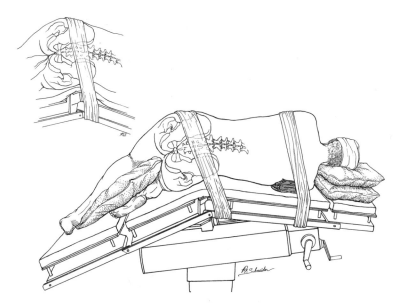

Figure 9–15

Restraining strap over up-side hip is positioned between the femoral head and the iliac crest to avoid compressing the vasculature crossing the hip joint and causing ischemic (aseptic) necrosis of the femoral head.

perhaps signaled by the preoperative weakness of the lower extremities.

Respiratory and Circulatory Complications

Acute respiratory and circulatory complications have been addressed in the course of this text as they occurred with changes in position from supine to lateral.

Impaired ventilatory function as reflected by reduced vital capacity occurs after both upper abdominal and thoracic surgery. Thoracotomies and pulmonary resections markedly impair active diaphragmatic excursions, potentially contributing to postoperative ventilatory dysfunction and requiring several weeks for recovery. Fratacci and associates[58] demonstrated that although thoracic epidural anesthesia improved other indices of pulmonary function through pain relief, it did not improve the inhibition of diaphragmatic contraction. The mechanism for inhibition of the diaphragmatic function is not clear but was thought to be related to postoperative reflex inhibition of phrenic neural activation.

The most common long-term respiratory complication associated with the lateral decubitus position is the frequent occurrence of postoperative atelectasis.[9, 62] Compression of the down-side chest wall and loss of functional residual capacity in the down-side lung is most often cited as a source of atelectasis.

Long-term circulatory complications are few if the same precautions used to prevent nerve damage are followed. The causes of vascular complications are similar because the vessels are found in the same neurovascular compartments.

- The standard lateral decubitus position does not predispose a patient to the development of venous thrombosis any more than any other surgical position provided venous occlusion or stasis is avoided.[47]
- Hyperabduction of the up-side arm, as might occur when the arm is suspended from the anesthesia screen, has resulted in peripheral gangrene.[11, 44, 73] Periodic palpation of the pulse in an abducted arm, particularly in an elderly or a diabetic patient, is suggested to prevent this complication.
- Acute and extreme rotation during positioning of the head in an elderly or atherosclerotic patient has been incriminated for central nervous system damage from occlusion of the vertebral artery.[11] A history of carotid artery disease, bruits, or temporary ischemic attacks should alert the anesthesiologist to this possibility.

Air embolus has occurred when the vena cava has been entered in the course of removing large renal tumors with the patient in the right lateral decubitus position. Maintaining the patient in the slight head-down position as in Figure 9–6C in the right lateral flexed position may prevent air embolus.

Ocular Complications

The lateral decubitus position places the down-side eye at risk of damage and permanent blindness from retinal artery thrombosis, one of the most devastating but preventable positional complications.[11, 44, 73] It can occur when the down-side eye has been subjected to external pressure such as an improperly placed head rest or pillow. Controlled or accidental hypotension may reduce retinal perfusion, maximize the effect of external pressure, and accentuate the possibility of thrombosis.[53] On examination, the affected pupil is dilated and reacts to consensual stimulation but not to direct light. The cornea is usually hazy, and the lids are edematous. Depending on the amount of retinal damage in the affected eye, the patient's complaints vary from blurring of vision to blindness.

Special efforts should be made to protect the down-side eye in the lateral decubitus position, and the precautions should be specifically described on the anesthesia record.

REFERENCES

1. Dorland WA: Illustrated Medical Dictionary. Philadelphia, WB Saunders, 1981.
2. Sims JM: In Silver Suture in Surgery. New York, Samuel S. and William Wood, 1857.
3. Thomas AN: The lateral decubitus position: Surgical aspects. In Martin JT (ed.): Positioning in Anesthesia and Surgery, 2nd ed. Philadelphia, WB Saunders, 1987, pp. 147–154.
4. Van Den Burgh R: Lateral-paramedian infratentorial approach in lateral decubitus for pineal tumors. Clin Neurol Neurosurg 92:311, 1990.
5. Butler VM, Dean LS, Little JR: Positioning the neurosurgical patient in the operating room. J Neurosurg Nurs 16:89, 1984.
6. Shah JL: Effect of posture on extradural pressure. Br J Anaesth 56:1373, 1984.
7. Cuschieri A: Thorascopic subtotal oesophagectomy. Endo Surg Allied Tech 2:21, 1994.
8. Gothard JWW, Branthwaite MA: Principles of anesthesia for thoracotomy. In Gothard JWW, Branthwaite MA (eds.): Anesthesia for Thoracic Surgery. Oxford, Blackwell Scientific Publishing, 1982.
9. Benumof JL, Alfery DD: Anesthesia for thoracic surgery. In Miller RD (ed.): Anesthesia. New York, Churchill Livingstone, 1994.
10. Alley RD: Thoracic surgical incisions and postoperative drainage. In Cooper P (ed.): The Craft of Surgery. Boston, Little, Brown & Co., 1964.
11. Lincoln JR, Sawyer HP: Complications related to body positions during surgical procedures. Anesthesiology 22:800, 1961.
12. Matlatinsky J, Kadlic T: Inferior vena caval occlusion in the left lateral position. Br J Anaesth 46:165, 1974.
13. Kropp KA: Unusual positions in urology: Surgical aspects. In Martin JT (ed.): Positioning in Anesthesia and Surgery. Philadelphia, WB Saunders, 1987.
14. Smith DR, Schulte JW, Smart WR: Surgery of the kidney. In Campbell MF, Harrison C (eds.): Urology. Philadelphia, WB Saunders, 1970.
15. Flocks RH, Culp D: Surgical Urology. Chicago, Year Book Medical Publishers, 1967.
16. Grayhack JT, Graham J: Renal surgery. In Glenn JF (ed.): Urologic Surgery. Hagerstown, MD, Harper & Row, 1975.
17. Horswell JL: Anesthetic techniques for thorocoscopy. Ann Thorac Surg 56:624, 1993.
18. Kirkwood CR, Clark L: Lateral Sims deliveries: A new application for an old technique. J Fam Pract 17:701, 1983.
19. Zimmerman CE: Endoscopy. In Techniques of Patient Care: A Manual of Bedside Procedures. Boston, Little, Brown & Co., 1976.
20. Willis RJ: Caudal epidural blockade. In Cousins MJ, Bridenbaugh PO (eds.): Neural Blockade. Philadelphia, JB Lippincott, 1988.
21. Iwa T, Nagai A, Yoshida C: Positioning for simultaneous intracardiac repair and/or ascending aorta and descending aorta surgery. Jpn J Surg 2:385, 1981.
22. Martin JT: Postoperative isolated dysfunction of the long thoracic nerve: A rare entity of uncertain etiology. Anesth Analg 69:614, 1989.
23. Kaplan JA, King SB: The precordial electrocardiographic lead (V5) in patients with coronary artery disease. Anesthesiology 45:570, 1976.
24. Noback CR: Intraoperative monitoring. In Kaplan JA (ed.): Thoracic Anesthesia. New York, Churchill Livingstone, 1983.
25. Stanley TE, Reves JG: Cardiovascular monitoring. In Miller RD (ed.): Anesthesia. New York, Churchill Livingstone, 1994, pp. 1161–1228.
26. Quill TJ: Blood pressure monitoring. In Ehrenwerth J, Eisenkraft JB (eds.): Anesthesia Equipment. St. Louis, CV Mosby, 1993, pp. 274–283.
27. Enderby GEH: Postural ischaemia and blood pressure. Lancet 1:185, 1954.
28. Mankowitz E: Blood pressure measurement during lateral tilt. Anaesthesia 34:84, 1979.
29. Kaye W: Invasive monitoring techniques. In McIntyre KM, Lewis AL (eds.): Textbook of Advanced Cardiac Life Support. Dallas, American Heart Association, 1983.
30. Reich DL, Kaplan JA: Hemodynamic monitoring. In Kaplan JA (ed.): Cardiac Anesthesia. Philadelphia, WB Saunders, 1993, pp. 261–298.
31. Kee LL, Simonson JS, Stots NA, et al.: Echocardiographic determination of valid zero reference levels in supine and lateral positions. Am J Crit Care 2:72, 1993.
32. Potger KC, Elliott D: Reproducibility of central venous pressures in supine and lateral positions: A pilot evaluation of the phlebostatic axis in critically ill patient. Heart Lung 23:285, 1994.
33. Kopman EA, Sandza JG: Manipulation of the pulmonary artery catheter after placement: Maintainence of sterility. Anesthesiology 48:373, 1978.
34. Kasten GW, Owens E, Kennedy D: Ventricular tachycardia resulting from central venous catheter tip migration due to arm position change: Report of two cases. Anesthesiology 62:185, 1985.
35. Salmenpera M, Peltola K, Rosenberg P: Does prophylactic lidocaine control cardiac arrhythmia associated with pulmonary artery catheterization. Anesthesiology 56:210, 1982.
36. Sessler DI: Temperature monitoring. In Miller RD (ed.): Anesthesia. New York, Churchill Livingstone, 1994, pp. 1363–1382.
37. Shinozaki T, Deane R, Perkins FM: Infrared tympanic thermometer: Evaluation of a new clinical thermometer. Crit Care Med 16:148, 1988.
38. Severinghaus JW, Kelleher JF: Recent developments in pulse oximetry. Anesthesiology 76:1018, 1992.

39. Eisenkraft JB, Cohen E, Neustein SM: Anesthesia for thoracic surgery. *In* Barash PG, Cullen BF, Stoelting RK (eds.): Clinical Anesthesia. Philadelphia, JB Lippincott, 1992, pp. 943–988.

40. Raemer DB, Francis D, Philip JH, Gable RA: Variation in P_{CO_2} between arterial blood and peak expired gas during anesthesia. Anesth Analg 62:1065, 1983.

41. Conrady PA, Goodman LR, Lainge F, Singer MD: Alteration of endotracheal tube position: Flexion and extension of the neck. Crit Care Med 4:8, 1976.

42. Lingenfelter AL, Guskiewicz RA, Munson ES: Displacement of right atrial and endotracheal catheters with neck flexion. Anesth Analg 57:371, 1978.

43. Toung TJK, Grayson R, Saklad J, Wang H: Movement of the distal end of the endotracheal tube during flexion and extension of the neck. Anesth Analg 64:1030, 1985.

44. Britt BA, Joy N, Mackay MB: Positioning trauma. *In* Orkin FK, Cooperman LH (eds.): Complications in Anesthesiology. Philadelphia, JB Lippincott, 1983.

45. Baraka A, Moghrabi R, Yazigi A: Unilateral pulmonary oedema/atelectasis in the lateral decubitus position. Anaesthesia 42:171, 1987.

46. Snoy FG, Woodside JR: Unilateral pulmonary edema (down-lung syndrome) following urological operation. J Urol 132:776, 1984.

47. Eggers GWN, DeGroot WJ, Tanner CR, Leonard JJ: Hemodynamic changes associated with various surgical positions. JAMA 185:1, 1963.

48. Baehrendtz S, Bindslev L, Hedenstiere G, Santesson J: Selective PEEP in acute bilateral lung disease: Effect on patients in lateral posture. Acta Anaesth Scand 27:311, 1983.

49. Werner O, Malmkvist G, Beckman A, et al.: Gas exchange and haemodynamics during thorocotomy. Br J Anaesth 56:1343, 1984.

50. Fessler HE, Brower RG, Shapiro EP, Permutt S: Effects of positive end-expiratory pressure and body position on pressure in the thoracic great veins. Am Rev Respir Dis 148:1657, 1993.

51. Klingstedt C, Hedenstierna G, Lundquist H, et al.: The influence of body position and differential ventilation on lung dimensions and atelectasis formation in anesthetized man. Acta Anaesthesiol Scand 34:315, 1990.

52. Meyhoff HH, Hess J, Olesen KP: Pulmonary atelectasis following upper urinary tract surgery on patients in the 25 and 45 degree jack-knife position. Scand J Urol Nephrol 14:107, 1980.

53. Courington FW: The role of posture in anesthesia. Clin Anesth 3:24, 1968.

54. Minamimoto T, Mutsuda T, Takaya N, et al.: Six cases of contralateral atelectasis immediately after thoracotomy in lateral position: Its mechanism and treatment (Japanese). J Jpn Assoc Thorac Surg 39:1112, 1991.

55. Henschel AB, Wyant GM, Dobkin AB, Henschel EO: Posture as it concerns the anesthesiologist: A preliminary study. Anesth Analg 36:69, 1957.

56. Jones JR, Jacoby J: The effect of surgical positions on respiration. Surg Forum 5:686, 1955.

57. Froese AB, Bryan AC: Effects of anesthesia and paralysis on diaphragmatic mechanics in man. Anesthesiology 41:242, 1974.

58. Fratacci MD, Kimball VVR, Wain JC, et al.: Diaphragmatic shortening after thoracic surgery in humans. Anesthesiology 79:654, 1993.

59. Rehder K, Sessler AD, Marsh HM: General anesthesia and the lung. Lung Dis 76:367, 1975.

60. Vellody VP, Nassery M, Druz WS, Sharp JT: Effects of body position change on thoracoabdominal motion. J Appl Physiol 45:581, 1978.

61. Pansard JL, Cholley B, Devilliers C, et al.: Variation in arterial to end-tidal CO_2 tension differences during anesthesia in the "kidney rest" lateral decubitus position. Anesth Analg 75:506, 1992.

62. Wulff KE, Aulin I: The regional lung function in the lateral decubitus position during anesthesia and operation. Acta Anaesth Scand 16:194, 1972.

63. Bach A, Atzberger M, Morar R, Krier C: Postoperative arterial oxygen saturation in children. Anasthesiol Intensivther Notfallmed 24:37, 1989.

64. Norton LC, Conforti CG: The effects of body position on oxygenation. Heart Lung 14:45, 1985.

65. Benumof JL: One-lung ventilation and hypoxic pulmonary vasoconstriction: Implications for anesthetic management. Anesth Analg 64:821, 1985.

66. Hayashi Y, Takaki 0, Uchida 0: Anesthetic management of patients undergoing bilateral unifocalization. Anesth Analg 76:755, 1993.

67. Frostell C, Blomquist H, Nilsson JA, et al.: Differential ventilation with selective PEEP in bilateral lung disease. Intensive Care Med 10:265, 1984.

68. Rivara D, Artucio H, Arcos J, Hiriart C: Positional hypoxemia during artificial ventilation. Crit Care Med 12:436, 1984.

69. Sonnenblick M, Melzer E, Rosin AJ: Body positional effect on gas exchange in unilateral effusion. Chest 5:784, 1983.

70. Dreyfuss D, Djedaini K, Lanore JJ, et al.: A comparative study of the effects of almitrine bismesylate and lateral position during unilateral bacterial pneumonia with severe hypoxemia. Am Rev Respir Dis 146:295, 1992.

71. Zach MB, Pontoppidan H, Kazemi H: The effect of lateral positions on gas exchange in pulmonary disease. Am Rev Respir Dis 110:49, 1974.

72. Polacek TL, Barth L, Mestad P, et al.: The effect of positioning on arterial oxygenation in children with atelectasis after cardiac surgery. Heart Lung 21:457, 1992.

73. Britt BA, Gordon RA: Peripheral nerve injuries associated with anesthesia. Can Anaesth Soc J 11:514, 1964.

74. Smith JW, Pellicci PM, Sharrock N, et al.: Complications after total hip replacement: The contralateral limb. J Bone Joint Surg Am 71:528, 1989.

75. Targa L, Droghetti G, Caggese R: Rhabdomyolysis and operating position. Anaesthesia 46:141, 1991.

76. Rommel FM, Kabler RL, Mowad JJ: The crush syndrome: A complication of urological surgery. J Urol 135:809, 1986.

77. Lawson NL, Mills NL, Oschsner JL: Occipital alopecia following open heart surgery. J Thorac Cardiovasc Surg 71:342, 1976.

78. Brown EM, Elman DS: Postoperative backache. Anesth Analg 40:683, 1961.

79. Clarke AM, Stillwell S, Paterson MEL, Getty CJM: Role of the surgical position in the development of postoperative low back pain. J Spinal Disord 6:238, 1993.

80. Jaffe TB, McLesky CH: Position induced Homer's syndrome. Anesthesiology 56:49, 1982.

81. Katayama T, Katou F, Motegi K: Unilateral parotid swelling after general anaesthesia. J Craniomaxillofac Surg 18:229, 1990.

82. Kimura H, Watanabe Y, Mizukoshi K, et al.: Six cases of anesthesia mumps. Nippon Jibiinkoka Gakkai Kaiho 96:1915, 1993.

83. Nambisan RN, Karakousis CP: Axillary compression syndrome with neuropraxia due to operative positioning. Surgery 105:449, 1989.
84. Kopoll HP, Thompson WAL: Suprascapular nerve. *In* Thompson WAL (ed.): Peripheral Entrapment Neu-ropathies. New York, Robert E. Krieger Publishing, 1976.
85. Lachiewicz PF, Latimer HA: Rhabdomyolysis following total hip arthroplasty. J Bone Joint Surg [Br] 73:576, 1991.

Ventral Decubitus Positions

Chapter **10**

The Ventral Decubitus (Prone) Positions

John T. Martin

BACKGROUND

The terms *prone, ventral recumbent*, and *ventral decubitus* are synonyms that describe a group of postures in which the patient is "face down," resting on some portion of the ventral thorax, abdomen, and ventral surfaces of the lower extremities. In the operating room these positions afford surgical access to dorsal aspects of the body. Singh[1] has stated in part that "the successful outcome of surgery on the thoracic and lumbar spine is largely dependent on the proper positioning of the patient before the operation begins." A similar statement can be made by the neurosurgeon who is operating on a patient's dorsal neck and head.

Concern about the safety of the prone patient during anesthesia and surgery is not new. The distinguished innovator Harvey Cushing[2] reported in 1909 that his full-time physician anesthesiologist, Dr. S. Griffith Davis, employed a simple safety device (then called a "phonendoscope") placed against the chest wall over the heart of the pronated patient and connected to Dr. Davis' ear to provide "continuous auscultation of cardiac and respiratory rhythm during the entire course of anesthesia. On several occasions, by the prompt appreciation of change in heartbeat or respiration thus acquired, it has been possible to avert what otherwise might have been surgical disasters, owing to the immediate

warning that led to the cessation of certain disturbing manipulations." Thus, before the era of endotracheal intubation, the hazards of anesthesia and surgery for the prone patient established the value of continuous cardiorespiratory auscultation and identified the precordial stethoscope, initially a canine cardiac monitor in Cushing's Hunterian Laboratory, as an important asset in the surveillance of anesthetized humans in the surgical theater.[3]

During normal sleep the prone position is preferred by many people with supple physiques. However, during general or regional anesthesia, changes associated with aging, plus drug-induced losses of normal protective reflexes and tissue tone, produce significant physiologic and functional hazards for the prone patient unless the anesthesia team is knowledgeable and vigilant. Satisfactory management of the prone position during anesthesia is the result of attention to a clutter of seemingly trivial details, each of which, if ignored, may lead to an avoidable problem. A well-documented review of the anesthetic management of vertebral column surgery has been published by Bagshaw and associates.[4] Anderton has also written a useful review of the prone position.[5] In the following discussion, the term *pronation* will refer to rotation of the patient's whole body about its longitudinal axis into the ventral decubitus position rather than indicating just the position of the forearm and hand.

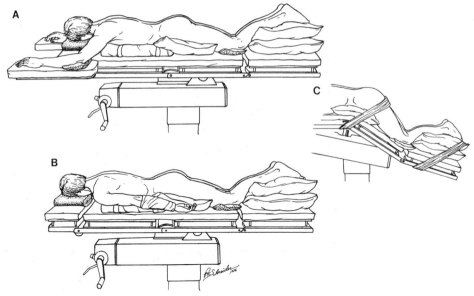

Figure 10–1

Classic prone position. *A.* Flat table with patient's arms above head. Note cephalad end of chest role just below clavicle with pillow across caudal end. Forearms are supported ventrad to transverse axis of thorax. Elbows and knees are padded; legs are flexed on thighs. *B.* Arms are snugged alongside torso. Head is turned on C-shaped face piece (see Fig. 10-16). *C.* Eventual flexed table top to minimize lumbar lordosis. Thrust of gluteal straps must be cephalad to retain torso against weight of lower extremities on tilted table.

VARIATIONS OF THE PRONE POSITION

When an individual is comfortably prone during normal sleep, the position is safeguarded by active reflexes that allow involuntary alterations of posture to offset atelectasis, ischemia, and skeletal stress. In the presence of an aged or abnormal vertebral column, sufficient mobility of the cervical spine may not be possible, and the position will be rejected or modified during sleep because torsion of the head produces significant neck pain. The posture may also be voluntarily or involuntarily avoided because of the existence of a thoracic outlet syndrome. None of these safeguards exists if the patient is anesthetized.

During anesthesia, compression of abdominal viscera against the table surface restricts caudad movement of the contracting diaphragm, hampers ventilation, and projects increased venous and cerebrospinal fluid (CSF) pressure into the spinal wound or cranial contents. Numerous mechanical devices and variations of the prone posture, described subsequently, have been proposed to redistribute body weight and keep pressure away from the abdomen. When the legs are significantly below the level of the heart, elastic compressive wraps are usually used to support venous return and limit pooling of blood in the extremities.

Horizontal Prone Position

This is the "classic" prone position with the patient resting on the ventral aspects of the torso, the legs extended, and the arms either raised beside the head on padded armboards (Fig. 10–1*A*) or retained at the sides of the body (see Fig. 10–1*B*). With arms alongside the head, the forearms should rest somewhat ventral to the transverse plane of the torso, not level with it, to avoid stretching the brachial plexus and its related vascular structures.

When the lumbar area is the surgical target, some form of elevating mechanism raises the torso off of the table surface to decompress the abdomen and relieve vascular congestion at the operative site. To aid surgical access to structures on the dorsal aspect of the vertebral column and their interspaces, the table surface can be angulated sufficiently to decrease lumbar lordosis (see Fig. 10–1 *C*) or the placement of legs relative to pelvic rests can be adjusted to tilt the pelvis and accomplish the same purpose. Subgluteal restraining straps should thrust significantly cephalad to prevent caudad slippage of the torso (see Fig. 10–1 C).

Because they found laparoscopic surgery involving structures in the dorsal abdomen to be time consuming and technically difficult in traditional dorsal decubitus positions, Bannenburg's group at the University of Amsterdam[6] investigated the feasibility of using the prone position with instruments inserted through the flanks of study animals. They found that the posture offered a clear and unobstructed view of the abdominal back wall and the large intestine.

Ophthalmologic Prone Position

The ophthalmologist occasionally repairs giant retinal detachments by vitreal injections of sulfur hexafluoride gas while the anesthetized patient is prone. In the course of the procedure the patient is initially supine, pronated for the injection, and returned to the supine position for the remainder of the operation. The postural change from the classic prone position is required by the need to provide surgical access to the face while the head is held firm by some means of fixation. Schepens and associates[7] report the development of a power-driven operating table for this purpose. Wollman and Newman[8] prefer to use the standard padded Mayfield neurosurgical head rest attachment to support the head at the level of the maxillae (Fig. 10–2). No reports of using the Mayfield-type skull

pin head holder for this purpose were located.

Head-Elevated Prone Position

In this modification of the "classic" prone position, the patient is usually placed flat on the table with the viscera freed and the chassis rotated sufficiently to place the head above the level of the heart. Because the head and cervical spine are the usual surgical sites, the arms are restrained alongside the body. Some form of holder is needed to keep the head stable relative to the trunk without compressing the eyes. Additional stabilization must keep the patient from slipping caudad if the head elevation is more than minimal (Fig. 10–3).

Many surgeons consider this posture to provide safer access to the cervical spine and posterior cranial fossa than does the sitting position. Gravity drainage helps avoid venous congestion at the wound. However, from the standpoint of the anesthesiologist, the head-elevated prone position has potential problems that may become critical. Depending on the degree of head elevation, a pressure gradient can exist between the operative site and the heart that provides the opportunity for hypoperfusion in the head and/or air entrainment into incised and patulous veins. Should resuscitation be needed, gaining access to the ventral chest for cardiac massage demands a change in the patient's position that chaotically disrupts the surgical field and consumes critical time. Recently,

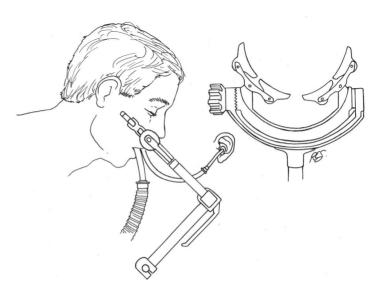

Figure 10–2

Ophthalmologic prone position with head extended and Mayfield neurosurgical (*inset*) rest supporting malar area to free eyes for surgeon. Malar rest depicted is thinned to improve display of relationship to face.

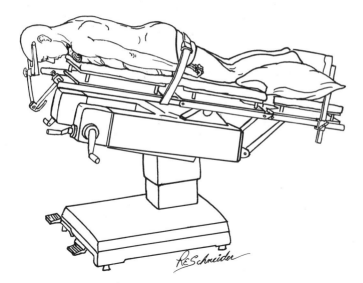

Figure 10–3

Head-elevated prone position for cervico-occipital exploration using Gardner skull clamp to retain head. Surgical field is above atrium and promotes venous drainage from wound. (Restraining arm wraps not shown for clarity.) Subgluteal strap thrusts cephalad against weight of torso.

however, Sun and colleagues[9] and Tobias and associates[10] have described successful cardiac resuscitation of neurosurgical patients using reversed precordial compression while the patients remained prone.

Sea Lion Prone Position

Iwabuchi and associates[11] arrange their conventional prone position by reverse-flexing the table top approximately 20 degrees at the hip break (Fig. 10–4A). Thereby the patient's back is arched (hyperlordotic), the head is above heart level, and the neck can be flexed as needed. The torso and lower extremities make equal dorsiflexed angles above the horizontal. They also use a modification of this head-elevated hyperlordotic prone posture in which the patient's head is maintained in the midline while the neck is extended to allow maximum access to the top of the skull. This extended-neck and back prone posture they term the *sea lion position* (see Fig. 10–4B).

Thoracic Prone (Overholt) Position

The head-down thoracic prone position was developed by Overholt and Langer.[12] It was intended to reduce lung soilage by permitting infectious material from the diseased lung, plus blood from the surgical site, to drain down the inverted tracheobronchial tree into the accessible upper airway and endotracheal tube where it could be removed by aspiration. A two-level operating table (Overholt-Compere Table, American Sterilizer Company, Erie, PA) was involved (Fig 10–5). The hips

of the patient were placed at one level, the sternum rested upon a lower adjustable table section, and the arms were extended ventrally and flexed at the elbow to remain on padded boards that were still closer to the floor. The advent of antibiotics and double-lumen endotracheal tubes circumvented the usefulness of this complicated posture. Because it required a stable chest wall, the Overholt position was dangerous for a patient of that medical era whose rib cage had been previously destabilized by a thoracoplasty designed to collapse an infected lobe or lung. A similar posture was independently developed by Sellor-Brown.[13]

Crouching or Kneeling Position

Several variations of this version of the prone position exist, and all are designed to remove pressure from the abdomen. The *crouching position*[14–16] (also referred to as the tuck, folded, or carpenter rule position) flexes thighs fully on trunk and legs fully on thighs (Fig. 10–6). The knees are spread apart to free the abdomen, and weight is borne principally on the thighs, knees, and lower legs. Restraining tapes are placed, and the table top is then tilted sufficiently to make the lumbar spine horizontal. Improved modifications of the tuck position have opened up the angulation at hips and knees and provided a gluteal support to retain the patient in place (Fig. 10–7, the Tarlov seat; Fig 10–8, the Hastings frame). In the *kneeling position*, the patient's thighs are flexed less acutely on the abdomen, the lower legs are often almost at right angles

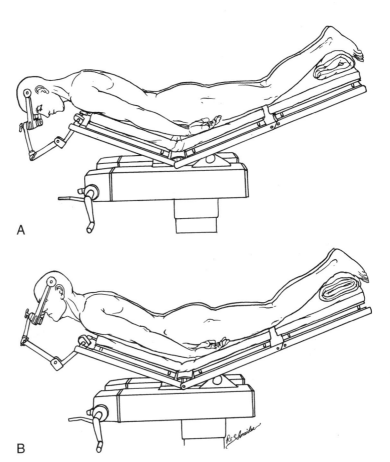

Figure 10–4

Iwabuchi's hyperlordotic prone position. *A.* Neck flexed. *B.* Neck extended in "sea lion" position. (Redrawn from Iwabuchi T, Sobata E, Suzuki M, et al.: Dural sinus pressure as related to neurosurgical positions. Neurosurgery 12:203, 1983.)

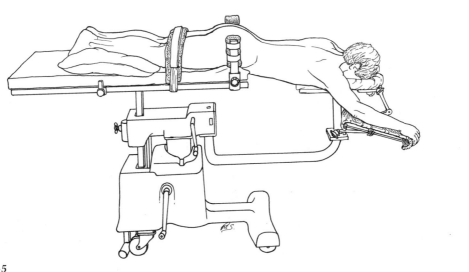

Figure 10–5

The Overholt-Compere table for prone position. (Redrawn from catalog circa 1952 of American Sterilizer Company, Erie, PA.)

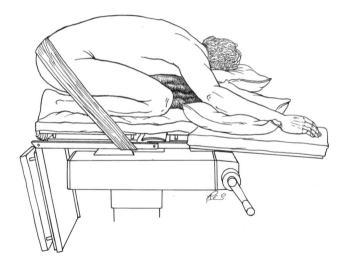

Figure 10–6

The tuck position. Weight rests on chest and legs; knees are lateralized to decompress abdomen. Note the severe angulation of hips and knees and the potential for toe injury from raising depressed foot section of table top. (Redrawn from Wayne SJ: The tuck position for lumbar disc surgery. J Bone Joint Surg 49:1195, 1967. *Note:* Dr. Wayne no longer uses this position.)

to the thighs, and weight is borne principally on the knees and chest (Fig. 10–9). The patient usually kneels on a step device placed on the depressed foot section of the table. The chest rests on the table (Buie position)[17]; on an appropriately thick stack of folded sheets (Georgia position)[18]; or on an adjustable elevator, such as the Wiltse jack.

In 1982, Cook and associates reported considerable experience with a variant of the kneeling position, curiously termed the *sitting prone position*, in which no rests compress the anterior iliac spines, the knees are on a shelf on the depressed leg section of the table, and the torso is stabilized by subgluteal supports that function as a modified seat (Fig. 10–10).[19] They use this modification of prone posture for posterior fossa procedures as well as for

operations at any level of the spine. Cook and associates' data for peak airway and central venous pressures from patients in this position compare favorably with similar data that they obtained while patients were supine and are better than their data from the same patients prone on a "laminectomy frame."

Taylor and colleagues[20] used an inguinal rest to elevate the abdomen off of the surgical table and added a bicycle-type seat applied to the buttocks to assure that caudad slippage of the torso did not occur if the table was tilted or flexed and the legs depressed farther (Fig. 10–11).

Whether crouching or kneeling, these positions are intended to flatten the lumbar curve of the spinal column. Each requires that the patient has an intact vertebral column. If the

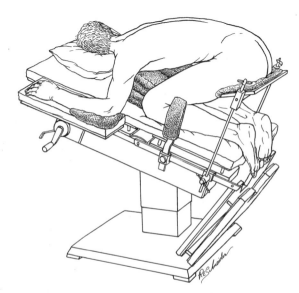

Figure 10–7

The Tarlov seat. Weight of torso is absorbed mainly by subgluteal rest and chest support. Knee brace retains separated knees on table. Note potential for toe injury from raising depressed foot section of table top. (Redrawn from Tarlov M: The knee chest position for lower spinal operations. J Bone Joint Surg 49:1192, 1967.)

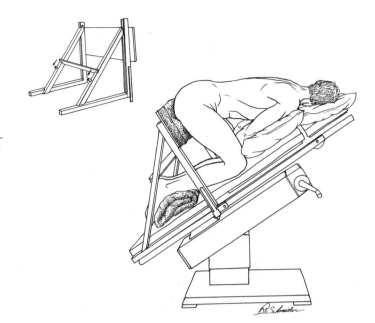

Figure 10–8

The Hastings frame. Weight of torso is absorbed by seat and chest support. (Reprinted from Hastings DE: A simple frame for operations on the lumbar spine. Can J Surg 12:251, 1969. By permission of the publisher.)

spine is unstable, the position is likely to cause a shearing, knife-like stress at the point of discontinuity that can crush or cut the contents of the spinal canal.

Semiprone Position

The semiprone position (see also Chapter 9) is a variation of a lateral decubitus position in which the patient's torso is allowed to rotate ventrad to some degree and is stabilized by suitable padding under its raised edge. It offers access to the posterolateral aspects of the thorax and spine (Fig. 10–12). It has been used by some to position the thorax so that the head can be rotated face down when the

full prone position is not desirable for some reason. Usually, however, the head is rotated toward the elevated shoulder and rests on padding under the down-side cheek that is sufficient to maintain a nonangulated cervical spine.

The up-side arm is usually rested alongside the head, either on a pad or on an adjustable arm holder. Access to the face is better for the anesthesiologist if the pad is used rather than the arm holder. A pad of sufficient thickness is placed under the anterolateral thorax just caudad of the down-side axilla to raise the torso off of the down-side shoulder. Its purpose is to prevent severe dorsal displacement of the shoulder girdle that would close the

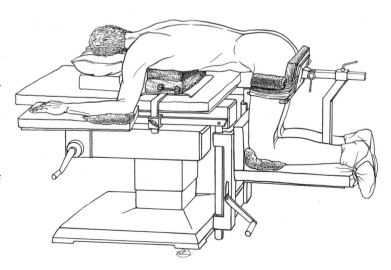

Figure 10–9

Andrews frame in use with Wiltse modification (elevatable chest jack). Weight of torso is borne by chest support and knees. Booties tied to kneeling ledge retain flexion. Ledge height is adjustable to level lumbar spine. (Redrawn from literature of Orthopedic Systems, Inc., Hayward, CA.)

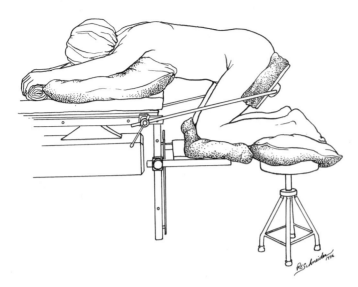

Figure 10–10

Cook's sitting prone position. (Redrawn from Cook AW, Siddiqi TS, Nidzgorski F, et al.: Sitting prone position for the posterior surgical approach to the spine and posterior fossa. Neurosurgery 10:232, 1982.)

retroclavicular space and compress the subclavian neurovascular bundle. The down-side arm should be placed behind the torso to prevent a traction neuropathy of the suprascapular nerve caused by the shoulder girdle being circumducted ventrally across the front of the torso.

Reverse Lithotomy Position

For simultaneous endoscopic access to intrarenal and transurethral sites in the urinary tracts of women for the removal of calculi, Lehman and Bagley[21] have employed a strangely named modification of the ventral decubitus position in which the legs of the pronated patient are almost fully extended, the knees are bent, and both lower extremities

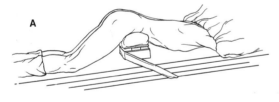

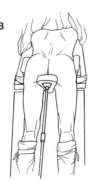

Figure 10–11

Taylor's iliac crest support (*A*) and cycle seat (*B*). Seat stabilizes patient against caudad displacement when table is tilted to level spine. (Redrawn from Taylor AR, Gleadhill CA, Bilsland WL, Murray PF: Posture and anaesthesia for spinal operations with special reference to intervertebral disc surgery. Br J Anaesth 28:213, 1956. BMJ Publishing Group.)

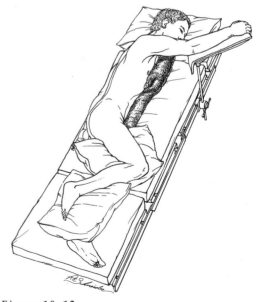

Figure 10–12

Semiprone position for costotransversectomy. Note down-side arm behind torso and hand by buttock. Firm rest under ventral chest prevents further pronation.

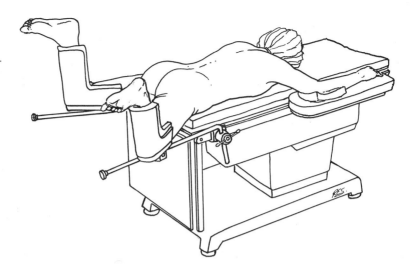

Figure 10–13

Lehman and Bagley's "reverse lithotomy" position for simultaneous endoscopic access to renal pelvis by means of a nephrostomy and to lower urinary tract through the urethra. (Redrawn from Lehman T, Bagley DH: Reverse lithotomy: Modified prone position for simultaneous nephroscopic and ureteroscopic procedures in women. Endourology 32:529, 1988.)

are abducted and secured in holders used traditionally for the lithotomy position (Fig. 10–13). The foot of the operating table is then lowered to allow a transperineal cystoscopic approach to the urethra, bladder, and ureters. Nephroscopy is accomplished through an existing nephrostomy tract that is easily accessible in the pronated flank. Grasso and colleagues subsequently reported successful use of the method in 111 additional patients.[22]

Prone Jackknife Position

The prone jackknife position is usually reserved for gluteal or anorectal surgery. The patient is placed prone on an operating table with the legs extended, the arms usually alongside the head, and the head turned to one side. Customarily a support of some type, most often a pillow, is placed beneath the pelvis. The inguinal crease is placed over the hinge between the back and thigh sections of the table top. Then the articulation between the thigh and back section of the table top is angulated until the two sections lodge against the ends of the table chassis and form an inverted "V" that has its apex at the patient's hips (Fig. 10–14). Finally, the chassis can be rotated head downward sufficiently to provide working access to the area of the buttocks and anus. Usually, adhesive tapes are applied to draw the buttocks laterally and improve perianal exposure. Urologists have used this gently flexed prone position with abducted lower extremities to provide dorsal access to the lower urinary tract when planning a prostatovesiculectomy.[23] Usually the angulation of the "V" is not severe because the extent to which most table tops will flex or reverse-flex is limited. Thus, the obvious physiologic trespasses of the posture are minimized. However, with some tables it is possi-

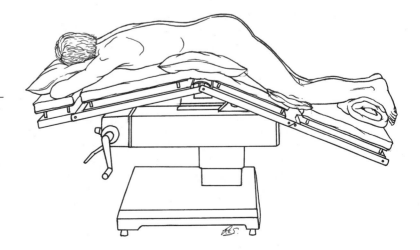

Figure 10–14

Low prone jackknife position with hips at back-thigh hinge of fully flexed table. Iliac pillow used for padding. (Gluteal tapes not shown for clarity.)

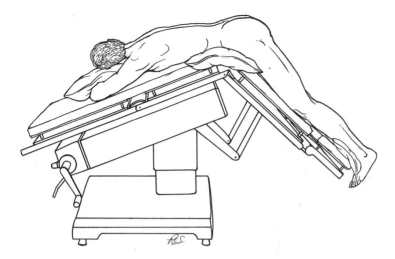

Figure 10–15

Steep prone jackknife position. Head section of table attached to foot section and hips flexed over thigh-leg hinge of table. Arrangement increases hip flexion and head-down tilt. (Gluteal straps not shown for clarity.)

ble to lengthen the foot section by adding the normal head section to it and then to use the thigh-leg hinge (knee hinge) as the flexion point (Fig. 10–15). With the chassis tilted maximally head down, this choice allows severe angulation of the patient across an acute inverted "V" and can constitute a more significant management problem if physiologic stability was precarious at the outset.

SUPPORT DEVICES FOR THE PRONE POSITION

Head Supports

Surgical Pillow and/or Foam Donut

In some anesthesiologic practices, experience has favored placing either a surgical pillow or a cutout made from a disposable foam ring (a "donut") under the down side of the rotated head. A *pillow* may be soft enough to gradually lose its thickness during use and allow the head to derotate toward a more midline position, moving the down-side eye into direct contact with the mattress of the head piece of the table. The opportunity then exists for either a corneal abrasion or compressive ischemia of the globe or both. Removing a section of the *foam donut* makes a C-shaped device that intends to allow the down-side eye to rest between lips of the "C." However, the remainder of most versions of that ring is rarely sturdy enough to prevent the weight of the head from separating the lips of the C and allowing the supposedly supported eye to settle against the surface of the mattress on the head piece of the table.

Then, despite adequate initial precautions taken when the patient was pronated, the opportunity develops for corneal abrasion or global compression of the down-side eye.

Despite the traditional use of pillows and modified rings in some practices, more reliable materials and techniques are available to support the head in such a way that injury to the down-side eye becomes highly unlikely.

The C-Shaped Face Piece

A simple protective support for the pronated, rotated head can be made rapidly from a thick piece of easily available, disposable Reston Foam (3M Company, St. Paul, MN). Folded in half at the midpoint of its length, the sticky side of the foam adheres to itself and produces a resilient pad that is twice as thick as the parent sheet. Cutting out the middle third of the rounded, folded edge of the pad, to a depth of one third of the width of the pad, forms an object that looks like a squared letter C (Fig. 10–16). Placing the resulting face piece on the mattress under the patient's head so that the tips of the "C" lie under the forehead and chin aligns the cutout area of the pad beneath the down-side eye, freeing it from compression. The upper limb of the C supports the forehead, its back supports the down-side cheek dorsally almost to the ear, and its lower limb supports the mandible. Almost invariably, in an average-sized adult head, the down-side ear lies behind the back edge of the pad and is free of pressure from the pillow or mattress. The resulting, firm but comfortably soft, disposable "C-shaped face piece" is sturdy enough to retain its thickness and is somewhat pli-

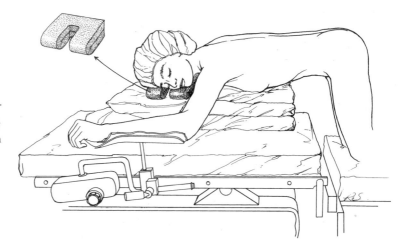

Figure 10-16

C-shaped face piece. Eye notch removes middle third of folded edge to one-third depth of pad. Ear lies behind back edge of pad.

able. However, it is sufficiently rigid so that the weight of the head will not separate its two limbs and allow the down-side eye to contact the mattress. I have used this device successfully for many years.

Ray Rocker-Based Face Piece

Ray[24] developed a rocker-based adjustable face rest with sponge pads to support the forehead and chin of a pronated patient. The device had considerable promise. He reported satisfactory experience with this face rest in over 100 routine surgical procedures. However, my personal experience with the unit included several instances of brawny supraorbital edema and postoperative anesthesia in the distribution of the supraorbital nerve that lasted beyond hospital discharge. Those several problems occurred during our first dozen uses of the rest and had not been encountered during more than three previous decades of using various types of support for the heads of pronated patients. Although the patients involved chanced to be men with large, heavy heads, the problem was frequent enough that I elected to cease using the device in my department. The experience of others may have been more positive.

Horseshoe Head Rest

Well-padded, adjustable horseshoe-shaped head rests that fit the face without compressing the eyes are traditional supports for the pronated head. Generally, they are satisfactory if the sagittal head position will not be disruptively tugged on during surgery and cause the head to be shifted enough to risk

ocular injury (Fig 10–17). Some surgeons and anesthesiologists prefer to reverse the horseshoe to support the pronated forehead with the face free. In either instance, the rest is clamped to a frame attached to the table and the padded "U" is fitted to the face of the

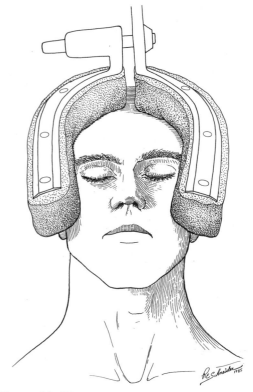

Figure 10-17

Adjustable horseshoe face piece for pronated face. Weight of head is distributed over forehead and malar regions with no compression of orbits. Anesthesiologist has clear access to patient's face.

patient or the reversed "U" is tilted to support the forehead or frontal portion of the skull depending on the degree of neck flexion desired. Tape restraints may be needed to retain the flexed head in the rest.

The patient's eyes and transoral devices can be viewed easily by using a hand-held mirror similar to one traditionally found on a lady's dressing table. Body restraints are needed to keep the patient's torso from shifting caudad and pulling the head off of the rest if the table chassis is tilted head up.

Three-Pin Head Holder

The most stable holder for the nonrotated prone head is undoubtedly one of the modifications of the device originally proposed by Gardner.[25] Spaced by an adjustable C-shaped frame, three pins penetrate the prepared skin to enter firmly into the outer table of the skull in a triangular fashion, two on one side of the head and one on the other (Fig. 10–18). After being carefully placed, the frame is tightened firmly to the skull, the device is locked onto a U-shaped frame that is clamped to the rails at the sides of the operating table, the posture of the patient is adjusted as needed, and the final head position is arranged.

The three-pin skull fixation device provides excellent immobility for the head, prevents

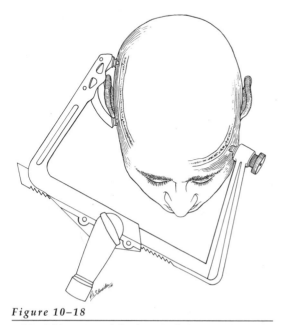

Figure 10–18

Mayfield version of Gardner skull clamp. Pins enter outer table of skull to produce firm grip with clamp. Unit may be adjusted on frame during procedure. (See also Fig. 10–3.)

caudad slippage of the tilted torso because of its unity with both skull and table, and permits almost unobstructed access to the patient's face and transoral devices. If desired, during the operation the attitude of the head can be changed easily by adjusting the joints of the table attachments for the C-shaped frame. Original fears about pin slippage, bacterial osteomyelitis of the skull from the transcutaneous pins, and postoperative pain at the pin sites have been either unrealized or negligible. Several models of the device have become widely available and have proved to be reliable head supports for a variety of surgical positions.

Parallel Longitudinal Devices

Sheet Rolls

A number of surgical sheets, symmetrically folded and wrinkle-free, can be rolled tightly and liberally taped to form a cylinder of uniform thickness that is the length of the patient's torso from clavicle to groin (Fig. 10–19). The key to usefulness of the cylinder is its minimal compressibility produced by the tightness with which it is rolled and taped; its proper construction is an unpopular process that demands considerable hand strength, usually from two people. One sheet roll is placed along each lateral aspect of the torso and each of its ends is tied, most often with roller gauze bandage, to the contralateral table rail. The rolls must be firm enough to absorb the weight of the torso and thick enough to lift the ventral body wall of the patient off of the table surface. The result should cancel any opportunity for the mattress to create enough intra-abdominal pressure to congest blood vessels at the dorsal surgical site. Although not strictly disposable, the rolls should be used only once and then disassembled for laundering of the sheets. Sheets of foam with one sticky side may be placed on the rolls to increase their comfort for the patient.

A pillow placed over the blunt caudad ends of the rolls spreads the pressure of the roll ends and dampens any thigh compression caused by modest flexion of the patient's hips. The cephalad end of each roll should almost reach but never cross the clavicle lest its pressure compresses the retroclavicular space and threatens the integrity of the neurovascular bundle into the upper limb. With the roll-supported patient arranged so that the

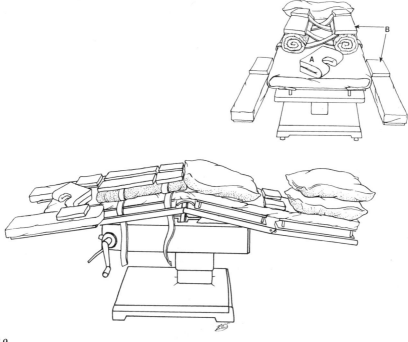

Figure 10–19

Prone position arrangement of a standard operating table. Longitudinal chest rolls are tied to contralateral edges of table. *Top.* View from head of table showing C-shaped face piece (A) and protective pressure point padding (B) made of adhesive foam sheeting (Reston Foam, 3M Co., St. Paul, MN). *Bottom.* Side view of final table angulation with rolls, pads, and pillows placed.

iliac crests are just over the back-thigh articulation of the operating table, the table top can be flexed as desired to lower the legs, decrease lumbar lordosis, and separate lumbar spinous processes.

Convex Frames

Reusable parallel arching frames have been available for many years.[26] Most have some degree of adjustable curvature that can be varied according to the physique of the patient and the requirements of the surgeon (Fig. 10–20, *inset*). The well-padded frame rests on the flat surface of the surgical mattress, and its arching capability is used to minimize or obliterate the patient's normal lumbar lordosis. Because they are reusable, these units demand careful cleaning between uses and equally careful removal of cleaning substances to prevent contamination of, or chemical injury to, the skin of a subsequent patient.

FORMED SUPPORTS

Cloward Surgical Saddle

A large, shaped pad (Fig 10–21A) of reusable plastic has been designed for pronated pa-

tients. Clipped to the operating table, it supports iliac crests, has an aperture that is intended to decompress the abdomen, and can be angulated sufficiently to establish a kneeling position. Although it is a successful device, the Cloward surgical saddle shares with all reusable pads the trait of losing some of its resilience over time and may eventually be a less effective support than when first constructed.

Bardeen Pad

With a history of many years of successful service, the Bardeen pad[27] (see Fig. 10–21B) is a reusable, adjustable, plastic device that is designed to support the thorax and hips of a pronated patient while reducing intra-abdominal pressure. Over time, however, a specific unit usually becomes compressible and the implied support is degraded or lost. At that point it needs replacement regardless of whether its cover is still intact. Although the Bardeen pad is a familiar item in most operating suites in North America, it is not thick enough to be of much use with an obese patient.

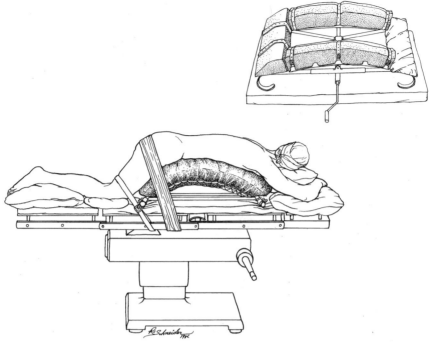

Figure 10–20

The convex saddle frame for spinal operations. (Redrawn from Moore DC, Edmonds L: Prone position frame. Surgery 17:276, 1950.) *Inset.* The adjustable Wilson frame for prone position. (Revised from Horton, 1977.)

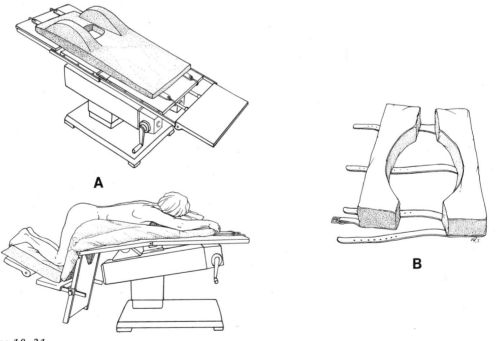

A

B

Figure 10–21

Reusable formed pads for pronation. *A.* Cloward surgical saddle. *Upper.* Pad applied to surgical table surface and hooked in place. *Lower.* Patient positioned on pad. (Redrawn from literature of Surgical Equipment International, Inc., Honolulu, HI.) *B.* Bardeen chest pad. (Redrawn from Bardeen A: A special pad for patients in the prone position. Anesthesiology 16:465, 1955; available from V. Mueller & Co., Chicago.) Note that any reusable foam pad may lose resilience with age and support can be less than anticipated.

Vacuum Packs

Large plastic "bean bags" are commercially available. Filled with tiny plastic spheres and vented to the outside through valves, they are designed to be shaped to various body parts and have all of the contained air removed by a vacuum line. When air free, they become quite firm, assuming a relatively unyielding cast-like structure that retains its molded shape until air is readmitted. Some have used these vacuum packs for shaped support of a pronated patient, but problems exist with them. The bags obviously contract when air is evacuated, and their surfaces wrinkle uncontrollably. Prolonged lying on those rather sharply uneven surfaces may damage thin or atrophic skin. A towel clip may inadvertently penetrate the surface of a supporting bag or a leaky valve may readmit air, causing the support to disappear at a totally inappropriate time during a procedure. Because they are relatively thin, and because separating them from the ventral body wall of a pronated patient can be tricky, effectively decompressing the abdomen of a sizable individual can be difficult. Generally, the "bean bags" are much more effective for purposes other than ventral support of a prone patient.

Pedestal Supports

Sandbags

Several sandbags can be taped together to produce a pedestal of desired height. These pedestals can then be placed on the operating table, one at the outer corner of each quadrant of the torso of a pronated patient. Although they are not fixed firmly to the table, they are heavy and the added weight of the patient usually retains the individual pedestals in place. However, bulky physiques may gradually shift them laterally during the procedure and obviate their usefulness.

Relton Frame

Relton and Hall[28] developed an adjustable four-pedestal frame that duplicated the arrangement of the sandbags but was significantly more stable (Fig. 10–22). Resting on the operating table, the frame could be adjusted to the dimensions of the pronated patient and did not allow the pedestals to shift because of the weight of the patient. Varying the position of the iliac pedestals could adjust the flexion of the hips and control the amount of lumbar lordosis. Variants of this basic design have been developed in various localities. Intraoperative adjustment of the iliac supports of the frame and the legs of the patient can control the amount of lumbar lordosis present during surgery.

Pedestal frames may pose a problem with obese patients. The high weight/body surface ratio for each supporting point may lead to pressure points or blistering of skin at the contact site. Some means of enlarging the surface of the supporting point, such as placing a folded blanket or other padding over the pedestal, may reduce the potential for tissue damage (Warner MA, personal communication, 1994).

Mouradian Modification of Relton Frame

To maintain longitudinal traction on the spine, Mouradian and Simmons[29] joined the Relton pedestals with the ventral half of a Foster frame (Fig. 10–23). With the intubated,

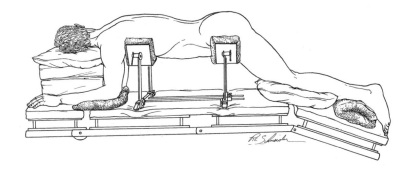

Figure 10–22

Relton adjustable pedestal frame in use. Padding and elevated leg section often used to flex knees further than shown. (Redrawn from Relton JES, Hall JE: An operation frame for spinal surgery. J Bone Joint Surg 49:327, 1967.)

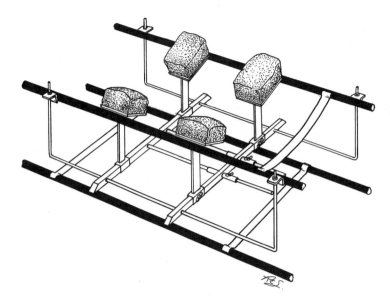

Figure 10–23

The Mouradian and Simmons modification of the Relton frame. (Redrawn from Mouradian WH, Simmons EH: A frame for spinal surgery to reduce intraabdominal pressure while continuous traction is applied. J Bone Joint Surg 59:1098, 1977.)

supine patient lying in traction on the dorsal shell of a Foster frame, the modified ventral section is attached and its supports adjusted to the physique of the patient. The entire unit is then pronated while traction is maintained. Because of the pedestals, the abdomen hangs free rather than being compressed by the standard ventral portion of the Foster frame.

Smith Iliac Elevator

Smith[30] developed a pair of curved metal iliac crest supports on a base that clamped to the elevatable transverse bar ("kidney rest") of the operating table (Fig. 10–24). With the thorax and rotated head of a prone patient resting on stacks of sheets, raising the bar could variably elevate the pelvis to decompress the abdomen. Because the lower extremities remained on the table surface, the hip elevation also angulated the thighs sufficiently to rotate the pelvis and decrease lumbar lordosis. The final configuration of torso and extremities closely resembled that produced by a Relton frame.

Kneeling Systems

These devices rest the weight of the patient on a chest support and on knees bent at approximately right angles to the long axis of the torso.

Kneeboards

This ancient version of the knee-chest position added considerable padding to the metal footboard of the operating table, affixed it to the rails of the leg section of the table, and angulated the leg section floorward approximately 90 degrees (Fig. 10–25). The board then acted as a ledge upon which the patient

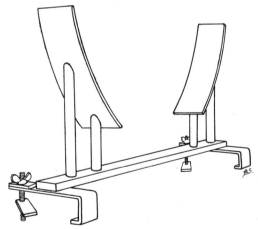

Figure 10–24

The Smith iliac elevator. Transverse plate can be bolted to elevatable kidney rest of operating table. Vertical rods holding curved supports insert into holes in plate according to width of ventral iliac crests. Lower extremities of patient rest on horizontal surface of operating table. (Redrawn from Smith RH: Hoist for the Georgia prone position. Anesthesiology 25:87, 1964.)

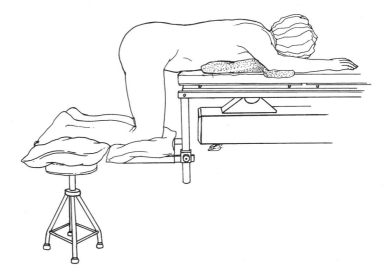

Figure 10–25

Standard operating table in kneeling configuration. Footboard of table becomes adjustable kneeling rest with padded operating room stool under ankles. (Thigh restraints not shown.)

kneeled during the procedure. Restraints around the dorsal thighs and padded supports under the chest and head completed the arrangement. Torque caused by the weight of the lower extremities on the kneeling ledge made its adjustment difficult if the posture needed to be changed during the anesthetic. However, the arrangement could be constructed with standard parts of the operating table.

Georgia Prone System

In 1964, Smith[31] constructed an early version of a kneeling device for the prone position. It consisted of a wheeled, adjustable knee hoist with iliac pads attached to it by metal rods (Fig. 10–26). The iliac pads acted as fulcrums

for the pelvis, allowing the dependent lower extremities to flatten the lumbar curvature.

Andrews Frame

A readily available version of a kneeling frame is accredited to Andrews. Attached to the vertical side rails of the down-angled foot section of the surgical table, the unit consists of a kneeling pad and a gluteal rest (see Fig. 10–9). Either a stack of sheets or an elevatable jack supports the patient's chest and the feet are held against the kneeling pad by straps from booties. A crank adjusts the elevation of the kneeling pad to alter lumbar curvature as desired. The device will support and manipulate the posture of a massively obese pronated

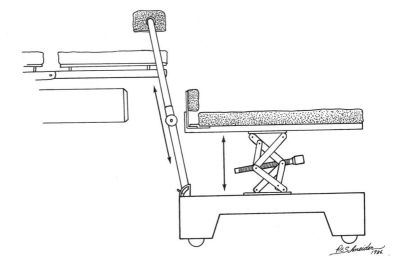

Figure 10–26

Smith mechanical hoist for the Georgia prone position. Height of both iliac pads and kneeling bench is adjustable to fit configuration of patient and degree of lumbar flattening desired. (Redrawn from Smith RH: Hoist for the Georgia prone position. Anesthesiology 25:87, 1964.)

patient with relative ease (see subsequent discussion on pathologic obesity).

ESTABLISHING THE PRONE POSITION

Preliminary Considerations

Regional or perispinal anesthesia used for surgery about the spine, sacrum, anus, or lower extremities often can be established after the patient has been suitably positioned prone on the operating table. However, if general anesthesia is intended as an adjunct, it is almost always started when the patient is still supine. Whether anesthesia is begun when the patient is still in a bed, on a wheeled cart, or on an operating table depends on the physical condition of the patient as well as the preference of the anesthesiologist. The choice is influenced by issues such as painful movement, presence of traction devices, accessibility of the airway for intubation, and stability of the cervical spine. For the sake of completeness, the following descriptions involve pronation from a cart or bed onto the operating table as well as pronation on the operating table itself. Each description assumes a patient with a normal vertebral column and neurologic examination unless otherwise stated.

Pronating an anesthetized patient requires a type and level of anesthesia that preserves autonomic compensation, allows sufficient analgesia to avoid abnormal sympathetic activity, and includes sustained relaxation to allow gentle positioning. Neither significant hypotension nor threatening hypertension should be permitted, and, should either appear, turning must be delayed until corrective measures become effective. The success of pronation should not be risked by vigorous paroxysms of coughing when the patient's head is manipulated on the endotracheal tube. No specific drugs or regimens are clearly superior for these purposes. Choices are based on the needs of the patient as well as on the experience of the team.

All monitoring leads, intravascular lines, and the urinary catheter should be placed and fixed securely while the patient is supine. They must be slack and long enough to sustain the position change. The corrugated breathing tubing of the gas machine should be longer than usual. For the brief duration of the turn the endotracheal tube is usually disconnected from the breathing circuit and reconnected immediately on preliminary stabilization of the head. Acceptable ventilation is assured, and all monitors are rechecked before final postural adjustments are made.

Either before or after the turn, lower extremities that are to be dependent should be encased in snug elastic stockings or wrapped with elastic material that is tight enough to minimize pooling of blood during the operation without simultaneously causing ischemia.

Pronating from Bed or Cart to Operating Table

When ready for the turn, the patient's bed or cart is moved parallel to and against the side of the operating table. The height of the table is adjusted so that the surface of its mattress is level with the one on which the patient is lying. Devices that have been selected to support the patient on the operating table are in place. Turning assistants are assembled and their duties defined. Two receivers stand against the free side of the operating table, two turners face them at the free side of the cart, and one turner is at the patient's foot. The anesthesiologist manages the head and airway (except as noted subsequently concerning an unstable spine) and coordinates the turn. The arms of the patient are kept alongside the body.

At a prearranged signal from the anesthesiologist, who has just disconnected the airway from the anesthesia machine, the receivers at the free side of the operating table extend their arms across the table top to receive the patient. The turners opposite them begin to rotate the patient slowly and smoothly from supine to lateral to prone onto the outstretched and table-supported arms of the receivers. The patient comes to rest on the receivers' arms on the operating table but is not yet symmetrically positioned. The anesthesiologist keeps the head of the patient firmly in the sagittal plane of the body until the turn is completed and then gently rotates the face toward the anesthesia machine unless a support has been previously arranged to maintain the head in the sagittal plane of the body. Once the patient rests on the arms of the receivers, no additional move is made until the airway is reconnected, ventilation is resumed, the cart or bed is taken away, and the various lines are determined to be intact. An effective method of gaining lifting purchase with minimal lumbar stress for the turning attendants is for the two turners to grasp the hands of the two receivers and together lift the patient into proper placement on the table supports while the anesthesiologist protects the head, face, and airway. The arms are positioned as desired, appropriate restraining tapes and straps are placed, the table top or kneeling rest is adjusted to achieve the desired prone position, and the turn is completed.

Pronating upon the Operating Table

Before turning the patient, all preliminary steps as described previously should be followed. If the patient is physiologically brittle, depressing the head of the operating table somewhat while deliberately slowing the turn and positioning may assist circulation. (An exception exists if the patient in question has an intracranial pathologic process with the potential for increased cerebral edema in the head-down position.) Both arms are alongside the torso.

Two turners are at the patient's "overgoing" side. Together they draw the patient toward them and simultaneously roll him or her into the lateral decubitus position so that the back rests against them. The anesthesiologist keeps the head in the proper plane and coordinates the maneuvers. The patient now rests on the "under-going" arm on the lateral half of the operating table. At least one receiver is present on the opposite side of the table.

The turning maneuver is continued until the patient is about three fourths prone. As the down-side arm emerges from beneath the patient, it is gently moved to a position behind the trunk and should be lowered over the side of the table as soon as possible without stressing the shoulder. The over-going arm is swung free to hang over the receiver's side of the table.

Next, the turners and receivers together lift the patient's shoulders and hips and move them sufficiently to center the trunk on the table. They support the chest above the table until the anesthesiologist can reposition the head, re-establish ventilation, and ascertain blood pressure.

At this juncture the patient is gently lifted by the turn/receive team and additional assistance places support devices beneath the patient. The arms are arranged on boards or alongside the trunk. Appropriate restraining tapes and straps are placed, and the table top is adjusted to achieve the final prone posture. Particular attention must be paid to the patient's neck during this final phase of the turn to prevent injurious manipulation as the trunk is tugged into position on the support devices.

Pronating a Patient Whose Cervical Spine is Unstable

A special circumstance applies when the cervical spine of the patient is unstable, the spinal cord is injured or at risk, or the neurologic status is precarious. Often the intended operation must be performed while some type of longitudinal traction device remains in place to stabilize the vertebral column. The patient is either turned prone onto an appropriately padded operating table or allowed to remain on the ventral shell of a bivalved frame that enhances nursing care by rotating supine to prone in the longitudinal axis of the body (a Foster or Stryker frame) or around the transverse axis of the body of the patient who is on a frame that rolls inside an attached circular track. On these types of specialized nursing beds, optimal support that decompresses abdominal viscera during anesthesia must be arranged on the ventral shell while the patient is still supine on the dorsal portion (see the previous discussion of the Mouradian modification of the Foster frame and Fig. 10–23). That support may be almost impossible to arrange after the turn into the prone position without distorting the traction forces on the spine.

Faced with these limitations, the anesthesiologist often chooses to intubate the patient awake after appropriate sedation and airway analgesia. Having the patient spontaneously ventilating, comfortable, and cooperative during the turn allows the neurologic function to be carefully and continuously checked throughout the move. Enough extra members should be added to the turning team so that spinal traction can be maintained during gentle repositioning. When the turn is completed and the stability of the patient is assured, general anesthesia is established in the usual fashion. Lee and associates[32] reported a successful technique using neuroleptanalgesia for intubation and pronation of awake patients, in a variety of conditions other than the need for cervical traction.

An alternative might be to administer general anesthesia and then monitor somatosensory evoked potentials or motor evoked potentials before, during, and after the turn.[33, 34] However, these are complex methodologies involving equipment and interpretive expertise not readily available in every location. Also, the physical maneuvers of turning the patient are potentially disruptive for monitoring leads and may compromise interpretation of the data.

When the continuity of the cervical spine is at risk, whether the patient is awake or asleep, it is prudent and customary to have the responsible surgeon (1) maintain the stable alignment of the head with the body during the turn, (2) position the pronated head to his or her satisfaction, and (3) personally assure that intact neurologic function has been retained once the patient is situated or that the position is optimized if neurologic function cannot be assessed.

Managing the Prone Head

Head posture is an important issue in the prone position. A significant inquiry in the preanesthetic visit is whether the patient can sustain head rotation while awake.

An arthritic or injured cervical spine that produces pain on rotation causes protective splinting of the neck in the awake patient and usually produces arousal due to pain when the patient moves improperly during sleep. Such a patient should not be subjected to unprotected head rotation under anesthesia, because severe and possibly prolonged postoperative neck pain is predictable. The same comment applies to the patient with a symptomatic cervical disk (see previous discussion of the unstable cervical spine).

When the operative site is caudad to the mid-thoracic vertebrae and the neck is supple, the head can usually be safely rotated to a position of comfort against a pillow or a soft supporting sponge that spares the downside eye and ear from compression (see previous discussion of face pieces). For more cephalad operative fields, head rotation may distort landmarks and sagittal alignment will be required. Several varieties of head holders have been described earlier in this chapter. Care must be taken to secure in place the transoral tubes and sensors that were placed when the patient was supine. The forces of gravity or unrecognized traction on these devices must not be allowed to dislodge them from the prone face.

Acceptable Arm Positioning

Deliberate questioning at the preanesthetic interview should determine how supple are the patient's arms.

- If sleeping with the arms over the head is avoided because of resultant dysesthesia, the posture cannot be used during an operation; the arms must be restrained alongside the trunk of the prone anesthetized patient.
- Partially ankylosed elbow or shoulder joints demand particular attention and assessment to avoid damage during positioning.
- An elbow that has had an ulnar nerve transplant is potentially at risk during pronation. Ample padding must be used to protect the relocated nerve regardless of the final arm position.

During the turn, the arms must be kept at the side of the patient and not be allowed to fall or be pushed toward either the dorsal or the ventral midline of the body. Losing an arm toward the ventral midline places it beneath the torso at the end of the turn and threatens continuity of vascular and monitoring lines until they can be retrieved. Losing an arm toward the dorsal midline can place serious stress on the anterior capsule of the shoulder joint and may cause subluxation.

When the turn is completed, arms that are to be placed above the head of the patient should be moved carefully from the turning position that retained them alongside the body. The arms can be allowed to dangle temporarily toward the floor. When ready to be placed on armboards, they should be rotated cephalad in a plane roughly parallel to the sagittal plane of the body. Extreme lateral hyperabduction that stresses the capsule of the shoulder joint must be scrupulously avoided even though it may be the easiest line of motion for the person tending the arm. The eventual position of the arms over the head of the patient should be supported by well-padded armboards located roughly parallel to the long axis of the table and placed sufficiently ventral to the transverse axis of the shoulders to allow gentle abduction and extension of the upper arm plus flexion of the elbow (see Fig. 10–1A). The head of the humerus must not be forced into the axillary neurovascular bundle, the axilla should be loose, the flexed elbow must be padded to protect the ulnar nerve, and effective pulses must be found at the wrist.

If the arms are intended to remain at the side of the patient during surgery, specific attention must be devoted to the patency and stability of intravascular lines in the forearms and hands. Mechanical disruption of any device buried beneath drapes can be expected unless adequate precautions are taken. Towels or sheets used to restrain the arms must be wrinkle free, snug enough to retain the arm in position, and not so tight as to restrict circulation (see Fig. 10–1B). When tucked beneath the patient, the restraints must not interfere with the freedom of the abdomen. An arm "toboggan" (properly referred to as a Wells Arm Protector [Mercury Enterprises, Inc., North Clearwater, FL]) or a similar device, insulated from the arm by a smooth folded towel or sheet, can be placed about the blood pressure cuff to shield it from the pressure of the body of a member of the surgical team. The broad flat body of the toboggan is designed to slip between the mattress and the top of the operating table, or between the mattress and the torso of the patient. The curved portion loosely encases the blood pressure cuff. However, if the toboggan is metallic, it may not be useful because its body will obstruct radiographs of the overlying structures that may be required during the operation.

Figure 18–6 in the second edition of this text shows the arms of the prone patient placed on armboards that are extended 90 degrees from the long axis of the table. This situation is capable of interfering with the access of the surgical team to incisions made in the thoracic dorsal midline. Unless the patient possesses an extremely supple physique, the posture can place severe subluxing stresses on the capsules of the shoulder joints and can fracture an osteoporotic or pathologic upper humerus. I have difficulty justifying the routine use of this position.

Postural Restraints and Padding

Bony prominences should be well padded to distribute pressure so that compressive, ischemic tissue damage becomes unlikely. Ribbed (corduroy) or pebbly (terry cloth bath towels and washcloths) padding should be avoided in favor of smoother and more gentle fabrics or plastic foam. This issue becomes particularly important for patients with atrophic skin or reduced subcutaneous tissue.

Gluteal strap restraints are designed to prevent the pronated patient from shifting caudad on the table. Properly applied, they are successful; thoughtlessly placed, they are useless or injurious. Their line of force must be against the thrust of the direction in which slippage can be predicted (see Fig. 10–1C). Illustrations in some texts often disregard this critical point, and the reader who has no operating room experience with patient positioning can gain an erroneous impression of what is required. If the table top is angulated or otherwise repositioned after the straps are placed, they may loosen or become excessively tight; the straps should be rechecked and may need to be replaced to assure their effectiveness.

PHYSIOLOGY OF THE PRONE POSITION

The ventral aspects of the human body are mobile relative to the dorsal surfaces and did not evolve as weight-bearing structures. Whereas they can serve as such during normal physiologic sleep, prerequisites are the presence of a flexible skeleton, normal muscle tone, intact circulatory reflexes, and the ability to increase spontaneous ventilatory effort sufficiently to expand the chest by lifting the dorsal torso off of the sternum. Anesthetic agents, muscle relaxants, and positive-pressure ventilation inflict major changes on the prone patient, producing a totally unfamiliar physiologic environment in which customary and adequate function is usually impossible without assistance.

Cardiovascular Dynamics

Identifiable cardiovascular problems are unusual when the average, otherwise healthy patient is positioned prone so that the inferior vena cava and femoral veins are not compressed. However, if pressure is exerted on these vessels, other avenues with lesser flow capabilities must provide venous return for cardiac refilling. As early as 1940 Batson[35] showed that inferior vena caval obstruction diverted blood flow from the distal parts of the body into perivertebral venous plexuses. McGregor[36] identified a valveless, low-pressure, reversible-flow system of thin-walled veins about the vertebral column and in the epidural space. Through intercostal and lumbar veins, those engorged plexuses are connected to vessels in the chest, abdomen, and pelvis. Engorgement of veins at the surgical wound makes hemostasis difficult and is visible immediately when intra-abdominal pressure increases. In a compressed abdominal cavity, great vessels and bowel are displaced dorsally against the vertebral column to increase their risk of injury by biting surgical instruments.[37-41]

Pearce[42] recorded inferior vena caval pressure with varying levels of abdominal compression in surgical patients who were anesthetized and pronated. Venous pressure responses to changed amounts of compression were abrupt, proportional, and dramatic (Fig. 10-27).

DiStefano's team[43] reported averages of inferior caval pressures measured in ten healthy adult male patients placed in several of the following postures: (1) prone on bolsters, (2) on a Wilson frame, (3) in the lateral decubitus position, (4) in a kneeling prone position, (5) in a tuck prone position, and (6) on a Hastings frame (see Fig. 10-8). They found the Hastings frame to offer the lowest caval pressures, least blood loss, easiest ventilation, and

Table 10-1

Venous Pressure Values in a Variety of Positions

Arrangement	Average Central Venous Pressure (cm H_2O)
Georgia prone	20.7
Prone, chest rolls	15.9
Lateral decubitus	11.1
Wilson frame	10.1
Tuck position	9.4
Hastings frame	1.4

From DiStefano VJ, Klein KS, Nixon JE, et al.: Intraoperative analysis of the effects of body position and body habitus on surgery of the low back. Clin Orthop 99:51, 1974.

best surgical exposure of the several varieties of prone position arrangements studied. Their average venous pressure values are presented in Table 10-1.

Using catheters in systemic and pulmonary arteries, Backofen and Schauble[44] monitored 16 patients (mean age, 65 years) who were turned prone during general anesthesia and carefully supported to prevent vascular obstruction. Parameters were measured in the

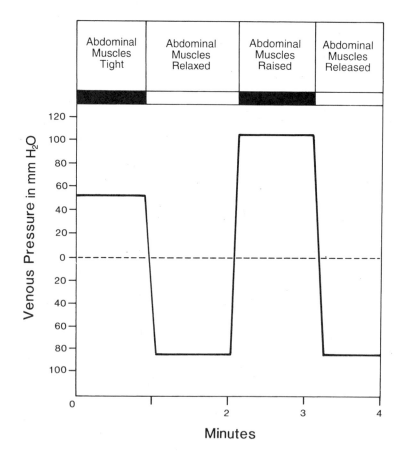

Figure 10-27

Venous pressure changes in the prone supported position. (Reproduced from Pearce DJ: The role of posture in laminectomy. Proc R Soc Med 50:109, 1957.)

supine position after induction of anesthesia and again after pronation. These workers found that the prone position did not alter heart rate or mean arterial, venous, and pulmonary artery occlusion pressures; however, the prone position was associated with significant increases in systemic and pulmonary vascular resistances that could not prevent decreases in stroke volume and cardiac index that also were significant. "Routine" measurements of arterial and central venous pressures would not have detected these changes, resulting primarily from reduced venous return to the right side of the heart. Backofen and Schauble recommended the use of pulmonary artery thermodilution catheters when patients with evidence of poor perfusion or cardiac failure are to be turned prone.

Yokoyama's group[45] evaluated the hemodynamic effects of the prone position on a convex frame in anesthetized patients. With the patients flat on the frame, no significant changes in hemodynamic variables were found. However, when the frame was arched into an operative configuration a significant decrease in cardiac index was encountered. The change would not have been detected if the capability of making cardiac output measurements had not been present.

McNulty and colleagues used longitudinal bolsters, the Cloward surgical saddle, and the Andrews frame as three varieties of supports for the prone position and compared their effects on venous pressure and blood loss during lumbar laminectomies.[46] They found central venous pressures to be least in the Andrews frame patients. Blood loss was about four times greater in the patients for whom the Cloward saddle was used than in those with either the bolster or the Andrews frame, but differences in surgical teams may have played a significant role in the disparity.

Respiratory Dynamics

The spontaneously ventilating patient of normal build lying flat on the entire ventral surface of the torso must raise the thoracic weight off the sternum to expand the chest. Viscera also limit inspiration when the weight of the dorsal trunk compresses the abdominal contents and forces the diaphragm cephalad. Effective spontaneous compensation can be expected to require an increase in the work of breathing. An exception involves the massively obese individual who, when supine, must expend great effort to inspire because

of the weight of the chest wall and the obstruction to the descent of the diaphragm caused by an overstuffed abdomen. These patients may ventilate more easily when prone if the abdomen is not compressed.

- Smith[18] reported a case involving an obese patient who required a threefold increase in inspiratory pressure for passive lung inflation after being turned prone without ventral supports. When supports were placed so that the abdomen hung free the inspiratory inflation pressures returned to the same values as in the supine position.
- Rehder and co-workers[47] noted that the weight of the freed abdominal contents had an "inspiratory effect on the diaphragm" when the pronated patient was properly supported by foam pads under the shoulder girdle and pelvis.

West and colleagues[48] and Hughes' group[49] have described the distribution of blood flow within the lung, according to relationships between vascular and alveolar pressures. Kaneko and colleagues[50] added the association of body posture. They believed that pulmonary blood flow in the prone position was almost as homogeneous as in the supine position, that is, the lung in the prone position was entirely a zone 3 of West with pulmonary venous pressure exceeding alveolar pressure and flow being dependent on the difference between pulmonary arterial and pulmonary venous pressures.

In an effort to identify the effect of the prone position on pulmonary shunting, Stone and Khambatta[51] studied 10 young, otherwise healthy, nonobese surgical patients scheduled for lumbar spinal surgery. Unlike the reports of others,[52, 53] their patients did not show persistent increases in shunting after induction of anesthesia in the supine position. After pronation was achieved these investigators noted no change in the magnitude of whatever shunting had occurred in the supine position. Their patients were placed on parallel rubber bolsters with the abdomen allowed to hang free.

Douglas and associates[54] studied mechanically ventilated respiratory failure patients in an intensive care unit. These workers found a consistent increase in arterial oxygen values after the patients were pronated (with ventilatory parameters unchanged) and supported so that the abdomens were hanging free (Fig.

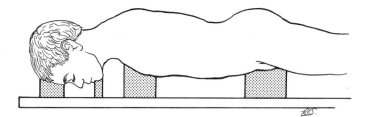

Figure 10–28

Prone support arrangement used in the study of Douglas. (Redrawn from Douglas WW, Rehder K, Beynen FM, et al.: Improved oxygenation in patients with acute respiratory failure: The prone position. Am Rev Respir Dis 115:559, 1977.)

10–28). Returning to the supine position reversed the improvement. The loss of functional residual capacity produced by the prone position was minimal and was less than had occurred in either the supine or lateral position.

Lumb and Nunn measured respiratory function in healthy awake volunteers first sitting and then in four horizontal positions common to anesthesia.[55] When the sitting subject assumed the supine position forced vital capacity decreased by 300 mL and functional residual capacity fell about 800 mL. Pronation increased functional residual capacity about 350 mL over the supine value. Mean rib cage contribution to ventilation was similar in all horizontal positions.

Pelosi and colleagues studied 17 normal, anesthetized, paralyzed patients undergoing lumbar disk surgery, measuring the effects of the prone position on the mechanical properties of the total respiratory system, the lung, and the chest wall as well as on functional residual capacity and gas exchange.[56] After base line measurements had been taken with the patients supine, they were turned prone on upper chest and pelvic supports as advocated by Smith.[30] Free abdominal motion was assured. Measurements repeated 20 minutes after pronation indicated that compliances of the respiratory system, lung, and chest wall were not significantly affected. Respiratory resistance values had risen slightly, mainly due to increased chest wall resistance. $PaCO_2$ was unchanged, whereas both functional residual capacity and PaO_2 increased markedly over values obtained with the patients supine. They concluded that the prone position improves lung volumes and oxygenation without adversely affecting respiratory mechanics.

Using healthy, awake volunteers, Mahajan and co-workers[57] established control values in the unsupported prone position and then examined three different prone postures: (1) knee-chest, (2) a frame with a hollowed interior, and (3) two separate supports under thorax and pelvis. Data were obtained for functional residual capacity, expiratory reserve volume, residual volume, and total lung capacity in each position while the subject was distracted by listening to music of his or her choice. The knee-chest position caused the least respiratory restriction of the three postures evaluated.

Seeking the mechanism by which the prone position improves oxygenation in the presence of the adult respiratory disease syndrome, Lamm and colleagues[58] reasoned that, when patients were supine, transpulmonary pressure would be less than airway opening pressure, that atelectasis would develop preferentially in dorsal lung units, and that the ventilation/perfusion ratios would improve in these regions after pronation. Measuring regional ventilation and perfusion and obtaining computed tomographic scans in subjects in both the prone and supine positions, they compared control dogs to those subjected to oleic acid–induced acute pulmonary injuries. After acute lung injury the prone position generated a transpulmonary pressure sufficient to exceed airway opening pressure in the dorsal regions where atelectasis, shunt, and ventilation/perfusion ratio heterogeneity become most severe in adult respiratory distress syndrome. Pronation improved oxygenation, median ventilation/perfusion ratios, ventilation/perfusion ratio heterogeneity, and the gravitational ventilation/perfusion gradient dorsally without adversely affecting ventral lung regions.

The necessary high airway pressures and large tidal volumes needed to ventilate a patient who is improperly positioned prone have several potential side effects that can be harmful.

- Pulmonary barotrauma is possible in the form of pulmonary interstitial emphysema leading to a pneumothorax or the spread of air as mediastinal, retroperitoneal, or subcutaneous emphysema.
- The back rises and falls with each infla-

tion, making the surgical field shift in and out of the shallow focus of the operating room microscope being used. The more caudad the field, the less annoying this issue becomes. It is difficult to eliminate the problem completely despite careful positioning.

- High venous and cerebrospinal pressures may be evident as fluid fluxes in the wound (see previous discussion).

Central Nervous System Dynamics

If the head of a prone patient is positioned below the level of the heart, the forces of gravity may cause a significant increase in the amount of blood and CSF that accumulates in and around the brain. As head-down tilt is increased, pressure in the carotid system rises and cerebral vascular resistance rises to maintain constant flow.[59] Pathologic areas of brain are thought to be vasoparetic, with flow being directly related to pressure, and subject to edema, as pressure increases in the microvasculature. A head with an open wound, whether surgical or traumatic, and a head containing a suspected intracranial pathologic process should not be positioned below heart level. Also affected by dependency, but to a less dramatic degree, are nonneural structures of the neck and head; edema and congestion may be evident in the conjunctivae, the nasal passages, and possibly the larynx.

Iwabuchi and associates[11] studied dural venous sinus (confluens sinuum) pressures in a group of surgical patients in various body positions. When the upper half of the body was raised 25 degrees, the confluens sinuum pressure fell to zero. When adults sat erect ($+90$ degrees), the pressure became -9 to -15 cm H_2O (average -12.7 cm H_2O). Children younger than 6 years old did not develop confluens sinuum pressures of less than zero even when sitting erect. Pressures were slightly above atmospheric (average 2.7 to 3.0 cm H_2O) in all patients placed in either version of their hyperlordotic prone position (see previous description). Although positive-pressure ventilation had no significant effect on dural venous sinus pressures, jugular compression elevated those pressures sufficiently to prevent air embolism. These workers confirmed their sea lion position as a favorable prone posture for cerebral venous drainage (see previous description).

Severe rotation of the head and neck has been shown to modify the flow patterns in both the carotid and the vertebral arterial systems.

- Toole[60] has stated that 60 degrees of head rotation begins to reduce flow through the contralateral vertebral artery and that 80 degrees of rotation obstructs the vessel. The mechanism is presumed to be compression of the artery as it passes cephalad through the transverse processes of the sixth through the second cervical vertebrae. If the vascular anatomy is normal and intact, compensation exists in the form of increased blood flow through the ipsilateral vertebral artery, as the head is rotated beyond 60 degrees. Also, as the pressure and flow in the vertebral system decrease, at some point compensatory retrograde (caudad) flow begins in the basilar artery because of its connections to the systemic perfusion through the circle of Willis. If the vertebral arterial anastomoses are abnormal, however, head rotation may threaten perfusion of the cervical cord, brain stem, cerebellum, and cochleovestibular apparatus. Occlusive disease in the vessels can be expected to intensify the problem.

- Flow through the carotid system can be altered by head position. The degree varies with the amount of arteriosclerosis in the vessels. If carotid flow is suspect, the head should probably be maintained in the midline after pronation rather than being turned to either side. Obviously, even anatomically normal carotid and jugular flows can be altered by compression of the down-side neck against poorly chosen support devices.

Computed tomography of vertebral columns has shown that the spinal cord relocates ventrad when the patient is placed in the prone position.[61] The ventral epidural space is compressed while the dorsal space is enlarged. This finding suggests that the shifted spinal cord makes the prone posture ideal for the establishment of lumbar epidural anesthesia.

Concerned that lumbar introduction of methotrexate into CSF produced erratic drug levels in cerebral ventricles in the treatment of meningeal leukemia, Blaney and colleagues[62] found that retaining nonhuman primates in the prone position for 1 hour after introduction of the drug into the lumbar CSF produced more than a 20-fold increase in the peak concentration and peak exposure of the compound in the CSF of the cerebral ventricles.

Perfusion of the spinal cord autoregulates in essentially the same manner as does perfusion of the brain,[63] with flow remaining grossly stable between mean systemic arterial pressures of approximately 50 and 135 mm Hg.[64] Blood flow to the cord was found to be decreased by hypocapnia and increased by hypoxia or hypercarbia or both; however, distribution of blood within the cord was not affected.

Increases in intrathoracic pressure from the inspiratory phase of intermittent positive-pressure ventilation are transmitted through venous channels to an open wound in the neuraxis. The fluxes of CSF volume in the surgical field are seen to be synchronous with the phases of ventilation.

POTENTIAL COMPLICATIONS OF THE PRONE POSITION

Injuries During the Turn

Dropping the Patient

Mentioning the possibility that a patient might be dropped during a turn is somewhat astonishing. However, it can happen as the result of the following:

- An uncoordinated or unskilled team of turning attendants
- Too few team members to accommodate the weight shifts of the turn
- The unexpected separation of operating table and transport cart just as the patient is in the lateral phase of the turn and is not well supported by the table, cart, or turning team

The opportunities for injury and litigation need little elaboration. Preventive measures required should be obvious.

Loss of Airway, Vascular Access Lines, Catheters, and Monitors

A careless turn, or one that must be accomplished rapidly with little time in which to prepare, can result in unexpected disruption of anything that is attached to the patient. Breathing circuit hoses of inadequate length can dislodge or extract an endotracheal tube with potentially fatal results. Vascular, uri-nary, and viscerostomy catheters require preliminary planning and specific attention throughout the turn if they are to remain in place and function as expected. Most monitor connections can be dispensed with during the turn but should be reattached and have their function verified as soon as the patient is stable in the new posture.

Injury to Arms

Life support protocols usually indicate that the arm over which the victim is rolled by a single rescuer should be placed alongside the victim's head as a support against a sudden lateral angulation of the neck. However, in the operating room where assistance is more adequate, most anesthesiologists prefer to protect the head and neck and turn over the arm after it is placed at the patient's side. The intention is to minimize stress on the anesthetized and relaxed shoulder joint while the anesthesiologist carefully manages the posture of the head during the turn.

Opportunities exist for the under-going arm to fall into any gap that might occur between the mattresses of the operating table and the cart during the turn. A shoulder dislocation, humeral fracture, or soft tissue injury could result. Preventing such an occurrence needs awareness of the possibility and watchful attention during the turn. The over-going arm should be protected from flopping toward either the ventral or the dorsal midline.

Injuries to the Turning Attendants

Properly accomplished, a supine-to-prone turn should pose no significant stress for the turning attendants. However, lumbar spine injuries are possible for those who are lifting, if the basic principles of handling heavy objects are ignored.

The two team members who are receivers have the most potentially threatening task. As noted previously, once the ventral aspect of the patient rests upon the arms of the receivers on the operating table, they must delay any further lift until the cart or bed can be taken away and the two opposite turners can move close to the side of the table. The four can then join hands under the patient and complete the lifting into the final operating position. By joining hands, none should have a significant or injurious burden even with the most heavy patient. By not joining hands, grips may slip and the weight of the patient can easily be damaging for the two receivers. Firm footing for each lifter is a critical issue. Slipping feet threaten the lumbar musculature of the lifter as well as the safety of the patient.

Accentuation of Multiple Trauma

The multiply traumatized patient with significant skeletal injuries is particularly susceptible to further injuries when moved. An unstable rib cage may make the prone position an unwise choice because of the potential for further lung injury or compression of the mediastinum. If the alternative of the lateral position is not realistic, the operation may need to be delayed until healing has stabilized the thorax.

When multiple trauma exists and traction appliances are in use, knowledgeable members of the surgical team should be involved in removing the appliances and assisting with the positioning maneuvers. The trauma patient or members of the immediate family should be made aware of the intentions and unavoidable hazards of positioning before surgery.

Injuries to the Eyes

Corneal Abrasion

Modern anesthesia rarely makes use of eye signs to assess anesthetic "depth." Progressive inequality of pupils can occur during anesthesia if a concomitant head injury exists and the prone position is used for rapid access to an injured spinal cord or posterior cranial fossa. In the vast majority of patients who are operated on in the prone position, however, eye signs are not major factors in the conduct of the anesthetic. Therefore, a practice of many is to protect the patient's eyes by instilling saline or an ophthalmic lubricant and taping the lids shut before pronation. This maneuver is deliberate protection against casual corneal abrasion or soiling of the eyes by solutions applied to the neck and occiput during cleansing of the skin. Patient goggles are available and are preferred for routine use by some anesthesiologists.

If the head is to be rotated laterally on a pillow or protective sponge, the down-side eye must be specifically protected against corneal injury. Vascular lines, monitoring cords, and various devices placed in the patient's mouth must not come to rest beneath the head and against the eyes.

Ocular Edema

Conjunctival edema, as well as edema of the dependent periorbital tissues, may occur when the head of the prone patient is below the level of the atrium or when the infusion volume of crystalloids is large. Apparently this type of edema represents a localized gravity-related accumulation of fluid and usually has no systemic significance. It also seems to pose little threat either to other ocular tissues or to the function of the involved eye.

Blindness

Racz (personal communication, 1986) reports the plight of a diabetic patient whose head was turned from side to side repeatedly by the anesthesiologist during a lengthy laminectomy in the prone position. Despite the precaution, unilateral blindness was present on arousal. Apparently the injury was caused by retinal ischemia from inadvertent pressure on the globe.

I have been made aware of several instances of blindness in the down-side eyes of pronated patients whose heads were turned onto a soft pillow, a folded blanket, or a foam ring from which a section had been removed. Each of these devices can fail to protect the eye by gradually becoming compressed and distorted by the weight of the patient's head during the course of the operation. The C-shaped face piece (see previous discussion and Fig. 10–16) offers more effective support when properly applied.

Katz and associates[65] reported four instances of ischemic optic neuropathy occurring after prolonged, multilevel lumbar laminectomies. Two were evident immediately after surgery, one appeared on the second day, and the other was noted on the twelfth day. Arteriosclerotic risk factors such as systemic hypertension, diabetes, coronary artery disease, and smoking were present in three of the cases. Deliberate hypotension and/or the anemia of uncorrected blood loss were implicated by the authors.

Historically, poorly sized horseshoe head rests that support a patient's head in the sagittal plane have been alleged to slip, resulting in compression of an eye, retinal ischemia, perhaps displacement of a crystalline lens, and blindness.[66] Wolfe's group[67] encountered an instance of unilateral blindness after their traditional use of a padded, adjustable

Mayfield head rest for a young adult who was pronated for correction of scoliosis. During the procedure there had been an episode of nodal rhythm that became complete atrioventricular dissociation before converting spontaneously to the previous normal sinus rhythm. Retrospectively, the authors thought that the dysrhythmic episode probably occurred at the time of the ocular compression that produced the retinal artery ischemia.

The skull pin head rest has minimized the risk of ocular compression, but its loose misapplication could potentially allow the patient's head to shift enough to cause an eye injury from one of the pins. Frequent inspection of the patient's face in its holder can be accomplished by the anesthesiologist by direct visualization or by viewing the reflection provided by a hand-held mirror similar to that traditionally a part of a lady's dressing table.

Williams and colleagues[68] have provided an extensive review of postoperative ischemic optic neuropathy that, while other factors were sometimes present, they found to be associated most often with hypotension and a low hematocrit. Their studies[69–71] indicated that autoregulation plays little part in choroidal or optic nerve circulation. According to Tsamparlakis, blood flow in these vessels is directly related to arterial pressure.[72] A clear inference is that systemic hypotension, causing perfusion deficits in these vascular beds, would be compounded by increased intraocular pressure produced by the weight of the head forcing a poorly supported eye against either the mattress of the operating table or the padding of an ill-fitted or slipped face piece.

Compression of the Ear

Pressure against the down-side ear comes from the surface against which the head rests or from the hands of the person turning the head. As noted previously, it may also be caused by some object carelessly left beneath the patient and unnoticed subsequently. A pillow beneath the head that is tugged at vigorously or a lateral movement of the torso after the head has been turned toward the contralateral shoulder may cause all or part of the external ear to be folded over. Whether from pressure or folding, cartilaginous damage may occur that is disfiguring. The final position of the down-side ear should be carefully evaluated after pronation has been com-

pleted. As noted earlier, the C-shaped face piece usually supports the head in such a way that the ear is not compressed.

Injuries to the Facial and Mandibular Nerves

Published reports of facial nerve injuries after pronation and head rotation are almost nonexistent. Most postoperative facial neuropathies have been attributed either to pressure on the angle of the mandible to open the airway during administration of anesthesia by mask or to pressure from a mask strap. Often, inflammation of the associated parotid gland has accompanied the neuropathy.[73, 74] I am aware of an instance in which a wrinkled sheet, against which the preauricular area was pressed by the weight of the pronated head, has been blamed for a postoperative facial nerve dysfunction.

Winter and Munro[75] reported a curious instance of postoperative unilateral sensory dysfunction of both the lingual and buccal branches of the mandibular nerve. A patient under general anesthesia was intubated, was pronated, and had his head rotated slightly toward the left shoulder and supported by an intact foam ring that was positioned to free the nose and dependent eye. Sensory deficits of the right side of the face and tongue were evident soon after the patient awakened. Motor function was intact. Facial sensation returned by the third postoperative day and tongue sensation had recovered fully by the end of 1 month. The authors speculated that the mandible was possibly retracted asymmetrically by the ring sufficiently to create tension on the down-side (right) pterygoid musculature and compress both nerves.

Neck Torsion, Flexion, and Extension

Skeletal stress from neck torsion has been discussed. Smith[76] contended that the neck should be flexed gently during the turn and in subsequent positioning. His concern involved the potential for neck extension to trap the greater occipital nerve as it emerges between the atlas and the axis, causing severe, protracted neck muscle spasm and headache in the postoperative period. Vascular problems may also arise from neck torsion (see previous discussion under Central Nervous System Dynamics).

When, and to what extent, neck torsion impairs cerebral function is difficult to determine. That it may do so is evident from the report of McPherson's group concerning a patient who was placed in the left semiprone (park bench) position and whose head was subsequently rotated leftward and the neck flexed.[77] Soon after positioning the cortical somatosensory evoked potentials disappeared. No changes were noted in the somatosensory evoked potentials derived simultaneously from the spinous process of the second cervical vertebra or in other monitored parameters. When the head was returned to the neutral position the cortical somatosensory evoked potential tracing returned to its previous normal configuration. Subsequent surgery was done with the patient in the lateral position, and no posture-induced somatosensory evoked potential changes were encountered.

When a narrowed cervical spinal canal exists due to some pathologic process, either flexion or extension of the neck may result in cord dysfunction. Hyperextension may produce a central cord syndrome[78] by pinching the cord in the confines of the narrowed canal.[79] Hyperflexion, possibly by stretching the spinal cord, has been described as the cause of midcervical tetraplegia.[80, 81] If midcervical abnormalities are suspected, a desirable protocol before the induction of the anesthetic includes awake intubation without neck extension, awake pronation with the head maintained in the sagittal plane, careful midline placement of the head without either flexion or extension of the neck, and detailed neurologic evaluations during and after the process. However, even these detailed and compulsive precautions are not foolproof.[82]

Vascular Disturbances

Head-Down Tilt

Any degree of head-down tilt added to the prone position increases venous congestion in the head proportionally. If intracranial pathology exists, the rise in intracranial pressure may become consequential. As a matter of principle, no form of the head-down position should be used in the presence of known or probable intracranial pathology.

Neck Rotation

As described previously, neck rotation may affect cerebral blood flow.

Effect of Intermittent Positive-Pressure Lung Inflation

A more common vascular disturbance associated with the prone position is intermittent relocation of blood volume into the veins of the operative site by the positive airway pressure used to inflate the lungs. The resulting congestion may be sufficient to interfere with the surgical dissection and hemostasis. To further complicate the problem, if the dura is opened, a simultaneous rhythmic bathing of the surgical field in boluses of CSF usually occurs. Assuring positioning that does not compress the abdomen and using the least permissible lung inflation pressures will minimize venous congestion and CSF surges in the operative field. However, the problem may continue to some degree as an irreducible background annoyance, particularly in very bulky patients.

Intravascular Volume Pooling

In the variants of the prone position in which a significant pressure gradient exists between the lower extremities and the right atrium, or when venous drainage from the legs is inadvertently obstructed by knee or hip flexion, sufficient amounts of blood may pool in the dependent structures to reduce atrial filling and cardiac output. The usual countermeasure against venous pooling is to encase the legs in compressive, nonischemic, supportive stockings or to wrap elastic bandages from feet to lower thighs before positioning. Should the problem persist, adding colloids or crystalloids to the circulating volume and promptly replacing shed blood is usually effective. However, repositioning the patient supine after the operative procedure may induce sufficient redistribution of infused supportive volume into the central circulation to overload the pulmonary circulation if cardiac output is impaired.

Compartment Syndrome

Sharp angulation of knees or hips can severely restrict circulation in the lower extremities, as can excessively tight leg wraps (see earlier discussion and also Chapter 6). Compartment syndromes may result during a lengthy procedure, producing rhabdomyolysis, distant organ failure, complicated fluid balance problems, secondary infections, a difficult or prolonged convalescence, and possibly death. Because the developing pathology is at the tissue level in the compartments, intraoperative monitoring of peripheral pulses such as the dorsalis pedis will rarely indicate the appearance and progress of compartmental ischemia.[83]

Venous Air Embolism

In the prone patient, venous air embolism is an entity to which little attention is usually paid. Sporadic consideration was initiated by Shenken's report of air being entrained by veins in an incision 10 cm above the heart of a prone patient.[84] The mechanical ventilator used for that individual included a subatmospheric expiratory phase, a technique subsequently abandoned that may have lowered mean pressure in veins of the lumbar area and enhanced entrainment. As a controversy developed about the value of right atrial catheters to detect and recover embolized air in the prone position, Tarlov[85] stated that there was no need for routine placement of a right atrial catheter for that purpose. He believed that, unlike the situation in the head where bony attachments can render an incised vessel patulous and aid air entrainment, the veins of the area of the lumbar spine are not similarly supported and are able to collapse in the presence of low venous pressure. Albin and co-workers[86] rebutted Tarlov's opinion, noting that 18% of the episodes of air embolus in an earlier study[87] occurred at the end of the procedure when closure was involving the veins in muscles of the neck. Albin and co-workers also made the point that a pendulous abdomen may help reduce venous pressure in perivertebral venous plexuses of kneeling patients and stated that venous air emboli had occurred in prone patients with wound-to-heart gradients of only 5.0 cm. They believed that atrial catheter placement was indicated in prone patients undergoing lengthy procedures and subsequently reported one patient in a Hastings frame and two patients on four-poster frames who developed definite intraoperative indications of venous air emboli.[88] Despite resuscitative efforts, both patients on the four-poster frames died, and considerable air was detected in their vascular trees at autopsy.

Artru[89] evaluated air recovery by either single-orifice or multi-orifice catheters placed in the right atria of anesthetized dogs that had been positioned to allow the abdomen to hang free. He showed that multi-orificed catheters recovered more of a measured amount of injected air than did the single orifice version. However, the survival of his animals was similar with or without aspiration of air. Tempelhoff and colleagues[90] found that the kneeling prone position decreased pulmonary capillary wedge pressures and central venous pressures to approximately 0 mm Hg and strongly agreed with Albin's opinion that prophylactic placement of an atrial catheter is indicated. Horlocker and associates[91] reported two cases of venous air embolism during spinal fusion, one of which could not be resuscitated. They advocated placement of a catheter for air aspiration during spinal fusion and suggested that its tip be located at the inferior cavo-atrial junction. Delaloye and Gerber[92] reported three cases of venous air embolism that developed millwheel murmurs during piston-impacted crumbled spongioid bone grafting in the lumbar spine, indicating that the technique inadvertently introduced air under high pressure into the disk space where it could decompress into venous channels that were opened by the dissection.

Although an uncommon entity, venous air embolism in pronated patients is documented and should be remembered when murmurs, arrhythmias, and hypotension develop without alternative explanations. No statistics are available about its incidence, but conversations have indicated that it is a more widespread event than the total number of reported cases would indicate.[93] Extensive neuro-orthopedic procedures on the lumbar spine may increase its risk. Under what circumstances full-scale prophylactic monitoring for venous air embolism is indicated for a pronated patient remains a personal judgment of the responsible anesthesiologist or surgeon. Disagreements among members of the care team about the necessity for catheter placement should be resolved in the light of patient safety.

Skeletal Distress

The principal skeletal distress for a patient who is placed in the prone position is neck pain, resulting from head rotation. Concerns about neck torsion, flexion, extension, and the precautions needed to manipulate an unstable cervical spine are discussed elsewhere in this text. Muscle relaxants used to facilitate turning an anesthetized patient may permit the process to place unrecognized stress on ligaments and joints. During the turn the hips and shoulders should be kept in the same plane at all times. Guadagni is quoted by Smith[76] as knowing that severe injury to the relaxed spine has developed in the course of improper turns.

A torsion injury of the lumbar spine is a potential consequence of a clumsy, uncoordinated turn from the supine to prone or the reverse. Although no statistics support this premise, one needs little imagination to contemplate the stresses capable of being applied to an unstable, relaxed anesthetized spine when hips and trunk are not kept in a constant, untwisted alignment during the turn.

Some of the kneeling prone postures place weight-bearing pressure on the patient's knees (see Fig. 10-8). Unyielding knee rests require careful padding to avoid producing painful knees postoperatively. Patients with significant arthritis of the knees should not be allowed to bear weight on them during surgery. The potential for the kneeling position or pedestal rests to inflict a scissoring injury on the spinal cord at the point where a vertebral column is unstable has been discussed earlier.

Pathologic joints that have restricted motion can also become painful if an extremity is forced beyond its permissible range of motion during positioning. Fractures of the long bones, the vertebral column, or the thoracic cage can easily destabilize during a turn; utmost vigilance must be applied to limit the capacity for damage.

Adequate padding is needed for evident bony prominences as a means of protecting overlying tissue from pressure necrosis. Point pressure applied to the infraclavicular area and sternum may be a source of persistent postoperative pain and tenderness and should be prevented by padding. Toes must be protected from pressure injury, preferably by a roll or a pillow placed under the ankles to hold them up and off the table surface.

Stressing the Brachial Plexus

The brachial plexus is vulnerable throughout its entire length in the prone position (Fig. 10-29). Should an arm be used as a lever during the turn, a stretch injury of the brachial plexus can occur, particularly if the patient's head is allowed to fall away from the arm that is being pulled. If the head of the humerus is thrust forcibly into the axillary neurovascular bundle the plexus can be damaged.

In the cubital tunnel at the elbow the ulnar nerve is susceptible to compressive injury. Careful attention to padding may lessen this hazard, but ulnar neuropathies have been present postoperatively despite deliberate protective measures at the time of position-

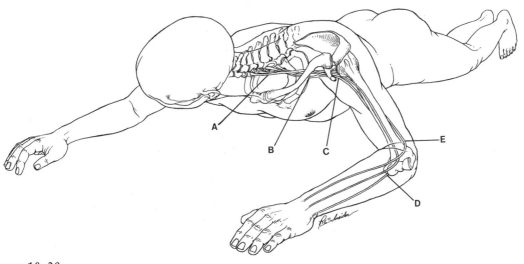

Figure 10-29

Sources of potential injury to the brachial plexus and its peripheral components in a pronated patient. Head position stretching plexus against anchors in shoulder (A). Closure of retroclavicular space by chest support with arms at side; neurovascular bundle trapped against first rib (B). Head of humerus thrust into neurovascular bundle if arm and axilla are not relaxed (C). Compression of ulnar nerve in cubital tunnel (D). Area of vulnerability of radial nerve to compression above elbow (E).

ing.[94] Pressure about 6 cm above the lateral epicondyle of the humerus may threaten the radial nerve as it courses around the upper arm (see subsequent discussion of closure of the retroclavicular space).

The Thoracic Outlet Syndrome

A variety of physical abnormalities have been recognized to cause compression of the brachial plexus and the subclavian vessels near the first rib and clavicle. Resulting plexus pain and paresthesias most commonly occur in the distribution of the ulnar nerve (C8-T1). Rotation of the head can be shown to produce pain and vascular upsets in the ipsilateral extremity if tension of the stretching anterior scalene muscle compresses the artery and plexus against the middle scalene muscle at the first rib. An anomalous cervical rib occurs in about 0.5% of the population and may compress the subclavian artery. The most consistent diagnostic finding is pain produced by re-creating the offending position.[95, 96]

Whatever the etiology, a patient who cannot raise the arms above the head (e.g., reaching toward a shelf, changing a light bulb, painting a ceiling) without experiencing paresthesias or who has numb extremities after sleeping prone with the head turned and arms alongside the head, may have severely debilitating upper extremity pain after being anesthetized and positioned prone in a standard head-turned, arms-elevated fashion (see Fig. 10–1A). Purposeful questioning during the preoperative visit helps identify potential thoracic outlet syndromes when the prone position is desired as the surgical posture (Fig. 10–30).[97–99] When an unanticipated thoracic outlet syndrome is discovered preoperatively, appropriate consultation must be considered before pronation. If the prone position must be used, the patient's head should be maintained in the sagittal plane, and each arm should be carefully restrained alongside the trunk in such a way that the shoulder mechanism is not stretched caudad and no dorsad pressure is placed on the clavicle. In

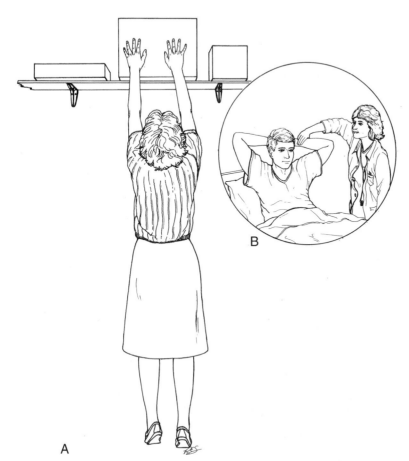

B

A

Figure 10–30

Assessment of a potential thoracic outlet syndrome. *A.* History of reaching or working overhead resulted in extremity pain. *B.* Provocative posture during interview with hands clasped on occiput, radial pulse repeatedly checked for damping. (From McLeskey CH [ed.]: Geriatric Anesthesiology. Baltimore, Williams & Wilkins, in press.)

the presence of serious obesity, however, such a placement of huge arms may create unavoidable problems for the surgical team trying to reach the dorsal midline of the patient's torso.

Closure of the Retroclavicular Space

The medial two thirds of the retroclavicular space is bounded dorsally, medially, and caudad by the curved ventrolateral wall of the upper thorax. When the shoulder mechanism is moved dorsad or caudad, the clavicle can compress the subclavian neurovascular bundle (composed of the subclavian artery, vein, and brachial plexus) against the upper ribs and disrupt its function (see Chapter 8 and Fig. 8–9). The radial pulse may be dampened or absent, and venous congestion of the arm is possible. An awake patient in this situation soon experiences multiple paresthesias into the arm and hand; strength may be reduced or lost in the extremity. At some point, anesthesia of a part or all of the upper extremity develops.

Because the anatomy of the retroclavicular space varies between patients, not all of the clavicles that are forced dorsocaudad compress the neurovascular bundle to the extremity. However, the possibility should be kept in mind for each patient and appropriate precautions should be routine.

In the prone positions, closure of the retroclavicular space can occur when a ventral support rests against the clavicle or the acromioclavicular joint. The final postural inspection after pronation should assure that the cephalad end of a longitudinal chest roll does not cross the clavicle and that pulses are present at the wrist. An unexpected prominence of the vertebral border of the scapula should alert the anesthesiologist to assess the possibility of unacceptable dorsal displacement of the shoulder. If shiftable thoracic supports, such as independent sandbag pedestals, are used, they should be checked at intervals during pronation as well as during the subsequent operation to assure that they have not migrated into a position that closes the retroclavicular space.

Alerted by pulse oximeters placed on fingers, Hovagim and colleagues[100] reported eight cases of arterial blood flow impairment produced by patient positioning, two of which occurred after pronation. In one, a parallel chest roll shifted laterally under the weight of a morbidly obese patient; repositioning the roll restored the pulse oximeter readings to baseline. In the other, stabilizing tapes had drawn a shoulder too forcibly against a supporting frame; releasing the tape restored the oximeter readings to normal. Their six additional instances occurred in several other positions. They consider pulse oximetry to be a valuable tool for the continuous assessment of patient positioning.

Breast Injuries

Breasts may threaten positioning, and positioning may inadvertently damage breasts. Despite the fact that this seemingly naive comment is well known to many, no definitive studies could be located to authenticate the impressions that experience has provided about the issue.

Abnormally large breasts offer an unstable and shifting platform when placed directly ventral to a prone thorax and may permit an unsettling change in the patient's posture after draping. Occasionally this instability is sufficiently troublesome to require that the prone position be abandoned in favor of the lateral position.

When Smith and colleagues developed the Georgia prone position,[18] they stipulated that females placed prone must have the breasts displaced laterally. However, comments made to me by older surgeons who had specialized almost exclusively in breast surgery during their careers, plus my own informal, nonstatistical questioning of female patients and nursing personnel who represented a variety of mammary physiques, have indicated that lateralizing traction on breasts is painful to many women, whereas medial and cephalad compression is not. Historically, women's clothing has been designed to thrust breasts medially and cephalad.

Clinical experience indicates that the pronated female patients whose breasts have been moved medially between postural supports rarely have ventral chest wall distress or breast tenderness postoperatively. If body contours or positioning devices force breast tissue laterally under considerable tension, the median (parasternal) breast margins may tear or bleed interstitially. Also, when a large patient with heavy breasts is prone with arms restrained at her sides, deliberately forcing bulky breast tissue laterally can, in turn, force her arms far enough away from the sides of her body to impede the surgeon's access to her dorsal midline structures (Fig. 10–31). Me-

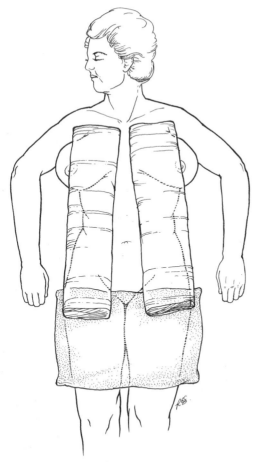

Figure 10–31

Obese prone patient with huge breasts forcing arms laterally and creating an obstruction for surgeons working in dorsal midline.

diad breast placement seems more satisfactory than lateral placement for most breast sizes during surgical procedures done with the patient in the prone position.

Longitudinal positioning frames or rolls, designed to relieve pressure on abdominal viscera, may occasionally damage breast tissue by direct compression. Ribbed (corduroy-like), pebbled (terry cloth), or wrinkled surfaces mark breasts after prolonged contact, and even soft plastic sponge pads can stretch mammary tissue or a nipple to the point of producing erythema, ecchymoses, or bleeding in susceptible individuals. Simply as a function of their extreme body weight, unusually heavy patients are at significant risk for breast injuries when placed prone.

Strong reasons occasionally exist to select a postural alternative to the prone position

because of breast abnormalities. The most common of these are listed below:

- True mammomegaly, because it provides an unstable base for a prone patient despite individualized positioning compromises
- The presence of extensive breast pathology, whether infectious or mitotic
- The engorged, painful breasts of a newly lactating mother

An unexpected complication of the prone position for a thin, small-breasted woman who has had an augmentation mammaplasty is rupture of a pliable breast prosthesis caused by unrecognized pressure or stretch-torsion from a chest support. Significant tissue damage may be caused by the escaped contents of the prosthesis.[101]

Infrequently a patient who has had a mastectomy will be a candidate for surgery in the prone position.

- Areas of the chest wall in the mastectomy site that are tender to touch or pressure may become painful after lying prone, particularly in an obese patient. Ischemic decubitus ulceration can occur as a result, may be difficult to treat, and may require graft replacement.
- If tissue induration secondary to surgery or radiation therapy is present in the subclavicular and acromioclavicular areas, the direct pressure of lying prone may be transmitted injuriously to the axillary and subclavian neurovascular bundle unless heavy foam padding is used to support the shoulder and adjacent thoracic cage.
- The presence of restricted shoulder motion because of postmastectomy tissue induration usually makes raising that arm alongside the head of the pronated patient difficult and undesirable. This problem is particularly troublesome in the massively obese prone patient because the presence of large arms restrained alongside the bulky torso moves the surgeon even farther away from the dorsal midline operative site.
- When a heavy-breasted patient who has had a unilateral mastectomy is to be positioned prone, thick foam padding may be needed to cushion the area of the missing breast if the torso is to be supported evenly on the table.

Occasionally a male with gynecomastia will

need to be placed in the prone position. The quantity of breast tissue induced by the condition is usually small to moderate, rather firm, minimally mobile, and infrequently tender. Apparently its presence does not influence the choice of sleeping posture for the patient. Positioning such a patient on longitudinal rolls may cause direct pressure on the breasts despite the best precautions. A kneeling frame with careful padding under the thorax might be less stressful. The potential for an injury to this aberrant tissue exists, but its magnitude is unknown because of the infrequency of the problem. However, the risk of injury to the abnormal male breast tissue should be discussed with the afflicted patient before pronation under anesthesia.

As a final step after positioning a prone patient, the breasts should be checked to assure that they are in a neutral or mediad configuration, that the nipples are not stretched, and that the supporting surfaces on the operating table are smooth and immobile.

Injuries to Coronary Arteries

Because the ventrodorsal dimension of a pliable thorax can be reduced in the prone position, mediastinal structures are theoretically at risk of compression between the sternum and the vertebral column. The structures can also be expected to shift ventrad in the prone position even though chest dimensions have changed only slightly. The significance of these events is difficult to determine and may depend somewhat on the weight of the patient and the condition of the mediastinal contents. Smith[76] wrote that he was unaware of impaired myocardial function due to prone positioning.

More recently, Weinlander and associates reported a case involving a patient who had a coronary artery bypass graft 8 years previously and, in the interim, had an uncomplicated anesthetic for a lumbar laminectomy in the prone position while supported by longitudinal chest rolls.[102] Needing a repeat laminectomy, he was anesthetized and placed in the knee-chest position. Venous congestion of the head and neck required relief by elevating the thorax on a sternal pad. Electrocardiographic evidence of myocardial ischemia followed placement of the pad, was refractory to drug therapy, and, at the conclusion of the laminectomy, required emergency intra-aortic balloon pump support and coronary artery revascularization. Although lacking conclu-sive proof, these investigators believe that the sternal compression caused by the pad obstructed the previously functional coronary artery graft and produced the ischemia. Apparently, the stresses of longitudinal chest rolls and a sternal pad can affect a revascularized myocardium differently.

Injuries to the Obese Abdomen

Morbidly obese patients occasionally must be positioned prone for operations on the back. Longitudinal chest rolls rarely can be arranged to provide enough lift to minimize high venous pressure in the surgical wound. Also, the massive amounts of breast tissue and abdominal panniculus adiposus usually create a shifting base that prevents firmly stabilizing the posture.

With adequate knee padding and reasonably firm chest support, such as the Wiltse jack or a stack of folded sheets (Georgia prone position system), a kneeling device similar to an Andrews frame (see Fig. 10–9) may permit satisfactory relief of abdominal compression. Frequently the pendulous abdomen will hang far down toward the patient's knees in this kneeling position and may actually intrude into whatever space exists between the edges of the thigh and foot sections of the angulated table top (Fig 10–32).

Two injuries threaten the pendulous and intrusive abdominal wall. First, unless insulated padding has been interposed, the flesh of the patient that invades the spaces between sections of the top of the operating table and comes to rest against metal parts of the table pedestal may permit a grounding burn when electrocautery is activated. Second, and more drastic, unless the patient is rolled carefully off of the prone frame onto a bed or transport cart while the foot section is still depressed, extreme caution must be exercised in terminating the position because returning the kneeling portion of the table to horizontal can easily trap the dangling, intruded abdominal wall between approximating edges of the foot and thigh surfaces of the table and produce a mangling, scissor-like wound of major consequence. The fat content of an extremely obese abdominal wall can make its recovery from either a burn or an unplanned and contaminated incisive injury very difficult to manage.

Viscerostomy Damage

Depending on their location, viscerocutaneous stomas on the abdominal wall can be

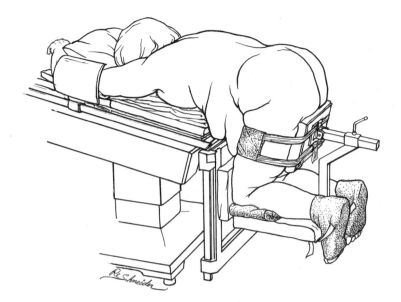

Figure 10–32

A pathologically obese patient can be successfully arranged on a kneeling frame. Pendulous abdomen protruding into the potentially irrigation-wetted hinging mechanism of table is susceptible to grounding burns with electrocautery use or scissoring injury if table sections are restored to horizontal plane at end of procedure.

compressed by prone supports, become ischemic, and require surgical revision (Fig. 10–33). Collection bags may be dislocated or penetrated during pronation, allowing unrecognized table soilage and inviting wound contamination during the subsequent procedure. Longitudinal rolls may be more of a problem in this regard than are pedestal devices. Kneeling systems seem potentially less threatening.

When a stoma is present it should be checked carefully once the final position is established and corrective measures instituted promptly if needed. Intraoperative position changes require similar checks. Discussing, either with the patient or with a responsible member of the patient's family, the possibility of problems with stomas is a wise addition to a preanesthetic interview.

Hypotension in a Pronated Patient

Nondeliberate hypotension may appear either slowly or with unexpected speed in a pronated patient. A slow onset of hypotension may be consistent with gradual pooling of blood volume in distensible, unsupported vessels of the dependent lower extremities that causes a significant reduction of inferior vena caval flow back to the heart. Applying compressive wraps or elastic stockings to the lower limbs before pronation minimizes the opportunity for dependent pooling. Underestimation of the amount of shed blood that needs to be replaced by crystalloids, colloids, or blood products can combine with unap-

preciated degrees of volume pooling to produce significant hypotension.

A rapid onset of hypotension in a prone patient, particularly in the presence of increased distention of veins in the dorsal surgical wound may indicate a shift of the ventral support sufficient to allow the weight of the patient to compress the abdomen and great vessels. Re-establishment of adequate support of the torso usually restores perfusion and decreases the vascular congestion at the surgical site.

A biting surgical instrument placed deep in an intervertebral disk space may incise the anterior longitudinal ligament of the spinal column and disrupt the dorsal wall of one of the great vessels, often the abdominal aorta.[38, 39] When sudden hypotension occurs in the presence of an otherwise stable anesthetic and little evidence of blood loss or congestion in the surgical field, and particularly when the low pressure responds poorly to volume replacement, such a possibility should be kept in mind. Rapid closure of the dorsal surgical wound and turning the patient supine for an emergency laparotomy to permit repair of the vascular injury may be the only means of restoring stable perfusion.

Injuries to Genitalia

In the classic prone position, the pillow placed over the caudad end of the longitudinal rolls to protect the ventral thighs (see Fig. 10–1) may trap the scrotum and penis. When retaining straps are placed, the genitalia and

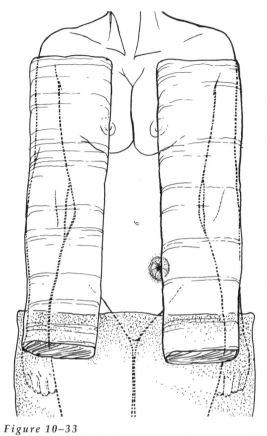

Figure 10–33

A longitudinal torso support impacts an unprotected viscerocutaneous stoma in the prone position. Surgical revision of the stoma may be needed. (From McLeskey CH [ed.]: Geriatric Anesthesia. Baltimore, Williams & Wilkins, in press.)

urinary catheter must be checked to assure their satisfactory position and patency. Straps and seats used to stabilize the kneeling prone patient can also compress the female perineum, and appropriate checks should be made to assure genital and catheter integrity once the final posture is attained.

Injuries to the Lateral Femoral Cutaneous Nerve

Smith[76] cautioned that the lateral femoral cutaneous nerve may be compressed by the devices that support the anterior-superior iliac spines. Resulting meralgia paresthetica can be extremely annoying to the patient. Padded iliac supports should combat this possibility. However, we can speculate that the most important etiologic factor might be hip flexion that forces dense fatty tissue into the area of the inguinal ligament just medial to the

anterior-superior iliac spine. Data supporting the occurrence of such an injury are not available, but the warning has merit.

Neurovascular Threats to the Legs

Extremes of lower extremity posture, as in the tuck or crouching variation of the prone position (see Fig. 10–6), can compress vessels and nerves in the popliteal fossa or in the inguinal region. After substantial ischemia, tissue hypoxia usually produces edema that increases pressures within fascial compartments enough to further compromise perfusion and cause severe pain on awakening. The resulting compartment syndrome[83] causes muscle necrosis and the release of myoglobin, a recognized cause of acute renal failure.[103] Fasciotomies may be needed to relieve compartment tension. Infections, pulmonary pathology, and difficult problems of fluid and electrolyte balance are often associated with compartment syndromes (see Chapter 6).[83] Amputation of one or both lower extremities is a possibility if vascular competence does not return and tissue damage is extensive.

When an anesthetized patient is placed in a kneeling posture on one of the various frames designed for the purpose, the resulting uphill gradient for venous return from the legs, combined with the lack of the normal vascular massaging action of the leg musculature that occurs while awake, can cause stasis accumulation of blood in the lower extremities. Consequent loss of circulating volume may be sufficient to reduce cardiac output. Before positioning, extremities that will be dependent usually should be wrapped in compressive, nonischemic bandages to minimize subsequent pooling of blood.

The use of an arching frame (see Fig. 10–20) or a set of parallel chest rolls (see Fig. 10–19) may reduce positional neurovascular threats to the dependent lower extremities because the limbs are more extended than with the tuck position and the vascular gradient is smaller than with the kneeling positions.

Thermal Homeostasis

Patients placed in any of the modifications of the prone position often remain there for long periods of time. Open surgical wounds that are extensive can lose significant amounts of body heat for a poikilothermic, anesthetized individual. The smaller the patient's body mass, the more critical this problem becomes. Because of the positioning devices, body contact with the surface of the operating table is much less than in the supine position. Obviously, therefore, a heat-exchanging water mattress is minimally effective for the prone patient. Also obvious is the need to constantly monitor body temperature throughout the anesthesia.

Combating hypothermia in the prone patient can be accomplished by altering the ability to radiate heat, by warming and humidifying gases in the breathing circuit, or by forcing warmed air over nonsurgical body surfaces.

- Simple plastic garbage bags can be wrapped around exposed body surfaces, specifically including the head, to minimize radiation.
- When the head or other body surfaces can be left exposed under a canopy of sterile drapes, a caged electrician's trouble light with a useful heat output can be hung near enough to the patient to become an effective radiant heat source without risking a surface burn. (The unit must be one that has been approved by the biomedical engineering group of the institution and is dedicated to this purpose.)
- Increased temperature and humidity in the patient's breathing circuit can be gained from one of the devices used for that purpose by respiratory therapists. When this method is chosen, the temperature of the inspired gases must be carefully and constantly monitored to avoid inflicting a thermal injury on the tracheobronchial tree. Breathing tubes that are long enough to be themselves sources of heat loss either may be wrapped with an insulating material or shortened to make the method effective.
- Radiant heat loss from an extensive wound during prolonged surgery may be sufficient to require warming the operating room. Routinely, and understandably, this maneuver is resisted by the surgical team, who can become quite uncomfortable as a result. However, prevention of hypothermia in an infant or in a person with a frail physique may be difficult unless environmental temperature is raised.
- Many anesthesiologists use forced heated air flowing over nonsurgical body surfaces to offset radiant losses during surgery. During protracted surgical procedures on the spine, warmed air can be blown over the exposed buttocks and lower extremities. For patients on pedestal devices, a forced air blanket can be attached to the ventral thorax and abdomen.

PREANESTHETIC EVALUATION

The preanesthetic interview with patients who are to be pronated should include a careful inquiry into several key issues. Responses that affect positioning should be carefully assessed when taking the patient's history in a manner that is informative and easily accessible to the anesthesia and surgical teams. When problems arise subsequently, the record of preanesthetic information is an important component of the demonstration of acceptable standards of care. Specific discussions between anesthesiologist and surgeon concerning significant positioning problems are prudent.

Head Rotation

Any history of a neck injury, cervical arthritis, a symptomatic cervical disk protrusion, or previous operations on cervical vertebrae requires a demonstration of the patient's ability to rotate the head. The extent of neck rotation or extension that produces pain should be gently demonstrated, described in the record of the interview, and not exceeded during the positioning process.

Arm Position

Patients with histories of being unable to work or sleep with one or both arms overhead because the posture is painful should be considered to have a thoracic outlet syndrome. At surgery, placing those arms alongside the head rather than at the sides of the torso and retaining the position throughout a lengthy operation may easily produce bilateral brachial plexus pain that will be intense, debilitating, and prolonged. Because placing obese arms alongside an obese torso may complicate the access of a surgeon to the dorsal midline of the torso, the surgical team should be alerted to arm positioning problems discovered in the preanesthetic workup.

Implanted or Mastectomized Breasts

When implants are present or a previous mastectomy site exists, particular care must be taken with padding of the pronated chest to cushion the pressure of elevating rests. A stack of folded sheets covered by heavy foam and the use of a kneeling system may be a better choice for the tight skin graft of an amputated breast than is either a pedestal rest or a longitudinal frame. The same may be true for massive mammomegaly. Often it is wise to discuss the risk of graft or implant injury with the patient during the interview. Mobility of the humerus on the mastectomized side must be evaluated because it may affect the choice of arm positioning after pronation.

Previous Coronary Artery Bypass Graft

While the evidence for this presumption is tenuous (see earlier), a longitudinal frame may be a better choice for the patient who has had previous myocardial revascularization rather than is a rest that places direct pressure on the sternum.

Unstable Chest Wall

When the chest wall is unstable after trauma, the weight of the thorax may force jagged rib ends apart and depress them into the substance of the lung. Depending on the urgency of the procedure, an alternate posture may need to be devised if surgery cannot be delayed until the chest wall can be stabilized. An anesthesiologic approach to urgent surgery in the presence of a pronated, unstable hemithorax might be a double-lumen endotrachial tube with the option of one-lung anesthesia after placement of chest tubes to prevent the occurrence of a tension pneumothorax.

Viscerostomies

When a viscerocutaneous stoma is present in a location that is likely to rest against ventral supporting frames or pedestals after pronation, the patient or family should be advised of the possibility of the stoma being injured in the positioning process despite the most careful preventive measures. Surgical repair of the compressed and ischemic stoma may be required.

Arthritic Knees

Patients who have a history of multiple injuries to the knee, have had repeated surgical procedures on the knees, or have active arthritis in knee joints are poor candidates for a kneeling version of the prone position that uses the knee-femur mechanism as a principal structural support for the posture. Their history usually includes an inability to achieve or sustain a kneeling posture while awake, either due to joint immobility or pain on compressing the area. An alternative version of the prone position with careful padding of the knees is a prudent choice.

REFERENCES

1. Singh I: The prone position: Surgical aspects. *In* Martin JT (ed.): Positioning in Anesthesia and Surgery, 2nd ed. Philadelphia, WB Saunders, 1987.
2. Cushing HW: Some principles of cerebral surgery. JAMA 52:184, 1909.
3. Shephard DAZ: Letter to the editor. Anesth Analg 65:1250, 1986.
4. Bagshaw RJ, Smith DS, Young MS, Bloom MJ: Anesthetic management of surgery in the vertebral canal. Anesth Rev 12:13, 1985.
5. Anderton JM: The prone position for the surgical patient: A historical review of the principles and hazards. Br J Anaesth 67:452, 1991.
6. Bannenburg JJ, Meijer DW, Klopper PJ: The prone position: Using gravity for a clear view. Surg Endosc 8:1115, 1994.
7. Schepens CL, Freman HM, Thompson RF: A power-driven multipositional operating table. Arch Ophthalmol 73:671, 1965.
8. Wollman SB, Neuman GO: Retinal surgery in the prone position: An inexpensive simple headrest. Anesthesiology 61:109, 1984.
9. Sun WZ, Huang FY, Kung KL, et al.: Successful cardiopulmonary resuscitation of two patients in the prone position using reversed precordial compression. Anesthesiology 77:202, 1992.
10. Tobias JD, Mencio GA, Atwood R, Gurwitz GS: Intraoperative cardiopulmonary resuscitation in the prone position. J Pediatr Surg 29: 1537, 1994.
11. Iwabuchi T, Sobata E, Suzuki M, et al.: Dural sinus pressure as related to neurosurgical positions. Neurosurgery 12:203, 1983.
12. Overholt RH, Langer L: Technique of Pulmonary Resection. Springfield, IL, Charles C Thomas, 1949.
13. Brair RHF: Operative surgery—thorax. *In* Surgery in Pulmonary Operations. London, Butterworths, 1968.
14. Ecker A: Kneeling position for operations on the lumbar spine especially for protruded intervertebral disc. Surgery 25:112, 1949.
15. Wayne SJ: The tuck position for lumbar disc surgery. J Bone Joint Surg 49:1195, 1967.
16. Wayne SJ: A modification of the tuck position for lumbar spine surgery—a 15-year follow-up study. Clin Orthop 184:212, 1984.
17. Buie LA: Practical Proctology, 2nd ed. Springfield, IL, Charles C Thomas, 1960.
18. Smith RH, Gramling ZW, Volpitto PP: Problems

related to the prone position for surgical operations. Anesthesiology 22:189, 1961.

19. Cook AW, Siddiqi TS, Nidzgorski F, et al.: Sitting prone position for the posterior surgical approach to the spine and posterior fossa. Neurosurgery 10:232, 1982.

20. Taylor AR, Gleadhill CA, Bilstand WL, Murray PR: Posture and anesthesia for spinal operations with special reference to intervertebral disc surgery. Br J Anaesth 28:213, 1956.

21. Lehman T, Bagley DH: Reverse lithotomy: Modified prone position for simultaneous nephroscopic and ureteroscopic procedures in women. Endourology 32:529, 1988.

22. Grasso M, Nord R, Bagley DH: Prone split leg and flank roll positioning: simultaneous antegrade and retrograde access to the upper urinary tract. J Endourol 7:307, 1993.

23. Eaton JM: Transsacral cystectomy. In Glenn J (ed.): Urologic Surgery, 2nd ed. Hagerstown, MD, Harper & Row, 1975.

24. Ray CD: Head and chin cushioned face rest for surgery in the prone position. Anesthesiology 64:301, 1986.

25. Gardner WJ: A neurosurgical chair. J Neurosurg 12:81, 1955.

26. Moore DC, Edmunds L: Prone position frame. Surgery 27:276, 1950

27. Bardeen A: A special pad for patients in the prone position. Anesthesiology 16:465, 1955.

28. Relton JES, Hall JE: An operation frame for spinal surgery. J Bone Joint Surg 49:327, 1967.

29. Mouradian WH, Simmons EH: A frame for spinal surgery to reduce intraabdominal pressure while continuous traction is applied. J Bone Joint Surg 59:1098, 1977.

30. Smith RH: One solution to the problem of the prone position for surgery. Anesth Analg 53:221, 1974.

31. Smith RH: A device for positioning the prone patient. Anesthesiology 25:87, 1964.

32. Lee C, Blarneys A, Nagel EL: Neuroleptanalgesia for awake pronation of surgical patients. Anesth Analg 56:276, 1977.

33. Lesser RP, Raudzens P, Luders H, et al.: Postoperative neurologic deficits may occur despite unchanged intraoperative somatosensory evoked potentials. Ann Neurol 19:22, 1986.

34. Edmonds HL, Paloheimo MPJ, Backman MH, et al.: Transcranial magnetic motor evoked potentials (tcMMEP) for functional monitoring of motor pathways during scoliosis surgery. Spine 14:683, 1989.

35. Batson OV: Function of the vertebral veins and their role in the spread of metastases. Ann Surg 112:138, 1940.

36. McGregor AL: A Synopsis of Surgical Anatomy, 7th ed. Bristol, John Wright & Sons, 1950.

37. Holscher EC: Vascular complications of disc surgery. J Bone Joint Surg 30:968, 1948.

38. Harbison SP: Major vascular complications of intervertebral disc surgery. Ann Surg 140:342, 1954.

39. Seely SF, Hughes CW, Jahnke EJ: Major vessel damage in lumbar disc operation. Surgery 35:421, 1954.

40. Smith RA, Estridge MN: Bowel perforation following lumbar disc surgery. J Bone Joint Surg 46:826, 1964.

41. Armstrong JR: Lumbar Disc Lesions, 3rd ed. Baltimore, Williams & Wilkins, 1965.

42. Pearce DJ: The role of posture in laminectomy. Proc R Soc Med 50:109, 1957.

43. DiStefano VJ, Klein KS, Nixon JE, et al.: Intraoperative analysis of the effects of body position and body habitus on surgery of the low back. Clin Orthop 99:51, 1974.

44. Backofen JE, Schauble JF: Hemodynamic changes with prone position during general anesthesia. Anesth Analg 64:194, 1985 (abstract).

45. Yokoyama M, Ueda W, Kirakawa M, Yamamoto H: Hemodynamic effect of the prone position during anesthesia. Acta Anaesthesiol Scand 35:741, 1991.

46. McNulty SE, Weiss J, Azad SS, et al.: The effect of the prone position on venous pressure and blood loss during lumbar laminectomy. J Clin Anesth 4:220, 1992.

47. Rehder K, Knopp TJ, Sessler AD: Regional intrapulmonary gas distribution in awake and anesthetized-paralyzed prone man. J Appl Physiol 45:528, 1978.

48. West JB, Dollery CT, Naimark A: Distribution of blood flow in isolated lung: Relation to vascular and alveolar pressures. J Appl Physiol 19:713, 1964.

49. Hughes JM, Glazier JB, Maloney JE, et al.: Effect of lung volume on the distribution of pulmonary blood flow in man. Resp Physiol 4:58, 1968.

50. Kaneko K, Milic-Emily J, Dolovich MB, et al.: Regional distribution of ventilation and perfusion as a function of body position. J Appl Physiol 21:767, 1966.

51. Stone JG, Khambatta HJ: Pulmonary shunts in the prone position. Anaesthesia 33:512, 1978.

52. Price HL, Cooperman LH, Warden JC, et al.: Pulmonary hemodynamics during general anesthesia in man. Anesthesiology 30:629, 1969.

53. Marshall BE, Cohen PJ, Klingenmaier CH, et al.: Pulmonary venous admixture before, during and after halothane:oxygen anesthesia in man. J Appl Physiol 29:653, 1969.

54. Douglas WW, Rehder K, Beynen FM, et al.: Improved oxygenation in patients with acute respiratory failure: The prone position. Am Rev Respir Dis 115:559, 1977.

55. Lumb AB, Nunn JF: Respiratory function and rib cage contribution to ventilation in body positions commonly used during anesthesia. Anesth Analg 73:422, 1991.

56. Pelosi P, Croci M, Calappi E, et al: The prone positioning during general anesthesia minimally affects respiratory mechanics while improving functional residual capacity and increasing oxygen tension. Anesth Analg 80:955, 1995.

57. Mahajan RP, Hennessy N, Aitkenhead AR, Jellinek D: Effect of three different surgical prone positions on lung volumes in healthy volunteers. Anaesthesia 49:583, 1994.

58. Lamm WJ, Graham MM, Albert RK: Mechanism by which the prone position improves oxygenation in acute lung injury. Am J Respir Crit Care Med 150:184, 1994.

59. Shenkin HA, Scheuerman WG, Spitz EB, et al.: Effects of change of position on the cerebral circulation in man. J Appl Physiol 2:317, 1949.

60. Toole JF: Effects of change of head, limb and body position on cephalic circulation. N Engl J Med 279:307, 1968.

61. Mustafa K, Milliken BA, Bizzarri DV: The advantages of the prone position approach to the lumbar epidural space. Anesthesiology 58:464, 1963.

62. Blaney SM, Poplack DG, Godwin K, et al.: Effect of body position on ventricular CSF methotrexate concentration following intralumbar administration. J Clin Oncol 13:177, 1995.

63. Marcus ML, Heistad DD, Ehrhardt JC, et al.: Regulation of total and regional spinal cord blood flow. Circ Res 41:128, 1977.

64. Kobrine Al, Doyle TF, Rizzoli HV: Spinal cord blood flow as affected by changes in systemic arterial blood pressure. J Neurosurg 4:12, 1976.

65. Katz DM, Trobe JD, Cornblath WT, Kline LB: Ischemic optic neuropathy after lumbar spine surgery. Arch Ophthalmol 112:925, 1994.

66. Walkup HE, Murphy JD: Retinal ischemia during unilateral blindness–a complication occurring during pulmonary resection in the prone position. J Thorac Surg 23:174, 1952.

67. Wolfe SW, Lospinuso MD, Burke SW: Unilateral blindness as a complication of patient positioning for spinal surgery: A case report. Spine 17:600, 1992.

68. Williams EL, Hart WM, Tempelhoff R: Postoperative ischemic optic neuropathy. Anesth Analg 80:1018, 1995.

69. Friedman E: Choroidal blood flow: I. Pressure-flow relationships. Arch Ophthalmol 83:95, 1970.

70. Bill A: Blood circulation and fluid dynamics in the eye. Physiol Rev 55:383, 1975.

71. Riva CE, Sinclair SH, Grunwald JE: Autoregulation of retinal circulation in response to decrease of perfusion pressure. Invest Ophthalmol Vis Sci 21:34, 1981.

72. Tsamparlakis J, Casey TA, Howell W, Edridge A: Dependence of intraocular pressure on induced hypotension and posture during surgical anesthesia. Trans Ophthalmol Soc UK, 100:521, 1980.

73. Britt BA, Gordon RA: Peripheral nerve injuries associated with anesthesia. Can Anaesth Soc J 11:514, 1964.

74. Glauber DT: Facial paralysis after general anesthesia. Anesthesiology 65:516, 1986.

75. Winter R, Munro M: Lingual and buccal nerve neuropathy in a patient in the prone position: A case report. Anesthesiology 71:452, 1989.

76. Smith RH: The prone position. *In* Martin JT (ed.): Positioning in Anesthesia and Surgery. Philadelphia, WB Saunders, 1978.

77. McPherson RW, Szymanski J, Rogers MC: Somatosensory evoked potential changes in position-related brain stem ischemia. Anesthesiology 61:88, 1984.

78. Schneider RC, Cherry G, Pantek H: The syndrome of acute central cervical spinal cord injury. J Neurosurg 11:546, 1954.

79. Peterson EI, Altman K: Central cervical spinal cord syndrome due to minor hyperextension injury. West J Med 150:691, 1989.

80. Grundy B, Gravenstein N, Reid SA: The central nervous system: Complications of positioning. *In* Martin JT (ed.): Positioning in Anesthesia and Surgery. Philadelphia, WB Saunders, 1987.

81. Wilder BL: Hypothesis: The etiology of midcervical quadriplegia after operation with the patient in the sitting position. Neurosurgery 11:530, 1982.

82. Deem S, Shapiro HM, Marshall LF: Quadriplegia in a patient with cervical spondylosis after thoracolumbar surgery in the prone position. Anesthesiology 75:527, 1991.

83. Martin JT: Compartment syndromes: Concepts and perspectives for the anesthesiologist. Anesth Analg, 75:275, 1992.

84. Shenkin HN, Goldfedder P: Air embolism from exposure of posterior cranial fossa in prone position. JAMA 210:726, 1969.

85. Tarlov E: Lumbar disk surgery in knee-chest position: Preanesthetic atrial catheter unnecessary: Question and answers. JAMA 238:253, 1977.

86. Albin MS, Newfield P, Paulter S, et al.: Atrial catheter and lumbar disk surgery: Correspondence. JAMA 239:496, 1978.

87. Albin MS, Babinski M, Maroon JC, Janetta PJ: Anesthetic management of posterior fossa surgery in the sitting position. Acta Anesthesiol Scand 20:117, 1976.

88. Albin MS, Ritter RR, Pruett CE, Kalff K: Venous air embolism during lumbar laminectomy in the prone position: Report of three cases. Anesth Analg 73:346, 1991.

89. Artru AA: Venous air embolism in prone dogs positioned with the abdomen hanging freely: Percentage of gas retrieved and success rate of resuscitation. Anesth Analg 75:715, 1992.

90. Tempelhoff R, Williams EL, Volmer DG: Is the "kneeling" prone position as dangerous as the sitting position for the development of venous air embolus? Anesth Analg 75:461, 1992 (letter).

91. Horlocker TT, Wedel DJ, Cucchiara RF: Venous air embolism during spinal instrumentation and fusion in the prone position: Correspondence. Anesth Analg 75:152, 1992.

92. Delaloye D, Gerber H: A special surgical technique leads to venous air embolism during neurosurgery of the spine: Correspondence. Anesth Analg 75:461, 1992.

93. Albin MS, Ritter RR, Bunegin L: Correspondence. Anesth Analg 75:153, 1992.

94. Kroll DA, Caplan RA, Posner K, et al.: Nerve injury associated with anesthesia. Anesthesiology 73:202, 1990.

95. Martin GT: First rib resection for the thoracic outlet syndrome. Br J Neurosurg 7:35, 1993.

96. Novak CB, Mackinnon SE, Patterson GA: Evaluation of patients with thoracic outlet syndromes. J Hand Surg 18:292, 1993.

97. Martin JT: The prone position: Anesthesiologic considerations. In Martin JT (ed.): Positioning in Anesthesiology and Surgery, 2nd ed. WB Saunders, Philadelphia, 1987.

98. Martin JT: Patient positioning. *In* Barash PG, Cullen BF, Stoelting RK (eds.): Clinical Anesthesia, 2nd ed. Philadelphia, JB Lippincott, 1992.

99. Anderton JM, Schady W, Markham DE: An unusual cause of postoperative brachial plexus palsy. Br J Anaesth 72:605, 1994.

100. Hovagim AR, Backus WW, Manecke G, et al.: Pulse oximetry and patient positioning: A report of eight cases. Anesthesiology 71:454, 1989.

101. Teuber SS, Ito LK, Anderson M, Gershwin ME: Silicone breast implant–associated scarring dystrophy of the arm. Arch Dermatol 131:54, 1995.

102. Weinlander CM, Coombs DW, Plume SK: Myocardial ischemia due to obstruction of an aortocoronary bypass graft by intraoperative positioning. Anesth Analg 64:933, 1985.

103. Keim HA: Acute renal failure: A complication of spine fusion in the tuck position. J Bone Joint Surg 52:1248, 1970.

Special Considerations

Chapter 11

Positioning the Extremities

David A. Nakata / Robert K. Stoelting

BACKGROUND

Current recommendations and practices regarding positioning and padding of the patient's extremities usually reflect attempts to prevent excessive stretch to nerves such as the brachial plexus and to avoid direct compression of superficial nerves like the ulnar nerve at the elbow. The protective effects of some recommendations (including rotational position of the abducted arms or use of additional padding around the elbow) remain unproven.[1] The historic notion that proper positioning and padding will prevent all perioperative peripheral nerve injuries is no longer tenable.[2–6] Indeed, despite use of accepted methods of positioning, padding, and monitoring of the patient's extremities, perioperative peripheral nerve injuries still occur, suggesting the distressing conclusion that some of these injuries are not completely preventable.[2, 4]

A recent American Society of Anesthesiologists Closed Claim Study reviewing nerve injuries showed that those related to anesthesia involved 227 (15%) of the 1541 claims reviewed.[4] Even though a number of limitations have been cited with regard to this form of investigation, it is extremely helpful in lending perspective to issues needing further study and research. In addition, this survey, unlike most others, assessed not only complications per se but those that led to litigation, reminding us that complications can adversely affect both patient and clinician.

It is hoped that numerous technical advances, such as pulse oximetry and end-tidal carbon dioxide monitoring, will lead to a significant decrease in the number of catastrophic events in anesthesia. Unfortunately, these advances will most likely have little effect on the incidence of perioperative injuries to nerves of the extremities. Unless the causes of injuries due to positioning are better understood, proper preventive measures cannot be implemented.

Patient positioning is optimum for the surgeon when it provides the easiest available access to the surgical target. However, a candidate for a surgical procedure may have pre-existing physical conditions that could disastrously complicate standard positioning maneuvers or make them impossible. An example is the patient with contracture secondary to an upper motor neuron lesion. Unfortunately, the physically normal individual is not completely safe from sustaining position-associated peripheral nerve injuries during an operative procedure despite the application of safeguards that are currently accepted as proper.[4]

What, then, is optimal positioning? The answer is thwarted by three factors that have impacted our ability to determine the etiologies of injuries ascribed to positioning:

1. Positioning-related complications are rare. Their scarcity makes their incidences and causative factors difficult to determine. When considering interpatient variables such as gender, age, weight, and coexisting diseases, determination of cause and effect becomes extremely difficult.

2. Appropriate animal models for studying the pathophysiology of various positions are lacking. Data from a rodent, or even a monkey, extrapolate poorly to humans.

3. Multiple different tissues can be injured, including soft tissue, joints, and nerves, making evaluation of injuries not only complex but also multidisciplinary.

Our purpose, then, is to make meaningful recommendations based on cause and effect by analyzing information that (1) is derived from different tissues, (2) is sporadic in frequency, (3) is historical and anecdotal, and (4) is gained from incomplete laboratory models. Considering these constraints, our discussion must be limited to areas that are well founded on scientific principles.

Consequently, we review pertinent aspects of the history and physical examination; discuss the anatomy, physiology, and pathology of the three most commonly injured tissues—soft tissues, joints, and nerves; and consider the three neural structures—the ulnar nerve, brachial plexus and lumbosacral trunk—most often involved in dysfunctions that appear postoperatively. Our purpose is not to make recommendations regarding every possible positioning maneuver. Instead, we attempt to offer information applicable globally to positioning strategies and support it with multiple references for the reader to pursue.

HISTORY AND PHYSICAL EXAMINATION

Because of the many life-threatening issues affecting surgical patients, information about optimizing the position of the extremities has not been recognized as an important part of the traditional history and physical examination. However, details elicited during a routine preoperative evaluation can be used to modify positioning techniques and minimize the risk of extremity complications.

Table 11–1 lists disease states that may contribute to positioning-related injury. Most of the information needed to diagnose the majority of these coexisting diseases should be obtained during a routine preoperative history.

Findings during the physical examination may also identify potential positioning problems. Table 11–2 lists physical findings that imply the possibility of positioning injury and allow the clinician opportunities to modify

Table 11–1

Patient History Data That May Influence Patient Positioning

Nerve entrapment syndromes (carpel tunnel)
Neuropathies
Diabetes mellitus
Osteoarthritis
Venous stasis
Pre-existing decubiti
Previous traumatic injury
Charcot-Marie-Tooth disease
Hereditary neuropathy with liability to pressure palsy
Alcohol abuse
Vitamin deficiencies
Malnutrition
Renal disease
Hypothyroidism
Previous joint fractures
Rheumatoid arthritis
Corticosteroid usage
Contractures

customary techniques. However, these findings are not always readily appreciated, especially in the case of the hereditary nerve palsies (Charcot-Marie-Tooth disease and hereditary neuropathy with liability to pressure palsies). Therefore, questioning about weakness, paresthesias, and numbness may be useful in identifying these rare conditions preoperatively. In addition, previously unappreciated nerve entrapment syndromes that can predispose patients to "double crush syndrome" may be discovered during the initial interview and examination.

Physical examination findings pertinent to positioning can be divided into three categories.

1. An asymptomatic irregularity that is not routinely detectable on physical examination.[7] For example, recurrent dislocation of the ulnar nerve that can be considered a "normal variant" may increase the risk of a perioperative injury to that nerve.

Table 11–2

Physical Findings That May Influence Patient Positioning

Range of motion of joints
Previous extremity surgery/trauma that may have
  injured nerves
Extremity edema
Skin turgor
Extremity weakness
Abnormal sensation
Decubitus ulcerations

2. An abnormality that is physically detectable but asymptomatic. For example, a healing surgical scar or traumatic, scar-producing injuries may cause abnormal stress on nerves and joints.

3. A symptomatic physical abnormality. For example, a fracture may impinge directly upon a nerve.

PRESSURE SORES AND SOFT TISSUE INJURIES

In the past, prevention of positioning-related injuries to the extremities has focused primarily on protecting peripheral nerves. However, soft tissues of the extremities are also at risk and can be exposed to many different types of destructive forces in the operating room. Some of these forces include compression and tissue shearing, which can lead to soft tissue injuries and pressure sores.[8–10]

All patients undergoing anesthesia and surgery should be considered at risk for development of pressure sores, a consequence of localized tissue compression that causes skin necrosis, blisters, and decubitus ulcers. They are most common in areas where soft tissue overlies bony prominences.

Anatomy

Bony prominences are covered by numerous heterogeneous layers of soft tissue that vary in thickness and type depending on the location and its nutritional needs. Skin is composed of two layers, an avascular epidermis and a dermis that contains blood vessels, nerve endings, hair follicles, and sweat glands. Skin serves many functions, including protection, sensation, temperature regulation, and excretion of water and lipids. Deep to the skin is a loose connective tissue layer, composed primarily of fat, that provides a degree of shock absorption and padding. This layer provides a plane upon which the more superficial skin is allowed to move with respect to deeper structures. However, owing to its composition, this loose connective tissue layer is susceptible to damage by lateral shear forces that can disrupt vascular structures and lead to tissue injury. Deep to this loose connective tissue layer is a plane of relatively avascular fascia overlying skeletal muscle. Despite its ability to generate and withstand significant levels of tension, skeletal muscle is poor at enduring prolonged compression, an

important fact in the development of pressure ulcers.[9] Deep to the muscle is periosteum that overlies bone.

Contributing Factors

Numerous factors influence the formation of pressure sores. These include age, nutritional status, systemic and local infection, moisture, chemical irritation, and thermal and electric burns. However, three factors are key to their development: *pressure, duration,* and *shear forces.*

Pressure

Types of Pressure. The pressure exerted on the structures within an extremity can be either extrinsic or intrinsic. Intrinsic pressure exists in the various compartments of an extremity due to hydrostatic and oncotic forces. These pressures can become pathologic in conditions such as compartment syndromes. Extrinsic pressure exists because of externally applied compression and can be due to the effects of a number of factors, including gravity, compressive tourniquets, and surgical retractors. In addition, factors such as the weight of the extremity or a pressure externally applied, such as that caused by a member of the surgical team, may add to the compression of soft tissues. Therefore, many different forces can potentially cause injury to soft tissue.

Amount of Pressure. The exact amount of pressure needed to cause an irreversible tissue injury is unknown. However, if pressure obstructs blood flow for a sufficient period of time, ischemia will occur.[7] In humans, studies have shown the mean capillary pressure to be approximately 35 mm Hg.[8, 11, 12] Therefore, if capillaries experience a sustained extramural pressure of greater than 35 mm Hg, ischemic tissue damage could be expected.[8] However, the elasticity of these tissues causes the formation of gradients that distribute pressure in a manner that dissipates force from the surface to the deeper structures.[13]

Numerous animal studies have been performed to determine the amount of external pressure required to produce tissue damage.[9, 14, 15] These studies suggest that a threshold pressure of 100 mm Hg sustained for 2 hours is needed to cause microscopic pathologic changes in tissues. However, the effects of extremely high pressures have also been evaluated and findings demonstrate that pressures greater than 1400 mm Hg can be applied for short intervals with minimal tissue damage.[14]

Whatever the amount of pressure required to produce a soft tissue injury, we can reasonably assume that the areas of the body that are subjected to the highest pressures for prolonged durations will be at greatest risk. Because not all parts of the body are subjected to the same degrees of pressure, knowing the distribution of pressure is important if proper intervention is to be taken to prevent pressure sores.

Distribution of Pressure. The distribution of pressure on various parts of the human body depends on a number of factors, including patient weight, height, lean body mass, and the presence of protective cushioning. Two percent of the body surface area of a normal individual in a supine position is subjected to a pressure between 60 and 70 mm Hg and 8% to a pressure between 40 and 60 mm Hg.[16] As noted earlier, unless the pressure exerted is sufficient to obstruct capillary blood flow, compression injuries are unlikely. Using this as the most conservative estimate, approximately 10% of the total body surface area in the supine position is likely to be at risk of pressure-induced injury.

In the supine position the calcaneus and occiput, and in the lateral position the greater trochanter, are subjected to the highest pressures.[17] These areas can experience pressure exceeding 100 mm Hg even when padding

materials are used. In the head, pressure under the occiput has been measured at 90 mm Hg, which, if sustained, has been shown to be associated with the formation of postoperative alopecia and frank decubitus ulcerations.[17] Because of this high degree of compression, consideration should be given to provide extra padding to at least the calcaneus, occiput, and greater trochanter.

The pressure applied to body surfaces, especially over bony prominences, can result in wide three-dimensional destruction of tissue (Fig. 11–1). Tissue necrosis is a time-dependent process. Consequently, a much larger area of eventual damage can result than might be appreciated on initial evaluation.[12] In addition, muscle has been shown to be more sensitive to ischemia than is skin.[18–20] Because of this, the initial superficial skin manifestations of pressure-induced soft tissue injury may not indicate the eventual extent of the destruction.[9] Significant undermining of soft tissue may have occurred despite what had appeared to be relatively minor skin trauma.

Shear Forces

Tissue shearing can also be a factor in the production of tissue damage. Shear stress is generated when parallel, but oppositely directed, friction forces are exerted on tissue. Certain positions are associated with greater amounts of shear than are others. These forces

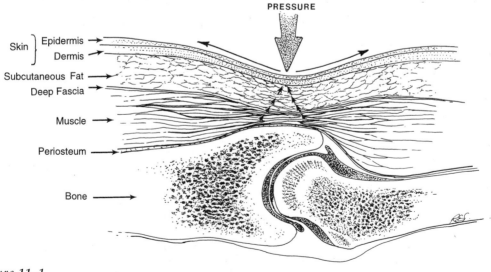

Figure 11–1

The various tissues affected by the application of externally applied pressure. Note the three-dimensional effect. (From Shea JD: Pressure sores. Clin Orthop Rel Res 112:89, 1975.)

can produce extensive tissue damage with disruption of tissue planes and thrombosis of vessels causing tissue necrosis.[10, 21] However, in instances such as the head-down tilt position, shearing forces provide the friction necessary to prevent patients from sliding off the operating table.[22] Intraoperative repositioning, particularly sliding patients to the desired location, may be associated with the development of shearing forces. Therefore, when moving patients, lifting the body may offer less potential injury than will sliding.

Classification of Pressure Damage

A ranking system for evaluating the extent of damage caused by the application of pressure has been devised by the National Pressure Ulcer Advisory Panel.[23, 24]

Stage I: Nonblanchable erythema of intact skin; the heralding lesion of skin ulceration. *Note:* Reactive hyperemia can normally be expected to present for one-half to three-fourths as long as the time that pressure had occluded blood flow to the area

Stage II: Partial-thickness skin loss involving epidermis and/or dermis. A superficial ulcer evolves and develops clinically as an abrasion, a blister, or a shallow crater.

Stage III: Full-thickness skin loss involving damage or necrosis of subcutaneous tissue that may extend down to, but not through, underlying fascia. The ulcer presents clinically as a deep crater with or without undermining of adjacent tissue.

Stage IV: Full-thickness skin loss with extensive destruction, tissue necrosis, or damage to muscle, bone, or supporting structures (e.g., the tendon of a joint capsule). *Note:* Undermining and sinus tracts may also be associated with stage IV pressure ulcers.

Owing to the insidious and progressive nature of the development of pressure ulcers, this classification may be less valuable early in their formation.

Prevention

Duration of pressure is probably the most contributive factor in the development of pressure lesions, and reducing the time of compression should decrease the incidence of pressure sores. Therefore, an argument can be made for repositioning extremities during prolonged operations whenever possible. Because the occiput and calcaneus in the supine

position and the greater trochanter of the femur in the lateral position are the areas that typically are subjected to the greatest degrees of compression, extra precautions should be taken for their protection. However, because a number of uncontrollable factors such as age, weight, coexisting disease, and duration of surgery may have overriding influences on protective measures, some patients almost certainly suffer pressure-induced injuries despite aggressive preventive measures.

JOINTS

Little emphasis has been directed toward describing what constitutes optimal joint positioning. Few complications involving joint positioning have been described, but whether this is due to our inability to recognize these complications or whether the incidence of injury is truly low is uncertain.

Optimal joint positioning requires an understanding of a number of different factors, including anatomic consideration of the joints and the impact of joint positioning on overlying structures such as muscles, tendons, and fascia. Kaltenborn[25] provides the most detailed insight into this complex subject and defines *resting joint position* as the position in which the joint capsule is most relaxed and joint laxity is greatest. It is the joint position used for prolonged immobilization in casts or splints and is the position most often adopted by pathologic joints because it allows for the greatest accumulation of fluid. Table 11–3 lists the resting position for the major joints and is provided as a starting point from which joint position can be considered.

Joint positioning is further complicated by the fact that many joints work in concert to facilitate particular extremity positions. Because of this the placement of one joint into a resting position may dictate that an adjacent joint be placed in a position not consistent with rest. An example is the elbow, which consists of the humeroulnar and humeroradial joints. These joints cannot be simultaneously placed at rest because it would require both elbow flexion and extension (see Table 11–3).

Surgical exposure may also mandate that joints be placed in positions other than rest. Multiple clinical examples exist, one being the placement of the upper extremity during abdominal surgery. Arranging the shoulder complex and humeroradial joint in resting

Table 11–3

Joint-Neutral Positions

Hand	
Carpometacarpal	Midway between abduction and adduction
	Flexion and extension 0°
Wrist	Longitudinal axis through radius and third metacarpal in straight line
Forearm	
Distal radioulnar	Supination 10°
Proximal radioulnar	Supination 35°, elbow flexed 70°
Elbow	Elbow flexed 70°, forearm supinated 10°
Humeroulnar	
Humeroradial	Elbow extended and forearm supinated
Shoulder	Abducted 55°, horizontally adducted 30°
Ankle	Plantarflexion 10°
	Midway between maximum inversion and eversion
Knee	Flexion 25°
Hip	Flexed 30°
	Abducted 30°, slight external rotation

Adapted from Kaltenborn FM: Mobilization of the Extremity Joints: Examination and Basic Treatment Techniques. Oslo, Olaf Norlis Bookhandel, 1980.

position would dictate placing the forearm and hand within the surgical field. Even though placement of joints into the resting position may not always be possible, consideration of what constitutes resting position of the joint may be helpful when positioning patients within the perioperative period.

NERVE INJURIES

Patients undergoing anesthesia may experience peripheral nerve injuries from stretch or compressive forces that cause neural ischemia. Anesthesia permits the assumption of postures that would not be tolerated in its absence. Coexisting diseases such as diabetes mellitus can further increase the likelihood of injury.[26]

Susceptible patients appear to develop nerve injuries "despite conventionally accepted methods of positioning and padding."[4] At present there is no evidence that padding around the elbow, in addition to that provided by a padded armboard, increases protection of the ulnar nerve,[1] nor do we have a model that tells us how to apply padding in an effective manner. Therefore, to understand how best to

protect against the appearance of perioperative neuropathies, we must first examine normal neural anatomy and physiology as well as the underlying mechanisms of nerve injuries.

Anatomy of Peripheral Nerves

Peripheral nerves are composed of bundles of neurons encased in a fibrous tissue meshwork composed of endoneurium, perineurium, and epineurium (Fig. 11–2). The endoneurium directly encases axons that are surrounded in turn by a layer of perineurium to form nerve fascicles. Nerve fibers that are bound by a collagen-rich epineurium often interconnect fascicles. The epineurium also contains arterial and venous plexuses, the "vasa nervorum," that run parallel to the long axes of nerves and receive occasional feeding vessels from surrounding connective tissue.[27]

The vasa nervorum, in conjunction with the other larger vascular structures, are vital to the proper functioning of peripheral nerves. Between individuals, as well as between extremities in the same individual, this complex, multiply anastomotic vascular network is highly variable (Fig. 11–3).[28] Endoneurial blood flow appears to be directly proportional to the number of endoneurial capillaries, and a decrease in the density of these capillaries increases the susceptibility of the nerve to ischemic neuropathies.[29] In addition, within the microcirculation discrete watershed areas exist that may predispose those portions of the peripheral nerve to ischemic injury.[30] Conceivably, therefore, positioning an extremity in one patient would yield an acceptable outcome, whereas this same posture applied to another patient, or to the opposite extremity of the same person, would lead to a nerve injury. With this variability in mind, it is hard to envision that all nerve injuries attributed to extremity positioning could be prevented by even the most careful protective measures.

Classification of Peripheral Nerve Injuries

Peripheral nerve injuries are classified into three distinct groups: *neurapraxia, axonotmesis,* and *neurotmesis* in ascending order of severity.[31, 32] These terms are important because they help to define both the extent of injury and the prognosis for recovery. Clinically, any

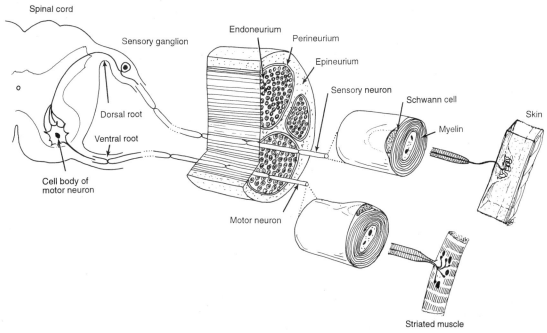

Figure 11–2

Diagram of the nerve and the various components that comprise its structures. (From Ham AW [ed.]: Histology, 8th ed. Philadelphia, JB Lippincott, 1979.)

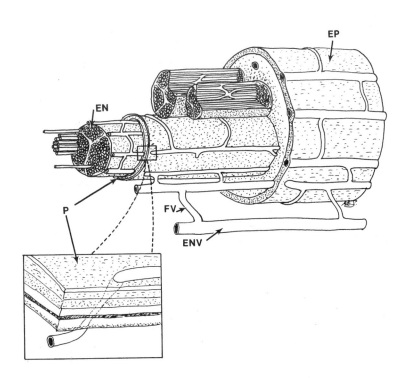

Figure 11–3

Schematic representation of the blood supply to a peripheral nerve. (EN = endoneurium, ENV = extraneural vessel, EP = epineurium, FV = feeder vessel, P = perineurium.) (From Butler DS. Mobilization of the Nervous System. New York, Churchill Livingstone, 1991; adapted from Lundborg G: Nerve Injury and Repair. Edinburgh, Churchill Livingstone, 1988.)

of these forms of injury may exist in a given nerve or all may be present simultaneously.

Neurapraxia: a nerve injury in which paralysis occurs in the absence of peripheral degeneration. Recovery is rapid and complete.

Axonotmesis: a nerve injury significant enough to cause peripheral axonal degeneration without complete destruction of the epineurium or the internal neural architecture. Recovery is ordinarily complete.

Neurotmesis: a nerve injury significant enough to cause a separation of the related parts of the nerves. An anatomic gap in the nerve is not mandatory, and the epineural sheath may appear to be intact. However, on healing, the nerve is replaced with fibrous tissue. Recovery is poor.

Anatomy Susceptible to Injury

Anatomic factors may play an important role in the formation of peripheral nerve injuries. Butler[33] has previously described five factors that are associated with "vulnerable anatomic sites." They include the following:

1. Osseous, fibro-osseous, or soft tissue tunnels. Two examples are the carpal and cubital tunnels, in which impingement upon neural structures can produce compression and friction with movement.

2. Areas of nervous system branching. With branching, the nerve becomes less mobile and probably more susceptible to injury.

3. Areas in which nerves are relatively fixed and immobile. Examples include the radial nerve at the head of the radius and the peroneal nerve at the head of the fibula.

4. Areas in which nerves are adherent to, or pass adjacent to, bone or other unyielding structures such as fascia. Examples include the radial nerve in the radial groove of the humerus and the brachial plexus as it passes over the first rib. The lateral femoral cutaneous and peroneal nerves pass close to fascial planes.

5. "Tension points," which are areas along the nervous system that apparently move little or not at all in relation to surrounding structures. These areas contain a high concentration of feeding vessels; therefore, injuries at these sites can produce neural ischemia. Examples of "tension points" are the tibial nerve in the posterior aspect of the knee and the nerves around the elbow.

Causes of Nerve Injury

Stretch

Stretch of a peripheral nerve causes injury by producing tension that can lead to nerve disruption or ischemia. Tension is produced at various rates within the different intraneural structures. Generally, peripheral nerves possess a high degree of laxity and elasticity. Initial stretching of a nerve produces straightening of the funiculus with elongation of the epineurium, the structure primarily responsible for the elastic characteristics of the nerve. If traction continues or increases and the elastic limit of the nerve is reached, rupture of the epineurium occurs. Stretching of the nerve up to the point of nerve rupture results in neurapraxia and axonotmesis. However, if this elastic limit is exceeded, neurotmesis is most likely to predominate.[34] Nerve stretch, in addition to causing elongation of the nerve, produces a decrease in cross-sectional area that can increase internal pressures (Fig. 11–4). If intraneural pressures becomes great enough, intraneural blood flow suffers and nerve ischemia results. Therefore, stretch can produce injury not only from mechanical trauma but also from internal compression due to increased intraneural pressure.

The degree of stretch that a peripheral nerve can withstand is unknown. Animal models have demonstrated that the elongation of peripheral nerves by 5% to 10% can result in a 50% decrease in intraneural blood flow and the appearance of microthrombi and granulocytosis.[35] If stretch is increased to 15%, intraneural blood flow ceases.[35, 36] If that amount of stretch is maintained for 30 minutes and then released, tissue hyperemia is noted but the integrity of the vascular and perineural structures appears to be maintained.[35]

Extreme stretching of peripheral nerves to 100% of their resting length is followed by complete paralysis even if rupture of the nerve does not occur. Microscopic examination exhibits either epineural hemorrhages or petechiae.[37]

If only petechiae are present, function usually returns within 1 month after injury, although histologic changes can be apparent for up to 5 months.[37] Although these extreme degrees of stretch are not encountered during extremity positioning, they highlight the remarkable regenerative capacity of peripheral nerves. Therefore, in most instances of nerve

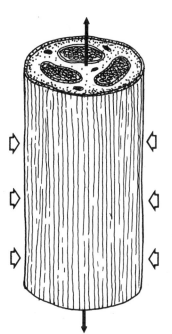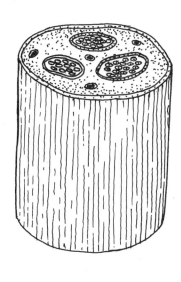

Figure 11–4

Nerve stretch associated with a decrease in cross-sectional area and increase in intraneural pressure. (From Butler DS: Mobilization of the Nervous System. New York, Churchill Livingstone, 1991.)

stretch, recovery of nerve function would be expected.

Compression

Pressure-induced injuries to peripheral nerves are dependent on both the quantity and the duration of pressure. Of these two variables, nerve injury is related more to duration than to quantity of pressure, although extremely high pressures may cause direct injury.[38] Both human and animal studies have been performed to assess the effect of pressure on nerves and have shown ischemia to be the common pathway to impaired nerve function.[39–42]

Pressure on peripheral nerves can produce four gradations of effect:[39]

1. None
2. Conduction loss with rapid, complete recovery
3. Conduction loss with delayed recovery without nerve degeneration (which is associated with preservation of gross sensation)
4. A complete anatomic lesion with nerve degeneration

Numerous animal studies have used pneumatic tourniquets to produce nerve injuries.[38–40] Strong evidence from both histologic and nerve conduction studies indicates that tourniquet injuries are similar to positioning-related nerve injuries.[43] Initially, compression shows nerve conduction with motor function being affected more often than sensation.[28, 43, 44] However, when sensory nerves are affected, full recovery of motor function is invariably prolonged. Despite the less resilient nature of the motor nerve, the rate of recovery of both motor and sensory nerves is comparable.[43] In addition, even after motor and sensory function appear to be clinically normal, nerve conduction tests can remain abnormal for a number of weeks.[45]

Compressive tourniquets have also been used to study the effect of direct compression versus ischemia on peripheral nerves. If nerve conduction velocities are measured at two sites, one directly under a tourniquet inflated to carotid artery pressure and the other distal to the tourniquet, nerve conduction is affected only in the area directly under the tourniquet.[40] However, if compression is increased sufficiently to cause obstruction of arterial blood flow, nerve conduction decreases at both locations. Therefore, nerve conduction appears to be dependent on maintained blood flow and the absence of ischemia.

Nerve conduction studies have also been used to determine the rate of recovery of nerve function after a compressive insult.[43, 46] The duration of ischemia has been shown to the most important factor in determining the rate of recovery of nerve function.[40] If compression sufficient to arrest blood flow for 1.5 hours is maintained and released, nerve conduction begins to return within 30 seconds and is fully recovered within 5 to 6 minutes. However, as tourniquet times approached 4 hours, 1 to 2 hours are necessary for return of normal nerve conduction. The ability of the peripheral nerves to tolerate these prolonged periods of ischemia may be due in part to the presence of the vasa nervorum, which may impart some protection due to extensive vascular networking.[28] Other factors, including hypothermia, also appear to protect against ischemic injury to peripheral nerves.[41, 42]

Additional Factors Associated with Peripheral Nerve Injuries

Factors other than compression and stretch during positioning are associated with the development of peripheral neuropathies. Examples include the "double crush syndrome," radial nerve palsies (Saturday Night palsies), and coexisting disease states such as diabetes mellitus. In addition, inherited primary peripheral neuropathies have been described, such as Charcot-Marie-Tooth disease and he-

reditary neuropathy with liability to pressure palsies.[47] These conditions may also affect the preoperative assessment and intraoperative management of patients.

DOUBLE CRUSH SYNDROME

Pre-existing subclinical peripheral nervous system conditions may play important roles in the development of perioperative nerve injuries. An example is the *double crush syndrome*. The term describes a peripheral nerve entrapment syndrome in which two lesions in the same nerve distribution act to potentiate the severity of either injury even though one is distal to the other.[48, 49] A carpal tunnel syndrome in conjunction with abnormalities of the cervical or brachial plexuses constitutes the most commonly described combination of events that leads to the formation of a double crush syndrome. The symptoms associated with this injury pattern are thought to be secondary to a decrease in axoplasmic flow (Fig. 11–5). Thus, patients with pre-existing subclinical peripheral nerve injuries may be at increased risk of manifesting symptoms of

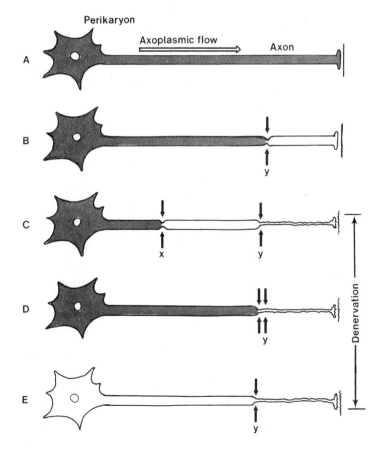

Figure 11–5

Nerve injuries associated with decreases in axoplasmic flow. The amount of axoplasmic flow is indicated by the degree of shading. *A*. Normal—no compression. *B*. Mild compression at "Y" is insufficient to cause denervation. *C*. Mild compression at two sites with the compression at "Y" being of insufficient intensity to cause denervation by itself. *D*. A single severe compression sufficient to cause denervation. *E*. Diseased nerve (e.g., diabetes) undergoes minimal compression that otherwise would not cause denervation but does so owing to the pre-existing pathologic process. (From Upton ARM, McComas AJ: The double crush in nerve entrapment syndromes. Lancet 2:359, 1973. © by The Lancet Ltd., 1973.)

injury after what would otherwise be insignificant injuries to the peripheral nervous system.

Numerous clinical observations have substantiated the existence of the double crush syndrome. Bilateral carpal tunnel syndromes have been found to be more prevalent in patients with cervical arthritis.[50] Also, the onset of a carpal tunnel syndrome has been associated with traumatic injuries to the cervical and brachial plexuses.[51, 52] Symptoms of cervical or brachial plexus nerve impingement are more often associated with carpal tunnel syndrome than might otherwise be expected.[53] In patients with this constellation of findings, proximal symptoms disappeared in 46 of 49 cases after surgical correction of the carpal tunnel syndrome.[54] A similar finding also has been made in connection with the thoracic outlet syndrome and with distal neuropathies.[55]

Electrical and histologic evidence of "double crush" also exists. Nemoto and associates[56] implanted low compressive force clamps on the sciatic nerves of dogs to produce an incomplete conduction block associated with mild axonal degeneration. If a second implantable clamp was then placed distal to the first, a complete conduction block and marked axonal degeneration could be induced in some animals. Furthermore, the loss of nerve function after the "double crush" was greater than the sum of the deficits separately. If the clamps were then removed, return of function could be demonstrated. These authors concluded that proximal nerve compression diminished the ability of the nerve to withstand further, more distal compression.[56] In addition, a synergistic effect was shown, suggesting that a second insult may only need to be minor to produce a clinically noticeable effect. Hence, previous subclinical nerve injury may predispose patients to double crush injuries.

RADIAL NERVE PALSY

Also known as "Saturday Night palsy," radial nerve palsy is a compression injury of the radial nerve that typically occurs during sleep. Electrophysiologically, it is a pressure-induced palsy.[57] In the majority of cases, sedative hypnotics, whether in the form of alcohol, illicit drugs, or anesthetic agents, have played a role in its development. However, radial nerve palsies have been reported to occur spontaneously despite the absence of any sedative hypnotic agents.[57] Therefore, if nerve injuries have been reported to occur in an unsedated, unanesthetized population, the familiar medicolegal contention that these injuries "cannot occur in the absence of anesthesia" becomes untenable. That fact also indicates a failure potential for our best-intended preventive measures.

NEUROPATHIES ASSOCIATED WITH OTHER DISEASES

Various metabolic conditions can also place nerves at increased risk. Some of these include diabetes mellitus, alcohol abuse, vitamin deficiencies, malnutrition, renal disease, and hypothyroidism.[58-63] Although the precise mechanism of nerve injuries secondary to metabolic conditions is usually unknown, a possible explanation is that these pre-existing conditions produce subclinical nerve injuries not dissimilar to those found in the "double crush" scenario. That possibility would cause the nerve to be placed at increased risk of damage from even routine nerve stretch and compression.

Diabetic neuropathy is the most well described of the peripheral neuropathies associated with underlying disease. For unknown reasons, peripheral nerves in patients with diabetes mellitus seem more susceptible to compression injuries. This neuropathic condition can affect virtually every part of the peripheral nervous system. Polyneuropathies involving the distal extremities are most often seen; however, mononeuropathies can also be present. Segmental demyelination and occlusion of nutrient arteries are common. This generalized decrease in blood flow to the nerves may predispose them to ischemia from passive compression associated with positioning of extremities.[26, 64]

INHERITED PERIPHERAL NEUROPATHIES

Inherited peripheral neuropathies have been well described and remain undiagnosed in a significant percentage of patients.[65-68] At least ten different disorders of this nature have been reported.[69]

Charcot-Marie Tooth polyneuropathy is an inherited autosomal dominant syndrome of the peripheral nerves characterized by a slowly progressive onset of weakness and mild sensory impairment. A less well-known autosomal dominant neuropathy, *tomaculous neuropathy* (also bearing the curious designation of *hereditary neuropathy with liability to pressure palsies*), is associated with demyelination and episodes of numbness and weakness that can progress to atrophy and nerve palsies after relatively minor trauma to peripheral nerves.

These patients, particularly if undiagnosed, are at markedly increased risk of complications secondary to the compressive forces associated with positioning. The introduction of DNA analysis has provided the diagnosis of some of these syndromes.

FACTORS AFFECTING SPECIFIC EXTREMITY NERVES

Traditionally, perioperative nerve injuries were commonly believed to be due to malpositioning.[70–73] Recent studies, however, refute much of the previously held dogma that all ulnar nerve injuries are secondary to errant actions of the surgical team.[2–5] Although neural ischemia appears to be the common mechanism in nerve injuries, other considerations include the anatomic relationship between a plexus or an individual nerve and adjacent structures such as tunnels, bones, and fascia. Besides our concepts of proper positioning of extremities, we need to examine associated factors such as anatomy, gender, extremes of body habitus, and the impact of prolonged hospitalization.

The Ulnar Nerve

Ulnar nerve injuries have been reported to occur in males as much as five times more frequently than in females undergoing similar operative procedures with comparable arm positions, clearly implying an anatomic predisposition to injury associated with the male body habitus.[3–5, 74] Kroll and associates speculate that the condylar groove is more shallow in males, rendering the ulnar nerve more vulnerable to damage from external compression despite the use of padded armboards with or without additional padding around the elbow.[4] Many patients who develop postoperative ulnar nerve injuries have been shown to have abnormalities of nerve conduction velocity at the elbow in both the affected arm and the opposite extremity.[75–77] The possibility exists that unavoidable events associated with anesthesia and surgery (including unavoidable external compression from positioning) may produce additive effects, exacerbating pre-existing subclinical neuropathies that may

be more vulnerable to focal ischemia or double crush than would be a normal nerve.[3, 5, 74]

For supine patients with arms abducted on padded support surfaces, palmar supination has been recommended by some authors as a means of placing the weight of the elbow on the olecranon process of the ulna rather than on the cubital tunnel and its contained ulnar nerve.[62] However, there is no evidence confirming that this practice decreases the likelihood of a postoperative ulnar nerve injury.[3, 5] In fact, there is evidence that ulnar nerve injury may occur despite the routine application of accepted positioning practices, including the use of additional padding around the elbows and placement of the supine patient's abducted forearms and palm in supination.[2, 4]

Incidence of Ulnar Neuropathies

A recent retrospective report, assessing 1,129,692 consecutive patients who underwent noncardiac surgery from 1957 through 1991 in a single institution, determined the rate of persistent ulnar nerve injuries to be 1:2729 (1 per 2729 patients.)[2] In addition to determining the incidence of injury, these data suggest that perioperative ulnar neuropathies are associated with factors other than general anesthesia and intraoperative positioning. In a smaller prospective study in 1987, Alvine reported the incidence of postoperative ulnar nerve injuries as 0.26%.[3] More recent closed claim studies have shown that ulnar nerve injuries account for 34% of all nerve injuries.[4] Despite these studies being performed under different conditions, they point collectively to other factors that are associated with ulnar nerve injuries, indicating the need and possible direction for further study.

Anatomy

The ulnar nerve originates from the C8 to T1 roots of the brachial plexus and travels medial to the axillary artery within the axillary sheath. It then passes along with the brachial artery between the coracobrachialis and triceps muscles. Separating from the neurovascular bundle, it passes under various fascial planes to arrive at the condylar groove (Fig. 11–6). The condylar groove is formed by the medial epicondyle and ulnar groove anteriorly and the ulnohumeral ligament laterally; it is roofed by the fibrous arcuate ligament, which connects the olecranon process of the

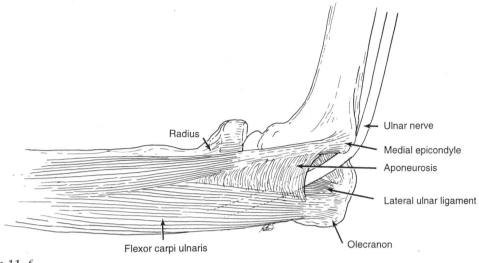

Radius

Ulnar nerve

Medial epicondyle

Aponeurosis

Lateral ulnar ligament

Flexor carpi ulnaris

Olecranon

Figure 11–6

Various bony and tendinous structures about the ulnar nerve as it passes through first the condylar groove and then the cubital tunnel. (From Kincaid JC: The electrodiagnosis of ulnar neuropathy at the elbow. Muscle and Nerve 11:1005, 1988. Copyright © 1988. Reprinted by permission of John Wiley & Sons, Inc.)

ulna to the medial epicondyle. From the condylar groove, the ulnar nerve enters the cubital tunnel. The roof of this tunnel is formed by the aponeurosis of the flexor carpi ulnaris muscle. After the ulnar nerve passes through the cubital tunnel it travels distally, giving off branches to the flexor carpi ulnaris and flexor digitorum profundus.

The vascular supply to the nerve is extremely variable along its length, with its distribution being inconsistent not only from patient to patient but between arms in the same individual.[78] This variability may be a factor when considering why, despite being provided with the same level of intraoperative care, some patients develop neuropathies whereas others do not.

Mechanism of Injury

The most likely site of isolated injury to the ulnar nerve is at the elbow, where its fibers pass through the condylar groove and then the adjacent cubital tunnel.[61, 75, 79–81] Shallowness of the condylar groove, in the absence of any other abnormality, may predispose the nerve to external trauma and compression. Because of the superficial, unprotected course of the nerve through the condylar groove (covered only by subcutaneous fat and skin), it is easily susceptible to external compression. Within the cubital tunnel, particularly under the edge of the flexor carpi ulnaris aponeurosis, compression and/

or entrapment of the nerve is a common cause of an ulnar neuropathy at the elbow. Clinically it is not possible to distinguish between ulnar nerve damage that occurs in the condylar groove versus entrapment in the cubital tunnel. Furthermore, it is not possible to differentiate these closely adjacent sites by electrophysiologic testing. Indeed, differing damage to fascicles within the ulnar nerve can make it difficult to accurately localize the site of ulnar nerve damage.

Anatomic and Congenital Causes of Ulnar Neuropathies

Anatomic and congenital reasons for ulnar nerve entrapment include cubital tunnel syndrome and recurrent dislocation of the nerve (Fig. 11–7).[82] Cubital tunnel syndrome is the most frequent ulnar nerve entrapment syndrome and is second only to carpal tunnel syndrome of the median nerve in frequency of entrapment syndromes. The exact incidence of the cubital tunnel entrapment syndrome is unknown; it can arise without any obvious compression injury. The patient with ulnar nerve compression typically complains of numbness of the little finger and the medial side of the hand. Pain and tenderness may also be noted about the medial epicondyle. Symptoms are often bilateral.[79] Numerous reports suggest that ulnar nerve entrapment plays an important role in the development of postoperative ulnar neuropa-

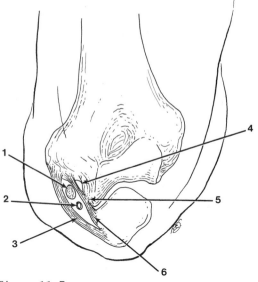

Figure 11–7

Cross-sectional view of the cubital tunnel. (1 = ulnar nerve; 2 = ulnar collateral artery; 3 = triangular arcuate ligament; 4 = medial epicondylar groove; 5 = medial aspect of the trochlea; 6 = medial ligament of the elbow) (From Perreault L, Drolet P, Farny J: Ulnar nerve palsy at the elbow after general anesthesia. Can J Anaesth 39:499, 1992.)

thies that are erroneously attributed to malpositioning and/or inadequate padding of the elbow region during surgery and anesthesia.[3, 61, 74]

Injured or diseased nerves are less able to withstand stretch and compression.[73] Double crush injury syndrome is a clinical example of such a process (see previous section). In this condition the ulnar nerve may be subclinically damaged by previous trauma or anatomic abnormalities. Because of this compressed state, the nerve no longer has the reserve to withstand even minor trauma and is at a significantly increased risk of suffering damage from otherwise normal compressive or stretching forces.[49, 56]

Recurrent dislocation of the ulnar nerve at the condylar groove, a common finding in the normal population, can also increase the risk of ulnar nerve trauma.[83] Dislocation of the ulnar nerve occurs when it leaves the postcondylar groove onto or across the tip of the medial epicondyle during elbow flexion.[58] The degree of ulnar nerve dislocation has been further subdivided into incomplete and complete dislocation. Incomplete dislocation of the ulnar nerve is defined to occur when the nerve moves out of the postcondylar

groove onto the tip of the humeral epicondyle during elbow flexion; complete dislocation involves ulnar nerve excursion beyond the incomplete version.[84] The majority of studies reviewing ulnar nerve dislocation have found it to be more common in men than women.[58] This suggests that anatomic differences about the condylar groove exist between the sexes and helps to explain why postoperative ulnar nerve injuries are more common in men. Complete dislocation of the ulnar nerve during elbow flexion has been reported to occur in approximately 4% of the population; whereas a mostly asymptomatic incomplete ulnar nerve dislocation can affect up to 25% of the population.[58] Whether either type of nerve dislocation is more susceptible to nerve injury than is the other or whether additional padding about the elbow is an effective preventive measure for either remains unclear.

Elbow Flexion

Studies at autopsy have determined the effect of elbow flexion on the intraneural pressures within the ulnar nerve at the cubital tunnel.[85] With the arm extended, the pressure within the cubital tunnel averages 7 mm Hg, a value well below normal capillary pressures. However, on extreme elbow flexion, pressures in the tunnel increase to an average of 46 mm Hg, exceeding capillary pressures with the capability of producing disturbances of intraneural blood flow that would cause ischemia if prolonged.[85]

Direct Compression

Prolonged application of pressure directly on the ulnar nerve has been shown to cause trauma and neuropathy.[39, 40–42] Injury to the ulnar nerve in the area of the condylar groove and cubital tunnel has been reported from compression of the nerve on the edge of the operating table.[6] Other less often considered potential causes of pressure-induced ulnar neuropathies include blood pressure cuffs, cables and tubing from monitoring and intravenous lines, irregularities of bed sheeting, and improperly placed padding materials.[86]

Postoperative Injury

Ulnar nerve dysfunction may also appear secondary to injuries that occur in the postoperative convalescent period. A significant number of ulnar neuropathies are not detected initially until more than 48 hours after surgery, with some being evident only after the first postoperative week.[2] This prolonged interval between surgery and the first nerve complaints suggests that in some patients nerve injuries are probably due to events that occur in the postoperative rather than the intraoperative period. Resting the condylar groove upon chair arms or bed mattresses, particularly in the sedated postoperative patient, may injure the ulnar nerve.[58, 87, 88] This may explain why prolonged hospitalizations of more than 14 days are associated with ulnar neuropathies.[2] Therefore, routine clinical evaluation and recording of peripheral nerve function before the patient leaves the postanesthesia care unit, or when first responsive in an intensive care unit, may help to better determine the time course of nerve injuries.

Evaluation of Ulnar Injuries

History taking and the physical examination are the first steps in evaluating ulnar nerve injuries. In general, the most reliable method of detecting an ulnar neuropathy is direct questioning of the patient to ascertain whether numbness of the fourth and fifth fingers has been experienced. On physical examination, two-point discrimination in these digits and weakness of the interosseous muscles of the hand may be detected. More indepth studies can then be performed using electrophysiologic techniques. However, these tests of nerve conduction can possess a relatively high degree of variability depending on factors such as arm position and temperature.[86] In addition, they are not always reliable in locating the precise site of damage along the nerve despite an obvious neuropathy on the physical examination.[76, 90]

Treatment of Ulnar Neuropathies

Prevention of an ulnar nerve injury is the most effective form of treatment.[74, 80] Prevention should be guided by the application of the information presented previously while taking into account both the surgical requirements for exposure and specific patient needs such as those due to contractures. If the practitioner is confronted by a patient with dysfunction of the ulnar nerve, neurologic consultation should, in most cases, be sought to determine the site and extent of the lesion. Nerve conduction studies may be helpful in both localizing the site of the lesion and de-

termining whether signs of denervation are present to imply that the pathologic process was present before surgery.[61, 74] In addition, if bilateral nerve conduction studies are performed, the detection of a subclinical neuropathy in the unaffected extremity possibly may suggest that these patients have a predisposition to ulnar neuropathies.[77] If the dysfunction is due to entrapment of the ulnar nerve within the cubital tunnel, ulnar nerve transposition has been suggested as therapy; however, the procedure has critics as well as supporters.[74, 91]

The Brachial Plexus

Brachial plexus injuries associated with the perioperative period were first reported over 100 years ago.[92] Initially, anesthetic agents were implicated as the cause because they were then thought to be neurotoxic. More recently, however, the most likely mechanism of injury in patients undergoing noncardiac surgical procedures has been attributed to positioning of the extremities. This realization has facilitated a change in the way that patient's arms are positioned and has helped to emphasize the importance of proper positioning despite the inconvenience that it may create for surgical exposure.

Incidence of Brachial Plexus Injuries

Studies suggest that the incidence of perioperative brachial plexus injuries has steadily decreased over the past 50 years. In 1950, two separate reports showed the incidence of postoperative brachial plexus injuries to be 0.4% and 1.2%.[72, 88] In 1973, the incidence of brachial plexus injury was reported as 0.06% in a retrospective study of 50,000 general surgical operations.[70] In 1988, the incidence of perioperative brachial plexus injuries was reported as 0.02%. Although these reports may not have similar sensitivities, they suggest that there has been a fivefold decrease in the occurrence of brachial plexus complications in the perioperative period.[93]

Despite this reduced incidence, injury to the brachial plexus due to stretch or compression can occur during virtually any procedure, even when correct intraoperative positioning procedures appear to have been maintained. The duration of the surgical procedure is important in the development of brachial plexus injuries; however, the injuries have occurred after procedures lasting as little as 40 minutes.[40, 88] A higher probability of injury has been associated with hyperabduction of the arm, use of shoulder braces to facilitate tilting the patient head down, and performance of a median sternotomy.[6, 72, 93–97]

Anatomy

The susceptibility of the brachial plexus to injury is due, in part, to its anatomic relationships with other structures in the neck and axilla. The plexus originates from the anterior rami of the lower four cervical and the first thoracic spinal nerves. Nerve roots pass through the intervertebral foramina where they form a plexus, bisect the anterior and middle scalene muscles, and divide into upper, middle and lower trunks (Fig. 11–8). As the trunks of the plexus travel between the clavicle and first rib, they form anterior and posterior divisions, which proceed into the axilla to become the lateral, medial, and posterior cords, which are named in relation to their anatomic location to the axillary artery.

As it migrates from the neck through the axilla, the brachial plexus comes into close proximity to a number of bony and relatively immobile soft tissue structures. The plexus is relatively fixed in at least two locations, namely, at the cervicothoracic spine and in the axillary fascia. These two areas of fixation are important in the production of brachial plexus injury because they decrease the mobility of the plexus and increase the likelihood of injury from both stretch and direct nerve compression. Rigid and semirigid structures neighboring the course of the plexus include the first rib, clavicle, head of the humerus, anterior and medial scalenus muscles, subclavius muscle, and pectoralis minor.[6, 70, 72, 98, 99] A number of factors, including anatomic abnormalities, hypertrophic musculature, arm and table position, and the presence of external immobilization devices (i.e., shoulder braces and wrist supports), can cause these structures to impinge on and injure the brachial plexus.[6, 72, 88, 93, 98–104]

Mechanisms of Brachial Plexus Injury

ARM ABDUCTION

Hyperabduction of the arm can stretch and injure the brachial plexus. The position of the cervical spine and head are important factors that can either decrease or exacerbate the extent of the injury.[94, 105] Because of these multiple factors, guidelines for positioning of the

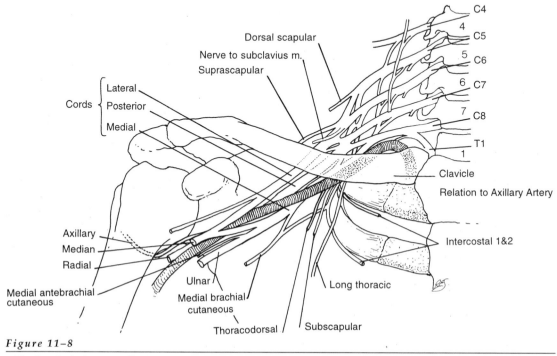

Figure 11–8

The brachial plexus in relation to the axillary artery. (From Pansky B: Review of Gross Anatomy. New York, Macmillan, 1979. Reproduced with permission of The McGraw-Hill Companies.)

upper extremities should be followed during abduction of the arm. They include the following:

1. If upper extremity abduction is necessary, it should be limited to a maximum of 90 degrees.[93]
2. Simultaneous abduction, supination, and extension of the upper extremity should be avoided.[6, 93]
3. The head and cervical spine should be maintained in neutral position.[98]
4. Dorsal extension and lateral flexion of the head to the side opposite the arm being positioned should be avoided.[6, 93]
5. Extension and abduction of the arms above the head should be avoided.[6, 93]

Placement of the patient into the prone position can also be accompanied by a stretch injury to the brachial plexus. The upper extremities of a pronated patient may be positioned either alongside the torso or extended above the head during anesthesia and surgery. In this regard, questions designed to detect the possible presence of a thoracic outlet syndrome (described by arm pain when arms are extended over the head or clasped behind the occiput) may be useful (see Chapter 10 and Figure 10–30). If these symptoms are present preoperatively, it may be prudent to place the arms alongside the torso rather than alongside the head when surgery in the prone position is planned.

SHOULDER BRACES

Historically, the use of shoulder braces has been an important factor in the development of brachial plexus injuries.[6, 93, 98, 102] When used for positioning a patient in head-down tilt, shoulder braces can cause injury by compressing the plexus against the numerous rigid and bony structures within the shoulder complex.[6] The fixed nature of the plexus at its insertion into the vertebral fascia and axillary sheath has been postulated as increasing the likelihood of plexus compression, presumably because of its decreased mobility.[98, 101]

When a brachial plexus injury occurs after the use of shoulder braces, it typically involves the upper segments of the plexus, in sharp contrast to injuries to the lower segments of the plexus that follow median sternotomies.[98] Other factors that may increase the risk of injury include the presence of congenital first ribs and coexisting diseases such as diabetes mellitus.[70, 93, 98] Despite the fact that

long-term disability can occur, the vast majority of these patients experience full recovery.[72, 93, 98, 100, 101, 104]

Shoulder braces are no longer used routinely, owing to the risk to the brachial plexus, the advent of nonslip mattresses for operating tables, and improvements in surgical techniques. However, they are still used on rare occasions to facilitate torso stability during extreme degrees of head-down tilt. Because of their infrequent usage, errors in proper positioning may be more likely to occur. Therefore, the following guidelines for their use are included:

1. Shoulder braces should be used only when absolutely necessary with the realization that brachial plexus injuries can occur despite the best of precautions.
2. If shoulder braces are used, they should be well padded and positioned so that they lie over the acromion and not the clavicle or the root of the neck.[95]
3. A nonslip mattress should be used when patients are tilted head down.[95] (In addition to mattress-to-table fixation by Velcro strips, numerous manufacturers are now producing supporting surfaces designed for restraining patients who are tilted head down.)
4. Use of wrist straps should be avoided.[6, 93, 95]
5. Arm abduction of greater than 90 degrees should be avoided.[95, 98]
6. The patient's arms should be tucked to the sides whenever possible.[93, 95, 98]
7. Shoulder braces should be adjusted before establishing head-down tilt.[98] After tilt is finalized, the positions of both the torso and the shoulder braces should be rechecked.

MEDIAN STERNOTOMY

In recent years, most brachial plexus injuries have been associated with median sternotomies. Even though they are not directly associated with positioning of the extremities, a review of these injuries is important because positioning can be implicated erroneously as their cause.

Prospective studies have reported the incidence of brachial plexus injuries after median sternotomy to be 5% to 19%.[97, 106] Numerous mechanisms of injury have been proposed, including (1) stretch, (2) compression, (3) trauma from insertion of central venous catheters, (4) anticoagulation, and (5) first rib fractures from mediastinal retraction.[107–109]

Stretch, Direct Nerve Trauma, and Nerve Compression. Nerve stretch and direct nerve trauma secondary to first rib fracture are believed to be the two most common causes of brachial plexus injury after median sternotomy.[105, 110] Autopsy studies have shown that sternal retraction leads to stretch of the brachial plexus by increasing the distance between the insertion of the plexus and the axillary fascia.[94, 96, 97, 103, 110] These studies also have shown that compression is not a major mechanism of plexus injury during median sternotomy.

First Rib Fracture. The same mechanical forces of sternal retraction that stretch the brachial plexus can also fracture the first rib and traumatize the plexus.[97] Autopsy studies have revealed direct penetration of the brachial plexus by broken sections of rib.[97, 111] Sternal retraction has been associated with first rib fracture in up to 33% of patients undergoing a median sternotomy.[97, 111] However, it may be difficult to diagnose fractures of the first rib after median sternotomy because 15% to 30% of these fractures are not appreciated on routine chest radiographs.[112] Therefore, recommendations have been made to obtain special oblique views of the cervical spine if a brachial plexus injury is noted after median sternotomy.[97, 111, 112]

Placement of the sternal retractor high up on the sternum appears to be the most important factor in the development of first rib fractures.[97, 113] However, the presence of a first rib fracture cannot be assumed to be the only mechanism of injury because neural deficits do not always accompany a fracture. Nonetheless, the high frequency of first rib fractures coupled with evidence from autopsy studies of direct brachial plexus trauma would support the fracture as being an important mechanism of plexus injury.[111]

Observations. Three clinically significant observations can be made about brachial plexus injuries after median sternotomies.

First, the more caudal components of the plexus are affected in greater than 80% of the cases and are described as the lower trunk, medial cord, and C8/T1 nerve distribution.[106, 113–116] When an injury occurs to the lower plexus nerve distribution it manifests itself in the ulnar nerve distribution. This localization is important to note because the American Society of Anesthesiologists closed claim study identified ulnar nerve injuries as the neuropathy most likely to be associated with litigation.[4] Therefore, injuries affecting the more caudal components of the brachial plexus could be mistaken for primary ulnar nerve injuries regardless of the cause.

Second, the contrast between lower plexus injuries due to median sternotomy and upper plexus injuries associated with shoulder braces emphasizes that more than one mechanism of brachial plexus injury exists. Appreciation of this duel mechanism of injury is important because prognosis and treatment may depend on an accurate anatomic diagnosis.

Third, the prognosis of brachial plexus injury after median sternotomy is typically good with a rapid return of nerve function within days to a few weeks in the vast majority of patients.[108, 117, 118] Serious complications occurred in less than 4% of the injuries.[106, 117] Closed claim data would also support spontaneous resolution in the majority of patients, especially considering the large number of cardiopulmonary bypass procedures performed and the high incidence (5%–19%) of brachial plexus injury after median sternotomy. In addition, the relative lack of litigation also implies a high degree of spontaneous resolution of brachial plexus injuries induced by median sternotomies.[4]

CENTRAL VENOUS CANNULATION

Use of the internal jugular vein to introduce a catheter into the central venous circulation has also been postulated as a potential mechanism of brachial plexus injury due to direct needle trauma.[106, 114] However, the relevance of this source of damage has been questioned by several investigators, and most would agree that internal jugular cannulation is not a proven cause of brachial plexus injury.[107, 117, 119–121] The lack of reports of injury in patients who have undergone this procedure supports the skepticism.[121, 122] However, the risk of central venous cannulation may be greater in patients undergoing a median sternotomy because anticoagulation is needed during cardiopulmonary bypass.

Anticoagulation. If trauma occurs during difficult central venous cannulation, anticoagulation might increase the likelihood of intraneural or extraneural hematoma formation.[95] Brachial plexus damage or first rib fracture from sternal retraction potentially could cause hematoma formation about the plexus. Plexus compression by hematomas has been reported after arterial puncture for axillary arteriography.[123] However, the lack of reports of compressive hematoma formation after venipuncture in anticoagulated patients tends to discount venous hematoma formation as a common mechanism of injury.

The Lateral Position and the Brachial Plexus

In the lateral position the brachial plexus of the down-side extremity may be compressed by the thorax and the head of the humerus.[93] A roll or pad of sufficient thickness should be placed under the lateral chest wall just caudad to the axilla to elevate the rib cage off of the table surface, free the down-side shoulder, and relieve stress on the brachial plexus. Proper positioning of the chest pad is critical if it is to function properly; its encroachment into the axilla will compress nerves and vessels, press against the humerus, and worsen stress on the brachial plexus. The commonly used term *axillary roll* improperly describes the pad, errantly suggests improper placement, and should be abandoned. Because patients are often repositioned after the initial placement of the chest pad, care should be taken to re-evaluate its location after the altered position is achieved.

The up-side brachial plexus is also at risk of injury because the position of the arm needs to be stabilized. Often the extremity is suspended from a movable "ether screen." Difficulty in assessing the position of that arm relative to the torso, particularly if it is moved after placement of surgical drapes, may lead to its inadvertent hyperabduction and injure the brachial plexus.

Evaluation of Brachial Plexus Injuries

Intraoperative somatosensory evoked potentials have been used to evaluate the effect of central venous cannulation and sternal retraction on nerve conduction of the brachial plexus during median sternotomy.[124] Transient changes in these evoked potentials have been noted during insertion of central venous catheters; however, in all cases, changes resolved within 5 minutes after completion of the insertion and no postoperative neurologic deficits were noted. Sternal retraction was associated with significant changes in somatosensory evoked potentials in 70% of the patients, with the majority returning toward baseline intraoperatively without the formation of postoperative neurologic deficits.[124] By contrast, all patients who did not have an intraoperative return of somatosensory evoked potentials demonstrated postoperative neuro-

logic deficits.[124] Therefore, intraoperative somatosensory evoked potential monitoring may be helpful in predicting those patients who are at highest risk for developing postoperative brachial plexus injuries.

Idiopathic Brachial Neuritis

Idiopathic brachial neuritis was first reported 40 years ago as a rare cause of brachial plexus dysfunction.[125, 126] Despite its rarity, it is important because it most commonly has been reported in the postsurgical population.[126] Findings include sudden onset, severe pain along the shoulder girdle, and atrophic paralysis of the muscles over the affected shoulder.[125] The pain usually subsides, but the paresis can persist for months or years; however, the prognosis is usually good in the majority of cases. Investigators in a recent study cited six examples and discounted the possibility of intraoperative brachial plexus injury due to the delayed onset of presenting symptoms and the multifocal pattern of nerve involvement demonstrated on electromyography. The etiology is unknown, but a number of causes have been postulated, including autoimmune disease, stress-induced activation of an unidentified dormant virus, and a possible genetic predisposition.

Lumbosacral Plexus

Evaluation of the American Society of Anesthesiologists closed claim database showed that more than 20% of their claims concerning nerve injuries involved the lumbosacral nerve root and sciatic nerves.[4] That study identified regional anesthesia and gender as two factors that may be important in the development of lower extremity nerve injuries. When neuropathy occurred, regional anesthesia was used in over 90%; 72% of those patients were females. However, after extensive review, the mechanism of nerve injury was deemed to be associated with regional anesthesia in only one third of the cases. That would suggest that other mechanisms may play important roles in the remainder. Possibilities include positioning, direct birthing trauma, and retractor-induced nerve injury.[127–131]

The five major lower extremity nerves, the common peroneal, tibial, sciatic, femoral and obturator, arise from the lumbosacral nerve roots (Fig. 11–9). The sciatic is the largest and divides into the tibial and common peroneal nerves. The femoral, obturator, and lateral

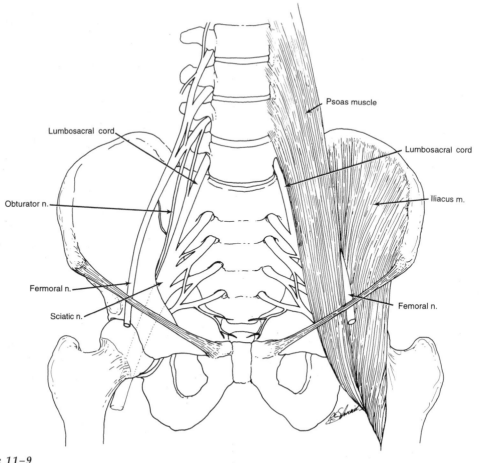

Figure 11-9

The lumbosacral plexus in relation to the structures within the posterior pelvis. (From Cole JT: Maternal obstetric paralysis. Am J Obstet Gynecol 52:372, 1946.)

femoral cutaneous nerves are derived primarily from the lumbar plexus. Neuropathies of each of these nerves have been noted within the postoperative period.[132-135] These conditions have been described elsewhere in this text (see Chapters 6 and 19).

Lithotomy Position

The development of lower extremity neuropathies after procedures involving patients in the lithotomy position has been well described by Warner and associates.[136] Their study reviewed 198,461 patients who had surgery while in the lithotomy position and reported the rate of postoperative neuropathies in lower extremities to be 1:3608. Risk factors included prolonged duration in the lithotomy position, very thin body habitus, and smoking in the perioperative period. They believe that a reduction in the time spent in the lithot-

omy position may be particularly beneficial in these patients with a preoperative smoking history and a body mass index of less than 20.

Regional Anesthesia

Epidural and spinal anesthesia, by themselves, cause a sensory and motor block not unlike that which accompanies traumatic peripheral sensory and motor nerve injuries. Therefore, to the uninformed person, trauma to the peripheral nerves after an epidural or spinal anesthetic may be interpreted as a direct consequence of regional anesthesia. This scenario emphasizes the importance of understanding the various mechanisms of injury so that correct explanations and intervention can be undertaken when these mishaps occur. As Dripps and Vandam[137] point out, "It is not scientific thinking always to attribute to the anesthetic a neurological complaint arising in a patient who has had spinal anesthesia." Major neurologic sequelae after epidural or spinal anesthetics are extremely rare.[138-141] A compilation of seven different studies reported the incidence of neurologic complications from epidural anesthesia as 0.09% (9/10,000) and that from spinal anesthesia as 0.05% (5/10,000), with the vast majority of cases enjoying full recovery.[142] However, case reports of neurologic deficits after regional anesthesia are not as encouraging, with some long-term injuries being reported.[143, 144] Some of the deficits included permanent paraplegia, adhesive arachnoiditis, and aseptic meningitis. However, definable events have been noted in many of these adverse outcomes, including infection, bleeding, and contamination of anesthetic agents. It is hoped that the resulting changes in the delivery of regional anesthesia will improve outcomes.

The presenting signs and symptoms associated with injuries to the lumbosacral trunk may help determine the mechanism of injury. Many of the complications associated with contamination of regional anesthetic agents and bleeding, either about the meninges or into the subarachnoid space, would be bilateral.[144] Bilateral symptoms distinguish these complications from positioning-induced injuries, which, except for compartment syndromes, would usually be unilateral. However, direct needle trauma to the lumbosacral trunk from placement of an epidural or spinal needle could be construed as being a complication of positioning of the extremity, owing to its likely unilateral presentation. Despite this possibility, direct needle trauma leading to neurologic deficit is an extremely rare event.[137, 145] In one study, only 17 instances of direct nerve trauma were noted in more than 10,000 patients undergoing spinal anesthesia. Complete recovery occurred, in most instances within 1 month.[146] In addition, review of the incidence of direct needle trauma to the spinal cord or peripheral nerves after diagnostic lumbar puncture finds no reports of such injury.

Obstetric and Gynecologic Procedures

Obstetric patients may develop paresthesias and motor dysfunction in the postpartum period for multiple reasons. They include (1) prolonged blockade by local anesthetics, (2) nerve entrapment, (3) prolapsing intervertebral disks, (4) trauma from delivery (both assisted and unassisted), (5) improper position-ing, and (6) uncommon etiologic events, such as adhesive arachnoiditis.[147] Ong and colleagues[147] found a rate of postpartum paresthesias and motor dysfunction of approximately 0.2% (2:1,000) in 23,827 consecutive deliveries in one women's hospital, whereas Abouleish[148] reported a rate of 0.4% (4:1,000) in 1,417 consecutive postpartum patients. In both studies, most of the deficits were transient numbness or tingling sensory disturbances. Motor dysfunction after obstetric procedures is unusual, often follows difficult forceps-assisted deliveries, and involves the femoral or sciatic nerves.[147]

The rate of sciatic and peroneal nerve injuries after vaginal surgical procedures ranges from 0.4% to 0.8% (4 to 8/1000).[127, 128, 149] Although the cause of injury may be improper positioning, direct trauma to intrapelvic nerves may occur. Abdominal wall retractors are often reported to be associated with postoperative femoral nerve injuries, although many other factors may be implicated. Blaming retractors assumes that the instrument has placed continuous pressure on the iliopsoas muscle and the femoral nerve passing through it. The pressure either stretches the nerve or renders it ischemic by occluding its penetrating nutrient vessels and/or the external iliac artery. Rosenblum and associates[150] have speculated that continuous pressure exerted by self-retaining retractors is more likely to produce a femoral neuropathy than is the more intermittent pressure of hand-held retractors.

Other factors may be associated with nerve injuries in patients undergoing gynecologic procedures. Vaginal retractors may compress the femoral nerve as it courses anteriorly out of the pelvic floor.[151] Patient factors, such as very thin body habitus and smoking in the perioperative period, may be associated with lower extremity nerve injuries.[136] Hemorrhage in the iliopsoas muscle or other structures of the pelvic floor may compress or decrease blood flow to nerves of the lower extremities.[152]

REFERENCES

1. Caplan RA, Posner KL, Cheney FW: Perioperative ulnar neuropathy. Anesthesiology 81:1321, 1994.
2. Warner MA, Warner ME, Martin JT: Ulnar neuropathy. Anesthesiology 81:1332, 1994.
3. Alvine FG, Schurrer ME: Postoperative ulnar-nerve palsy. J Bone Joint Surg Am 69:255, 1987.
4. Kroll DA, Caplan RA, Posner K, et al.: Nerve injury

associated with anesthesia. Anesthesiology 73:202, 1990.

5. Stoelting RK: Postoperative ulnar nerve palsy–Is it a preventable complication? Anesth Analg 76:7, 1993.

6. Britt BA, Gordon RA: Peripheral nerve injuries associated with anaesthesia. Can Anaesth Soc J 11:514, 1964.

7. Brook B, Duncan G: Effects of pressure on tissue. Arch Surg 406:696, 1940.

8. Elliot TM: Pressure ulcerations. Am Fam Phys 25:171, 1982.

9. Daniel RK, Priest DL, Wheatley DC: Etiologic factors in pressure sores: An experimental model. Arch Phys Med Rehabil 62:492, 1981.

10. Reichel SM: Shear forces as a factor in decubitus ulcers in paraplegics. JAMA 166:762, 1958.

11. Guyton AC: Textbook of Medical Physiology, 7th ed. Philadelphia, WB Saunders, 1986.

12. Agris J, Spira M: Pressure ulcers: Prevention and treatment. Clin Symp 31:1, 1979.

13. Shea JD: Pressure sores. Clin Orthop Rel Res 112:89, 1975.

14. Brook B, Duncan G: Effects of pressure on tissue. Arch Surg 406:696, 1940.

15. Husain T: An experimental study of some pressure effects on tissue with reference to the bed sore problem. J Pathol Bacteriol 66:347, 1953.

16. Lindan O, Greenway RM, Piazza JM: Pressure distribution of the surface of the human body: I. Evaluation in lying and sitting positions using a "bed of nails." Arch Phys Med Rehabil 46:378, 1965.

17. Souther SG, Car SD, Vistnes LM: Pressure tissue ischemia and operating table pads. Arch Surg 107:544, 1973.

18. Harman JB: The significance of local vascular phenomena in the production of ischemic necrosis in skeletal muscle. Am J Pathol 24:625, 1948.

19. Strock PE, Majno G: Vascular response to experimental tourniquet ischemia. Surg Gynecol Obstet 129:309, 1969.

20. Milton SH: Experimental studies on island flaps. Plast Reconstruct Surg 49:444, 1972.

21. Conway H, Griffith BH: Plastic surgery for closure of decubitus ulcers in patients with paraplegia: Based on experience with 1000 cases. Am J Surg 91:946, 1956.

22. Hewer CL: Maintenance of the Trendelenburg position by skin friction. Lancet 1:522, 1953.

23. Pressure Ulcers in Adults: Prediction and Prevention. US Department of Health and Human Services publication No. 92-0050. Washington, DC, US Government Printing Office, May 1992.

24. Preventing Pressure Ulcers. US Department of Health and Human Services publication No. 92-0048. Washington, DC, US Government Printing Office, May 1992.

25. Kaltenborn FM: Mobilization of the Extremity Joints: Examination and Basic Treatment Techniques. Oslo, Olaf Norlis Bookhandel, 1980.

26. Massey W, Pleet B: Compression injury of the sciatic nerve during a prolonged surgical preocedure in a diabetic patient. J Am Geriatr Soc 28:188, 1980.

27. Rosenburg D: Peripheral neuropathy. In Neurology. New York, Grune & Stratton, 1980.

28. Sunderland S: Blood supply of the nerves of the upper limb in man. Arch Neurol Psychiatry 53:91, 1945.

29. Kozu H, Tamura E, Parry GJ: Endoneurial blood supply in peripheral nerves is not uniform. J Neurol Sci 111:204, 1992.

30. Kelly CJ, Augustine C, Rooney BP, Bouchier-Hayes DJ: An investigation of the pathology of ischemic neuropathy. Eur J Vasc Surg 5:539, 1991.

31. Seddon HJ: Three types of nerve injury. Brain 66:237, 1943.

32. Seddon HJ: A classification of nerve injury. BMJ 2:237, 1942.

33. Butler DS: Mobilization of the Nervous System. New York, Churchill Livingstone, 1991.

34. Haftek J: Stretch injuries of peripheral nerve: Acute effect of stretching on rabbit nerve. J Bone Joint Surg Br 52:354, 1970.

35. Lundborg G, Rydevik B: Effect of stretching the tibial nerve of the rabbit: A preliminary study of the intraneural circulation and the barrier function of the perineum. J Bone Joint Surg Br 55:390, 1973.

36. Ogata K, Naito M: Blood flow of peripheral nerves: Effects of dissection, stretching, and compression. J Hand Surg [Br] 11:10, 1986.

37. Denny-Brown D, Doherty MM: Effect of transient stretching of peripheral nerve. Arch Neurol Psychiatry 54:116, 1945.

38. Ochoa J, Fowler TJ, Gilliatt RW: Anatomical changes in peripheral nerves compressed by a pneumatic tourniquet. J Anat 113:433, 1972.

39. Denny-Brown D, Brenner C: Paralysis of nerve induced by direct pressure and by tourniquet. Arch Neurol Psychiatry 51:1, 1944.

40. Bentley FH, Schlapp W: Experiments on the blood supply of nerves. J Physiol 102:62, 1943.

41. Gerard RW. The response of nerve to oxygen lack. Am J Physiol 92:498, 1930.

42. Lewis T, Pickering GW, Rothchild P: Centripetal paralysis arising out of arrested bloodflow to the limb, including notes on a form of tingling. Heart 16:1, 1931.

43. Trojaborg W: Rate of recovery in motor and sensory fibres of the radial nerve: Clinical and electrophysiological aspects. J Neurol Neurosurg Psychiatry 33:625, 1970.

44. Giliatt RW: Disorders of peripheral nerves. J R Coll Phys 1:50, 1966.

45. Mayer RF: Conduction velocity in peripheral nerve during experimental demyelination in the cat. Neurology 14:714, 1964.

46. Vargo MM, Robinson RR, Nicholas JJ, Marvin RC: Postpartum femoral neuropathy: Relic of an earlier era? Arch Phys Med Rehabil 71:591, 1990.

47. Lupski JR, Chance PF, Garcia CA: Inherited primary peripheral neuopathies. JAMA 270:2326, 1993.

48. Upton ARM, McComas AJ: The double crush in nerve-entrapment syndromes. Lancet 2:359, 1973.

49. Osterman AL: The double crush syndrome. Orthop Clin North Am 19:147, 1988.

50. Hurst LC, Weissberg D, Carroll RE: The relationship of the double crush to carpal tunnel syndrome: An analysis of 1,000 cases of carpal tunnel syndrome. J Hand Surg [Br] 10:202, 1985.

51. Guyon MA, Honet JC: Carpal tunnel syndrome or trigger finger associated with neck injury in automobile accidents. Arch Phys Med Rehabil 58:325, 1977.

52. Dyro FM: Peripheral entrapments following brachial plexus lesions. Electromyogr Clin Neurophysiol 23:251, 1983.

53. Massey EW, Riley TL, Pleet AB: Coexistent carpel tunnel syndrome and cervical radiculopathy: Double crush syndrome. South Med J 74:957, 1981.

54. Cherington M: Proximal pain in carpel tunnel syndrome. Arch Surg 108:69, 1974.

55. Wood VE, Biondi J: Double-crush nerve compression in thoracic-outlet syndrome. J Bone Joint Surg Am 72:85, 1990.

56. Nemoto K, Matsumato N, Tazaki K, et al.: An experimental study on the "double crush" hypothesis." J Hand Surg [Am] 12:552, 1987.

57. Gassel MM, Diamantopoulos E: Pattern of conduction times in the distribution of the radial nerve. Neurology 14:222, 1964.

58. Sunderland S. Ulnar nerve lesions. *In* Sunderland S (ed.): Nerves and Nerve Injury. New York, Churchill Livingstone, 1978.

59. Folberg CR, Weiss AP, Akelman E: Cubital tunnel syndrome. Orthop Rev 23:136, 1994.

60. Wadsworth TG, Williams JR: Cubital tunnel external compression syndrome. BMJ l:662, 1973.

61. Cameron MGP, Stewart OJ: Ulnar nerve injury associated with anaesthesia. Can Anaesth Soc J 22:253, 1975.

62. Wadsworth TG. The cubital tunnel and the external compression syndrome. Anesth Analg 53:303, 1974.

63. Jones HD. Ulnar nerve damage following general anaesthics. Anaesthesia 22:471, 1967.

64. Stoelting RK, Anesthesia and Co-Existing Disease, 3rd ed. New York, Churchill Livingstone, 1993.

65. Dyck PJ, Thomas PK, Griffin JW, et al.: Peripheral Neuropathy, 3rd ed. Philadelphia, WB Saunders, 1993.

66. Earl CJ, Fullertom PK, Wakefield GS, Schutta HS: Hereditary neuropathy, with liability to pressure palsies. Q J Med 132:481, 1964.

67. Staal A, de Weerdt CJ, Went LN: Hereditary compression syndrome of peripheral nerves. Neurology 15:1008, 1965.

68. Davies DM: Recurrent peripheral-nerve palsies in a family. Lancet 2:266, 1954.

69. Asbury AK: Diseases of the peripheral nervous system. *In* Braunwald E, Isselbacher K, Petersdorf RG, et al (eds.): Harrison's Principles of Internal Medicine. New York, McGraw-Hill, 1987.

70. Parks BJ: Post-operative peripheral neuropathies. Surgery 74:349, 1973.

71. Lincoln JR, Sawyer HP: Complications related to body position during surgical procedures. Anesthesiology 22:800, 1961.

72. Westin B: Prevention of upper-limb nerve injuries in Trendelenburg position. Acta Chir Scand 108:61, 1954.

73. Nicholson MJ, Eversole UH: Nerve injury incident to anesthesia and operation. Anesth Analg 36:19, 1957.

74. Perreault L, Drolet P, Farny J. Ulnar nerve palsy at the elbow after general anaesthesia. Can J Anaesth 39:499, 1992.

75. Payan J: Electrophysiological localization of ulnar nerve lesions. J Neurol Neurosurg Psychiatry 32:208, 1969.

76. Tackmann W, Vogel P, Kaeser HE, Ettlin T: Sensitivity and localizing significance of motor and sensory electroneurographic parameters in the diagnosis of ulnar nerve lesions at the elbow. J Neurol 231:204, 1984.

77. Alvin FG, Schurrer NE: Postoperative ulnar nerve palsy. J Bone Joint Surg Am 69:255, 1987.

78. Sunderland S: Peripheral nerve trunks. *In* Nerves and Nerve Injuries. New York, Churchill Livingstone, 1978.

79. Miller RG: The cubital tunnel syndrome: Diagnosis and precise localization. Ann Neurol 6:56, 1979

80. Miller RG, Camp PE: Postoperative ulnar neuropathy. JAMA 242:1636, 1979.

81. Kincaid JC, Phillips LH, Daube JR: The evaluation of suspected ulnar neuropathy at the elbow. Arch Neurol 43:44, 1986.

82. Dawson DM: Entrapment neuropathies of the upper extremities. N Engl J Med 329:2013, 1993.

83. Eisen A: Early diagnosis of ulnar nerve palsy: An electrophysiologic study. Neurology 24:256, 1974.

84. Childress HM: Recurrent ulnar nerve dislocation at the elbow. J Bone Joint Surg Am 38:978, 1956.

85. Pechan J, Julis I: The pressure measurement in the ulnar nerve: A contribution to the pathophysiology of the cubital tunnel syndrome. J Biomech 8:75, 1975.

86. Sy WP. Ulnar nerve palsy possibly related to use of automatically cycled blood pressure cuff. Anesth Analg 60:687, 1981.

87. Winer JB, Harrison MJG: Iatrogenic nerve injuries. Postgrad Med J 58:142, 1982.

88. Dhuner K-G: Nerve injuries following operations: A survey of cases occurring during a six year period. Anesthesiology 11:289, 1950.

89. Checkles NS, Russakov AD, Piero DL: Ulnar nerve conduction velocity: Effect of elbow position on measurement. Arch Phys Med Rehabil 52:362, 1971.

90. Bralliar F: Electromyography: Its use and misuse in peripheral nerve injuries. Orthop Clin North Am 12:229, 1981.

91. Mawk JR, Thienprasit P: Postoperative ulnar neuropathy. JAMA 246:2806, 1981.

92. Budinger K: Ueber lahmungen nach Chloroformnarkosen. Arch Klin Chir 47:121, 1894.

93. Cooper DE, Jenkins RS, Bready L, Rockwood CA Jr: The prevention of injury to the brachial plexus secondary to malpositioning of the patient during surgery. Clin Orthop Rel Res 228:33, 1988.

94. Jackson L, Keats AS: Mechanism of brachial plexus palsy following anesthesia. Anesthesiology 26:190, 1965.

95. Po BT, Hansen HR: Iatrogenic brachial plexus injury: A survey of the literature and of pertinent cases. Anesth Analg 48:915, 1969.

96. Kirsh MM, Magee KR, Gago O, et al.: Brachial plexus injury following median sternotomy incision. Ann Thorac Surg 11:315, 1971.

97. Vander-Salm TJ, Cereda J-M, Cutler BS: Brachial plexus injury following median sternotomy. J Thorac Cardiovasc Surg 80:447, 1980.

98. Clausen EG: Postoperative ("anesthetic") paralysis of the brachial plexus. Surgery 12:933, 1942.

99. Wright IS: The neurovascular syndrome produced by hyperabduction of the arms. Am Heart J 29:1, 1945.

100. Trojaborg W: Electrophysiological findings in pressure palsy of the brachial plexus. J Neurol Neurosurg Psychiatry 40:1160, 1977.

101. Raffan AW: Post-operative paralysis of the brachial plexus. BMJ 2:149, 1950.

102. Ewing MR: Postoperative paralysis in the upper extremity. Lancet 1:99, 1950.

103. Graham JG, Pye IF, McQueen INF: Brachial plexus injury after median sternotomy. J Neurol 44:621, 1981.

104. Dawson DM, Krarup C: Perioperative nerve lesions. Arch Neurol 46:1355, 1989.

105. Kwaan JHM, Rappaport I: Postoperative brachial plexus palsy. Arch Surg 101:612, 1970.

106. Hanson MR, Breuer AC, Furlan AJ, et al.: Mecha-

nism and frequency of brachial plexus injury in open-heart surgery: A prospective analysis. Ann Thorac Surg 36:675, 1983.

107. Hanson M: Reply. Ann Thorac Surg 38:661, 1984.

108. Keates JRW, Innocenti DM, Ross DN: Mononeuritis multiplex. J Thorac Cardiovasc Surg 69:816, 1975.

109. Breslin FJ: Fracture of the first rib unassociated with fracture of other ribs. Am J Surg 37:384, 1937.

110. Honet JC, Raikes JA, Kantrowitz A, et al.: Neuropathy in the upper extremity after open heart surgery. Arch Phys Med Rehabil 57:264, 1976.

111. Vander Salm TJ, Cutler BS, Okike ON: Brachial plexus injuries following median sternotomy: II. J Thorac Cardiovasc Surg 83:914, 1982.

112. Curtis JA, Libshitz HI, Dalinka MK. Fracture of the first rib as a complication of midline sternotomy. Radiology 115:63, 1975.

113. Roy RC, Stafford MA, Charlton JE: Nerve injury and musculoskeletal complaints after cardiac surgery: Influence of internal mammary artery dissection and left arm position. Anesth Analg 67:277, 1988.

114. Lederman RJ, Breuer AC, Hanson MR, et al.: Peripheral nervous system complications of coronary bypass graft surgery. Ann Neurol 12:297, 1982.

115. Treasure T, Garnett R, O'Connor J, Treasure J: Injury of the lower trunk of the brachial plexus as a complication of median sternotomy for cardiac surgery. Ann R Coll Surg Engl 62:378, 1980.

116. Shaw PJ, Bates D, Cartlidge NEF, et al.: Early neurologic complications of coronary artery bypass surgery. BMJ 291:1384, 1985.

117. Tomlinson DL, Hirsch IA, Kodali SV, Slogoff S: Protecting the brachial plexus during median sternotomy. J Thorac Cardiovasc Surg 94:297, 1987.

118. Sotaniemi KA: Brain damage and neurological outcome after open heart surgery. J Neurol Neurosurg Psychiatry 43:127, 1980.

119. Wang LP, Hagerdal M: Reported anesthetic complications during an 11 year period: A retrospective study. Acta Anaesth Scand 36:234, 1992.

120. Horrow JC: Brachial plexus injury. Ann Thorac Surg 38:660, 1984.

121. Vander Salm TJ, Welch G: Brachial plexus injury after open heart surgery. Ann Thorac Surg 38:660, 1984.

122. Sylvestre DL, Sandson TA, Nachmanoff DB: Transient brachial plexopathy as a complication of internal jugular vein cannulation. Neurology 41:760, 1991.

123. O'Keefe DM: Brachial plexus injury following axillary arteriography. J Neurosurg 53:853, 1980.

124. Hickey C, Gugino LD, Aglio LS, et al.: Intraoperative somatosensory evoked potential monitoring predicts peripheral nerve injury during cardiac surgery. Anesthesiology 78:29, 1993.

125. Magee KR, DeJong RN: Paralytic brachial neuritis. JAMA 174:1258, 1960.

126. Malamut RI, Marques W, England JD, Sumner AJ: Postsurgical idiopathic brachial neuritis. Muscle Nerve 17:320, 1994.

127. McQuarrie HG, Harris JW, Ellsworth HS, et al.: Sciatic neuropathy complicating vaginal hysterectomy. Am J Obstet Gynecol 113:223, 1972.

128. Burkhart FL, Daly JW: Sciatic and peroneal nerve injury: A complication of vaginal operations. Obstet Gynecol 28:99, 1966.

129. Batres F, Barclay DL: Sciatic nerve injury during gynecologic procedures using the lithotomy position. Obstet Gynecol 62:92, 1983.

130. Brown JT, McDougall A: Traumatic maternal birth palsy. J Obstet Gynaecol 64:431, 1957.

131. Johnson EW: Sciatic nerve palsy following delivery. Postgrad Med 30:495, 1961.

132. Bergqvist D, Bohe M, Ekelund G, et al.: Compartment syndrome after prolonged surgery with leg supports. Int J Colorectal Dis 5:1, 1990.

133. Reddy PK, Kaye KW: Deep posterior compartmental syndrome: A serious complication of the lithotomy position. J Urol 132:144, 1984.

134. Khakuk IM: Bilateral compartment syndrome after prolonged surgery in the lithotomy position. J Vasc Surg 5:879, 1987.

135. Paschal CR, Strzelecki LR. "Lithotomy positioning devices" AORN J 55:1011, 1992.

136. Warner MA, Martin JT, Schroeder DR, et al.: Lower extremity motor neuropathy associated with surgery performed on patients in a lithotomy position. Anesthesiology 81:6, 1984.

137. Dripps RD, Vandam LD: Long-term follow-up of patients who received 10,098 spinal anesthetics. JAMA 156:1486, 1954.

138. Crawford JS: Lumbar epidural block in labour: A clinical analysis. Br J Anaesth 44:66, 1972.

139. Hellman K: Epidural anaesthesia in obstetrics: A second look at 26,127 cases. Can Anaesth Soc J 12:398, 1965.

140. Eisen SM, Rosen N, Winesanker H, et al.: The routine use of lumbar epidural anaesthesia in obstetrics: A clinical review of 9,532 cases. Can Anaesth Soc J 7:280, 1960.

141. Moir DD, Davidson S: Postpartum complications of forceps delivery performed under epidural and pudendal nerve block. Br J Anaesth 44:1197, 1972.

142. Kane RE: Neurologic deficits following epidural or spinal anesthesia. Anesth Analg 60:150, 1981.

143. Nicholson MJ, Eversole UH: Neurologic complications of spinal anesthesia. JAMA 123:679, 1946.

144. Greene NM: Neurologic sequelae of spinal anesthesia. Anesthesiology 22:682, 1961.

145. Vandam LD, Dripps RD: Exacerbation of pre-existing neurologic disease after spinal anesthesia. N Engl J Med 225:843, 1956.

146. Vandam LD, Dripps RD: Long-term follow-up of patients who received 10,098 spinal anethetics. JAMA 172:1483, 1960.

147. Ong BY, Cohen MM, Esmail A, et al.: Paresthesias and motor dysfunction after labor and delivery. Anesth Analg 66:18, 1987.

148. Abouleish E: Neurologic complications following epidural analgesia in obstetrics. Reg Anes 7:119, 1982.

149. Pratt JH: Sciatic neuropathy complicating vaginal hysterectomy. Am J Obstet Gynecol 113:231, 1972.

150. Rosenblum J, Schwarz GA, Bendler E: Femoral neuropathy: A neurological complication of hysterectomy. JAMA 195:409, 1966.

151. Hill EC: Maternal obstetric paralysis. Am J Obstet Gynecol 83:1452, 1962.

152. Wooten SL, McLaughlin RE: Iliacus hematoma and subsequent femoral nerve palsy after penetration of the medial acetabular wall during total hip arthroplasty. Clin Orthop 191:221, 1984.

Chapter 12

Positioning the Head and Neck

Mark A. Warner

BACKGROUND

Proper positioning of the patient's head and neck is a key issue in all surgical postures. Although most anesthesia personnel are meticulous in their positioning and care of the head, neck, and facial structures for patients placed in the sitting, lateral decubitus, and prone postures, less attention is often devoted to these structures when the patient is supine or in a lithotomy position. Proper establishment of the various positions is addressed in specific chapters of this text. However, a number of basic principles apply to arrangement of the head and neck in any surgical posture. They include avoidance of extremes of ranges of motion; prevention of compression injury to nerves, organs, and soft tissues; and avoidance of positions that may occlude blood and lymph flow.

NORMAL RANGE OF MOTION

The head and neck complex, when taken as a unit, is able to bend and move in a variety of directions. Its mobility is primarily attributed to the atlantoaxial-occipital segment with the remainder of the cervical spine being involved to a lesser extent.[1] Except for anteroposterior flexion in the sagittal plane of the occiput on the atlas (C1) and simple rotation of the atlas on the axis (C2), motions of the head and neck complex are dependent on the combined interactions of each vertebra-to-vertebra segment. These motions include anteroposterior flexion and extension, lateral flexion, and rotation. Pure rotation in a horizontal plane does not occur in the cervical spine. All rotary movement in the cervical spine is accompanied by some degree of lateral flexion.[1, 2]

Flexion

Flexion of the head and neck occurs first with anteroposterior motion of the external occipital condyles on the atlas,[2, 3] the movement of "nodding" up and down in a sagittal plane. The occiput can flex approximately 10 degrees on the atlas. An additional 5 degrees of flexion occurs between the atlas and axis. The cervical spine provides the remainder of the anteroposterior angulation. Within the cervical spine, the greatest degree of flexion occurs in the midcervical region at the C4–5 and the C5–6 interspaces.[4] Very little anteroposterior flexion occurs at the C7–8 and C8–T1 interspaces. Although there is wide variation in the maximum flexion of the head and neck in healthy volunteers, the atlanto-occipital and midcervical regions account for most of the range of flexion.

The kinetics related to flexion of the head and neck have important implications in various patient positions. Of these, the effect of flexion on the cervical canal should receive the greatest attention. Ventral bending of the cervical spine causes the cervical facets to glide on each other and elevates the posterior elements of the vertebrae until the interspinous ligaments are stretched to their maxi-

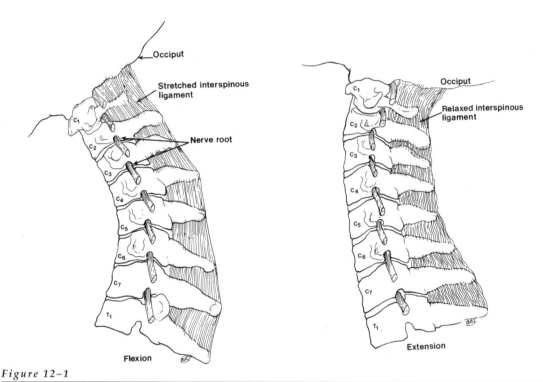

Figure 12–1

Flexion of the head and neck (*left*) elongates the spinal canal's posterior wall more than the anterior wall, especially in the midcervical region. The spinal cord is stretched and the nerve roots are pulled cephalad against the undersurface of the intervertebral foramina. In contrast, the anatomic changes associated with extension (*right*) are more evenly distributed over the entire length of the cervical vertebrae. The spinal cord does not stretch and the nerve roots are not pulled cephalad within the foramina.

mum and stop further flexion. The posterior wall of the cervical canal elongates more than its anterior wall (Fig. 12–1, *left*). Because the spinal cord is tethered in position by its nerve roots, the cord and its dura elongate. In extremes of flexion the cervical nerve roots are pulled cephalad against the undersurface of the intervertebral foramina (see Fig. 12–1, *left*). Although these foramina open somewhat during flexion, the resulting stretch may injure specific roots, especially in the presence of pathologic conditions that narrow foramina. The spinal cord is most elongated at the C4–5 level because the C4–5 segment of the cervical spine is the site of maximum anteroposterior flexion. Extreme tension on the cord and dura may cause the cord to become ischemic.[5, 6] Midcervical tetraplegia from cervical hyperflexion has been reported and is discussed in greater detail later in this chapter.

Extension

Like flexion, extension of the head and neck usually occurs first with anteroposterior extension of the occiput on the atlas.[1] The nor-

mal range of extension at this level is 25 degrees. Approximately 10 degrees of extension occurs in the atlantoaxial segment. The midcervical region is the cervical spine's most mobile region during extension. Extension of the cervical spine is a more diffuse motion than flexion, but like flexion, the maximum angulation of extension occurs at the C4–5 level.[4]

The effects of hyperextension on the spinal cord and cervical nerve roots are the reverse of those of hyperflexion. Hyperextension effectively shortens the cervical canal and does not place cephalad tension on cervical nerve roots (see Fig. 12–1, *right*). Each nerve root usually occupies 20% to 25% of the lumen of an intervertebral foramen.[7] Extension minimizes the angulation of the nerve roots as they enter the foramina and may protect the nerves from trauma against the undersurfaces of the foramina. Unfortunately, anteroposterior extension also narrows the vertebral foramina. In a normal spine the degree of narrowing of the foramen is not enough to compress nerve roots; in abnormal spines, however, the foramina can become constricted and impinge on the roots. Foraminal narrowing may be increased by inflammatory and osteophytic involvement of the soft tissues that occupy the remainder of its lumen. Rotation, especially to the ipsilateral side, may further decrease the foramen's caliber, adding to the risk of nerve root injury.[8]

Hyperextension in the atlanto-occipital and atlantoaxial segments of the head and neck may entrap the occipital nerves as they transit these structures. The C1–3 nerve roots form the occipital nerves as they emerge through the ligamentous and muscular tissue in those areas. Unlike those in other segments of the cervical spine, these nerve roots are not protected by bony foramina. Entrapment of the greater and lesser occipital nerves by hyperextension of the neck may result in paresthesias or pain in their distribution areas. The pain associated with mild or moderate degrees of occipital nerve entrapment may be misinterpreted as a symptom of other causes of perioperative headache.[9]

Rotation

Half of the horizontal rotation in the head and neck occurs between the atlas and axis.[1] Between these two vertebrae, approximately 90 degrees of rotation is possible from extreme left to extreme right. The atlas rotates around the odontoid process of the axis, with its range of motion being limited by attachments of ligamentous and muscular structures. Rotation within the cervical spine occurs only after rotation within the atlantoaxial segment has occurred. Because the external occipital condyles only move sagittally on the atlas, no rotation occurs in the atlanto-occipital segment.

Caudad to the axis, rotation of any cervical vertebra on the neck is limited by a bony locking mechanism in which the anterior tip of the upper articular process of the caudad vertebra impinges on the posterolateral corner of the cephalad vertebra's body (Fig. 12–2). The lateral extension of the transverse process forms the lateral margin of the vertebral artery foramen. In normal cervical spines this locking mechanism prevents excessive rotation and safeguards the vertebral artery as it ascends through the transverse processes to the foramen magnum.[8] Despite this protective mechanism, extremes of rotation in the cervical spine may impinge on vertebral blood flow, a problem that is discussed in greater detail subsequently.

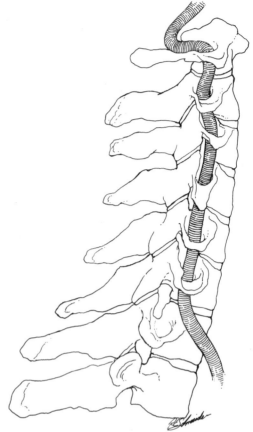

Figure 12–2

The vertebral artery passes through a foramen of the transverse process in the cervical vertebrae. The anterior tip of the superior articular surface of the lower vertebra locks against the body of the upper vertebra and prevents excessive rotation that would entrap the vertebral artery as it passes through the foramina.

Lateral Flexion

Lateral flexion and rotation never occur as isolated movements in the cervical spine below the atlantoaxial segment.[1, 2] Lateral flexion (side bending) cannot occur without rotation, and any rotation of the cervical spines initiates lateral flexion. The combined motion narrows the foramina on the side to which the head laterally bends and toward which the head turns. On the side from which the head rotates, the foramina simultaneously widen.

As noted earlier, extension of the cervical spine may narrow the intervertebral foramina. The combination of extension, rotation, and lateral flexion of the head and neck may especially decrease the lumen of a foramen. In addition, as they proceed along the foramina, the nerve roots consist of distinct motor and sensory components. The dorsal roots contain sensory fibers. These fibers lie in close proximity to the facet's articular processes and their joint capsules that form the lateral walls of the foramina. Extension, lateral flexion, and rotation cause these articular surfaces to twist and can stretch the joint capsules. This stretch can cause inflammation and edema of the capsules and impinge on the sensory fibers of the nerve roots.[10] In surgical positioning, this combination of motions may occur when placing a patient in the prone position if the head and neck are extended, laterally flexed, and rotated toward one side.

PATHOLOGIC PROCESSES

A number of pathologic processes increase the risk of perioperative problems with the head and neck. Many of these processes may be symptomatic and identifiable during a preoperative evaluation.

Rheumatoid Arthritis

This systemic process often results in weakened ligamentous structures and severe degeneration of cervical spinal joints. The most common site of instability of the cervical spine in patients with rheumatoid arthritis is the atlantoaxial segment. Within this segment, the cervical spine is usually stable in extension but may be markedly unstable in flexion.[11] A strong correlation exists between atlantoaxial subluxation and rheumatoid interstitial lung disease.[12] The destructive processes of rheumatoid arthritis on ligaments and bones may be augmented by administration of high doses of corticosteroids, although the corticosteroids paradoxically relieve the symptoms of joint inflammation. Corticosteroids directly inhibit osteoblastic activity within the vertebral bodies and stimulate osteoclasts.[13] These effects lead to osteoporotic changes and subsequent vertebral compression. Rheumatoid nodules, the most common extra-articular manifestation of rheumatoid arthritis, often develop in the soft tissues of the cervical spine and in the dural coverings of the cervical cord and its nerve roots. The nodules decrease the range of motion of the head and neck and also occupy space in the narrowed cervical spinal canal and foramina.[14]

Ankylosing Spondylitis

Pathologic processes that accompany the arthropathies of ankylosing spondylitis affect multiple organs, especially the lungs (fibrosis), heart (aortic regurgitation), and eyes (uveitis). Inflammation of the articular surfaces of the vertebral bodies promotes osteoblastosis and consolidation of the vertebral bodies. Although the spinal column is usually first affected in sacral and lumbar areas, the cervical spine is soon afflicted.[15] Exercise and mobility appear to retard the progress of ankylosis.[16] Because the atlantoaxial joint is rarely immobile, the constant motion within this segment may account for its rare involvement by ankylosis. Although the cervical spine often develops ankylosis later than the sacral and lumbar spine, its general mobility and lack of protection by other body supporting structures make it particularly vulnerable to trauma and fracture. In trauma, especially when forces result in hyperextension of an ankylosed spine, the cervical region is usually the first to fracture.[17] In osteoporotic cervical vertebrae, the extension forces applied during jaw thrust and head extension during airway manipulation may increase the risk of vertebral fracture.

Meningismus

Viral and bacterial meningeal involvement can cause inflammation that ranges from piaarachnoiditis to extensive inflammation of the dura and supportive structures. The cranial nerve roots may also be involved. Headache and a stiff neck are common signs and symptoms of meningeal irritation. Meningeal irritation activates protective flexor reflexes that shorten and immobilize the spine.[18] Patients with these signs have limited cervical spine range of motion during the preoperative evaluation, but anesthetic induction agents and neuromuscular blocking drugs block these protective flexor reflexes. Meningeal irritation often is associated with dural edema, and the cord and nerve roots may be compressed in a narrow spinal canal or intervertebral foramina.[19]

Cervical Trauma

Cervical spine trauma may result in bony instability of the spinal canal and increase the risk of spinal cord damage. In addition, trauma and pain often trigger protective flexor reflexes that shorten and immobilize the cervical spinal column.[8, 20] An edematous spinal cord and nerve roots may be compressed and made ischemic in narrowed spaces. The best method to manage an airway in a patient with cervical trauma is controversial.[20-22] Regardless of whether the patient is endotracheally intubated through the nose, mouth, or a surgically obtained airway (e.g., cricothyroidotomy), most anesthesia personnel agree that the head and neck should be maintained in a neutral position within a sagittal plane. For the patient who will be moved into a position other than supine, intubating the trachea while the patient is still awake is a useful technique. It allows the patient to cooperate with neurologic evaluations performed during and after the move into the final position and is a rapid method of identifying position-induced neural complications.[23]

Cervical Disk Disease

A defect in a cervical intervertebral disk can distort the relationship of the vertebral components of segmental joints and alter the size and shape of an intervertebral foramen.[24] The contents of the foramen may become inflamed from pressure, traction, and angulation. The pain and dysfunction associated with cervical disk disease may limit head and neck mobility.[25] In general, nerve root compression from herniation of a cervical disk is unusual. The annulus fibrosus is much thicker and more dense in the posterior lateral portion of the disk and thus more resistant to distention into the intervertebral foramen. More commonly, the cervical disk degenerates, allowing the vertebral articular surfaces to approximate.[26, 27] Periosteal sites that become raw from wear and tear develop osteophytes.[28] Osteophytic activity associated with disk disease is most likely to occur in the most lordotic segment of the cervical spine, C4–C5, where static and kinetic stresses are greatest. Within the cervical (and also lumbar) spine, where lordosis produces greatest pressure in the concave side of the curve, osteophytes most commonly form in the posterior spine. These osteophytes are most likely to encroach on the cervical nerve roots during extension of the neck. For this reason, prudence mandates that positions requiring prolonged cervical extension be avoided to any extent possible for patients with known cervical disk disease.

Other Conditions

Many other conditions may increase the risk of head and neck problems during positioning. These include congenital and acquired anatomic deformities, traumatic and burn injuries, and anatomic distortion due to radiation therapy, spinal column fixation, and other surgical procedures. Each condition requires a careful preoperative assessment of its effect on the mobility and stability of the head and neck.

AVOIDING POSITIONING TO THE LIMITS OF MOTION

The extremes of range of motion for flexion, extension, lateral flexion, and rotation of the head and neck vary dramatically from patient to patient. A good rule to follow when positioning patients is to avoid any position that would place the head or neck at the limit of a particular motion. At the extremes of range of motion, either bone-to-bone interfaces or connective tissues that are stretched to their maximum flexible length must support any weight bearing. Prolonged immobilization in this type of position causes discomfort and may damage these support structures.

Two examples demonstrate the problems associated with positions in which the head and neck are placed at the extremes of motion. In the first example, a patient undergoing a parathyroidectomy is positioned supine with a blanket or roll under the shoulders. The head and neck are hyperextended to permit maximal exposure of the anterior neck. In this case, the head must be supported. The cervical spine should not be placed into maximal extension; certainly, the head must not be allowed to hang unsupported (Fig. 12–3). The anterior ligamentous and muscular supports of the cervical spine may be stretched beyond their normal limits. Prolonged stretch can cause ischemic pain and edema.[29] Most of the ligaments and muscles of the neck are attached to the bone by myofascial tissue that blends into the periosteum. Traction exerted on the periosteum causes minute tears and painful edema. The posterior portions of intervertebral disks, especially in the midcervical region, are compressed. This pressure produces lateralized pain that may project into the shoulder and upper arm. Because disks are avascular and relatively free of nerve endings, controversy exists regarding the ability

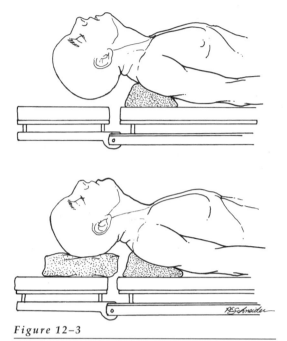

Figure 12–3

A roll or pad placed under the shoulders to maximize surgical exposure to the anterior surface of the neck may lift the head sufficiently (*top*) to subject the cervical vertebrae, spinal cord, and cervical nerve roots to injury unless the occiput is supported also (*bottom*).

of pressure on a disk to cause pain.[30] However, Holt has shown that cervical diskography and the injection of small amounts of saline (0.2 mL) into the posterior disk nucleus produces lateralizing pain.[31] Additional risks in this example are entrapment of the occipital nerves by the occiput as they exit the C1–2 and C2–3 segment interspaces and compression of the cervical nerve roots within the narrowed intervertebral foramina.

In the second example of problems associated with positioning at the extremes of motion, a patient is placed into a sitting position for surgery on the posterior cervical spine. To provide maximal surgical exposure of the dorsum of the neck, the patient's chin is flexed forward to the chest (Fig. 12–4*A*). At this maximum limit of flexion, the cervical cord stretches, especially at C4–5 where the cervical spine is maximally flexed. The cord becomes ischemic during a prolonged period of stretch, and the patient is paralyzed below the C5 level. Whether the cord ischemia is secondary to direct compression of small vessels that penetrate the cord or to the stretching of those vessels until their lumina become too narrow to provide adequate blood flow

is uncertain. The resulting lesion, *midcervical tetraplegia,* is most commonly reported to occur after prolonged head flexion during intracranial surgery performed on patients who were in a sitting position, but it also has been reported in patients who have had their head and necks flexed while supine.[32, 33] In neurosurgical patients who underwent their procedures while placed in a "park bench" position, McCallum and co-workers[34] and McPherson and colleagues[35] have reported the use of somatosensory evoked potentials elicited by stimulation of the median nerve to detect abnormal changes that have subsequently been reversed by reducing the degree of neck flexion. However, the sensitivity of somatosensory evoked potentials to detect midcervical tetraplegia has been questioned. Cottrell and his team[36] found that this modality was not sensitive enough to reliably detect tetraplegia in a primate model. In a separate experimental model, Levy and colleagues[37] noted a similar lack of sensitivity and suggested that motor evoked potentials may be better suited for this purpose.

TECHNIQUES TO AVOID COMPRESSION INJURIES

Soft tissues, nerves, and organs of the head and neck should be well padded to widely distribute any compressive forces; and, if appropriate, the head should be moved or turned frequently to avoid prolonged pressure on the same tissues. When the patient is prone, however, intermittent head turning may not be advisable because of potential danger to the eyes, the nose, and transoral instrumentation. Nevertheless, frequent checks of the position of the pronated head should be accomplished to assure that the originally safe arrangement has not been altered. The head and neck should be placed in as neutral a position as possible to avoid extremes of motion that might compress superficial nerves such as the occipital nerves (see earlier). The eyes should be padded and positioned to avoid pressure being placed directly on them.

Pressure Alopecia

Prolonged compression of hair follicles may produce hair loss.[38] The depilation is not immediate, often beginning 3 days or more after surgery. It has been noted in medical patients who have been paralyzed and ventilated dur-

Figure 12–4

Maximal flexion of the head and neck by placing the chin on the chest in the sitting position may evoke cervical spinal cord ischemia and venous outflow obstruction of the tongue and neck. *A.* Severe head and neck flexion is shown with chin pressing firmly against surface of anterior chest. *B.* Moderate flexion, permitting insertion of thumb or fingers of attendant between chin and chest, still provides excellent surgical exposure of structures in the posterior cranial fossa and posterior cervical spine.

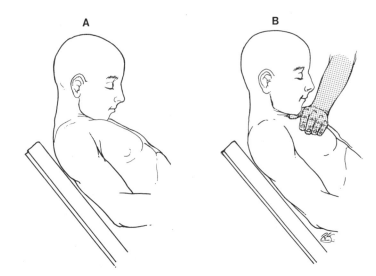

ing prolonged stays in intensive care units as well as in surgical patients.[39] In most patients there is a slow and sparse regrowth of hair after several months, but if prolonged pressure causes necrosis of the hair follicles, the alopecia is permanent. Frequent turns of the head to relocate the points of contact between hair-bearing tissue and supportive surfaces during prolonged anesthesia may be the best method to decrease the risk of alopecia. In a randomly selected group of cardiopulmonary bypass patients, Lawson and associates[40] prospectively evaluated the efficacy of repositioning their heads every 30 minutes during surgery and the recovery phase until endotracheal extubation. Using this simple technique, they nearly eliminated the occurrence of occipital alopecia in their patient population. In contrast, alopecia occurred in 21% of the patients in their control groups. A more detailed description of pressure alopecia is found in Chapter 5.

Eye Protection

Eyes are at risk in all of the perioperative positions, and eyelids should always be closed. Many anesthesia personnel prefer to tape the eyes shut for all procedures, but others argue that the use of tape increases the risk for corneal abrasion if the lids partially open under the tape or if the tape is removed without first confirming that the lids are shut. Some anesthesiologists prefer to use protective goggles for their patients. Regardless of the mechanism in use, the intent is to close the eyelids to prevent chemical or mechanical damage to the cornea and sclerae and to

avoid drying of the corneal epithelium.[41] The use of lubricants for the surface of the eye is also controversial. Those who prefer lubricants use them to keep the eyes from drying.

External pressure on the globe of the eye may result in blindness from increased intraocular pressure that inhibits central retinal artery perfusion or produces central retinal artery occlusion. Unilateral blindness has been reported in anesthetized supine patients in whom badly fitting facemasks resulted in pressure against one eye.[42] External pressure on the eyes is more likely, however, in patients who are placed in the prone or lateral decubitus position.[43–45] Padded head rests, towels, blankets, or other equipment that was initially placed so as to not endanger the eye may shift to compress the globe, increase intraocular pressure, and occlude the central retinal artery. Monitoring wires and intravenous tubing should be checked to confirm that none have migrated into a position that could harm the eyes. The position of the head should be checked frequently to confirm that no shifting has occurred that would place pressure on the eye.

Precautions similar to those taken to prevent compression and damage to the eyes also should be taken for the ears. The ears should be checked frequently, especially in the lateral decubitus or prone position, to confirm that the pinna and its helix have not been doubled over or pinched.

Compression Syndromes

Several compression syndromes involving the head and neck can be exacerbated during the perioperative period. The anterior scalene syndrome, the claviculocostal syndrome, and the pectoralis minor syndrome are similar and have one common denominator: their symptoms and signs are attributed to compression of the neurovascular bundle in the region of the cervical thoracic dorsal outlet.[46-48] The neurovascular bundle consists of the brachial plexus nerves and the subclavian vessels. Symptoms associated with the compression of the neurovascular bundle within the cervical thoracic dorsal outlet include pain and paresthesias. With repeated episodes of compression, patients usually describe their pain as deep, dull, vague aching in the arm and hand that appears during the early morning hours and may cause awakening. The distress may also occur after prolonged sitting or after extended periods of seated activities such as sewing or keyboarding.[46] The presence of a cervical rib or a large transverse process of C7 has been implicated in the etiology of these syndromes. The neurovascular bundle may be entrapped between the rib and clavicle. (See also the discussion of the preoperative evaluation of a patient with a thoracic outlet syndrome in Chapter 10.)

Either a cephalad shift of a patient's body, while the upper extremity is anchored alongside the trunk by wristlets, or caudad depression of the clavicle, as may occur when a patient relaxes in the sitting position, may diminish the retroclavicular space and compress the neurovascular bundle. Theoretically, a stiff pillow or blanket pressed firmly against the down-side clavicle of a patient in the lateral position may diminish the space within the thoracic outlet and compress the neurovascular bundle. These syndromes may be detected during the preoperative examination by having patients hyperabduct their arms. Bringing the hands together behind the head is one way to perform this maneuver (see Fig. 10–30, Chapter 10). Patients who are identified as having an outlet obstruction should be positioned carefully to avoid compression of the clavicles. Pulses in their upper extremities should be evaluated at frequent intervals if the arms must be placed alongside the head during surgery.

PREVENTING VASCULAR OBSTRUCTION

Placement of the head and neck at the limits of motion may produce anatomic changes that compress blood vessels and lymphatic vessels, causing ischemia or edema that may be life threatening. The two main vascular obstructions that may compromise blood flow or produce severe edema involve (1) the vertebral arteries and (2) venous and lymphatic drainage of the face, tongue, and oropharynx.

Vertebral Artery Obstruction

Excessive rotation with varying degrees of lateral flexion of the cervical spine can compress and occlude the vertebral artery on either the ipsilateral or the contralateral side. Faris and co-workers[49] found that the contralateral vertebral artery could be completely occluded with extreme rotation (and some obligatory lateral flexion) of the head and neck in healthy young male volunteers. As noted previously, there is a bony locking mechanism in the cervical spine by which the anterior tip of the upper articular process of the caudad vertebra impinges on the lateral process of the cephalad vertebra. This locking mechanism normally prevents excessive rotation and protects the vertebral artery as it ascends to the foramen magnum, but active assistance with rotation or forced passive rotation can overwhelm and eliminate the protection of the interlocking facets.[8] The facets may override one another and compress the vertebral artery as it passes cephalad through the foramina in the transverse processes of the first six cervical vertebrae.

Compression of the vertebral artery has been reported during chiropractic manipulations of the neck.[50, 51] Other abrupt changes in head position may lead to its compression and thrombosis, which, if not recognized and treated, may lead to progressive brain stem infarction.[52]

Venous and Lymphatic Obstruction

Excessive flexion of the head and neck may obstruct the venous and lymphatic outflow from the face, tongue, and oropharynx and cause severe perioperative edema of these structures.[53-56] In some cases of tongue and oropharyngeal edema, the use of oropharyngeal airways and other intraoral and pharyngeal appliances and tubes may contribute to the obstruction,[53] but a factor common in these cases is the placement of the head and neck in sufficient flexion to cause the chin to touch the chest. Several of these cases required tracheostomy. If possible, excessive flexion of the head and neck should not be used unless *absolutely necessary* to facilitate surgical exposure, and then only for shortest possible period of time. In most instances, neck flexion can be sufficient to provide adequate dorsal exposure for the surgeon when an examiner's finger can be passed easily between the mentum and the chest wall (see Fig. 12–4).

Postural Changes in Anatomic Relationships of Vessels in the Neck

Perioperative cannulation of central vessels in the neck may be complicated by altered anatomic relationships that occur as the position of the head is changed. Sulek and co-workers[57] demonstrated that rotation of the head during internal jugular vein cannulation markedly changes the relationship between the internal jugular vein and the ipsilateral carotid artery. Heads of volunteers were rotated from the vertical midline to 40 and 80 degrees contralateral to the side of the study. Reference points were located in the neck 2 and 4 cm cephalad to the clavicle. Using ultrasound images, they found that with the head in the sagittal plane of the torso the internal jugular vein overlapped the more dorsal carotid artery in the anteroposterior view by the same minimal degree at each of the two reference points. When the head was rotated, however, the degree of turn could change the anteroposterior overlap significantly. Vessel overlap was negligible with the head midline, evident with 40 degrees of rotation, and maximal with 80 degrees. Whereas most head rotation also involves some degree of rotation and flexion of the cervical spine (see earlier), the effect of lateral flexion on the anatomic relationships between the two vessels was not measured. The investigators speculated that the increased overlap of the internal jugular vein over the carotid artery that is caused by head rotation greater than 40 degrees increases the risk of inadvertent puncture of the carotid artery for the following reasons:

- The internal jugular vein is frequently collapsed by the maneuver of needle insertion.
- Collapse of the vein may enhance needle puncture of its posterior wall and penetration of the underlying carotid artery.

They recommended that the head be kept as close as possible to a midline position during catheterization of the internal jugular vein and that needed rotation not exceed 40 degrees during the procedure.[57]

PREOPERATIVE EVALUATION

The preoperative evaluation of every anesthetized patient should include a review of historical and current problems that may limit or impair head and neck motion and a physical examination that includes determination of comfortable ranges of motion and symptoms related to various positions of the head and neck.

A variety of problems may signal potential difficulties with positioning the head and neck of an anesthetized patient. Pertinent inquiry includes the following:

- Does *rheumatoid arthritis* extend to the cervical spine, temporomandibular joints, or cricoarytenoid interfaces? Is there evidence of pulmonary fibrotic interstitial lung disease? (As noted earlier, a strong correlation exists between the presence of lung involvement and atlantoaxial subluxation.)
- Has the spinal involvement of *ankylosing spondylitis* progressed to include the cervical spine? Have there been previous osteoporotic fractures of vertebral bodies? Are cervical nerve roots symptomatic for compression or entrapment?
- Does scarring from previous *head and neck surgery, burns, or radiation* impair range of motion? Is the cervical spine stable? Has it been fused?
- Are there symptoms of pain or numbness in the upper extremities that might be due to *compression syndromes*? Can they be exacerbated by abduction and elevation of the arms as when painting or changing a light bulb?
- Is there evidence of *limited range of head and neck motion*? What position(s) is usually used during night-time sleeping? With a pillow(s)? Is there difficulty with head turning to back up a car while driving? Does putting on a pullover sweater cause a problem? Has endotracheal intubation been difficult in the past?

Positive findings in a detailed physical examination of the head and neck may lead to additional tests. Simple screening maneuvers include the following:

- *Range of motion*: The comfortable limits

of range of motion for flexion, extension, lateral flexion, and rotation should be determined. At each end of the range of comfortable movement, does further movement provoke symptoms such as pain, paresthesias, or a change in consciousness? Any limitations should be carefully and clearly documented in the patient's chart.

- *Compression syndromes*: Can patients place their hands behind their heads comfortably (see Fig. 10–30)? Does the hyperabduction associated with this maneuver evoke symptoms of neurovascular compression?
- *The anticipated surgical position*: If questions exist about the propriety of the proposed surgical position, the patient should be asked to assume the intended posture as closely as possible during the preoperative evaluation. Can it be achieved with comfort? Does it evoke symptoms such as pain or paresthesias?

REFERENCES

1. Cailliet R: Functional anatomy. *In* Cailliet R (ed.): Neck and Arm Pain. Philadelphia, FA Davis, 1964.
2. Fielding JW: Cineroentgenography of the normal cervical spine. J Bone Joint Surg 39:1280, 1957.
3. Werne S: The possibilities of movement in the craniovertebral joints. Acta Orthop Scand 28:165, 1959.
4. Jones MD: Cineradiographic studies of the normal cervical spine. Calif Med 93:293, 1960.
5. Wilder BL: Hypothesis: The etiology of midcervical quadriplegia after operation with the patient in the sitting position. Neurosurgery 11:530, 1982.
6. Cottrell JE, Hassan NF, Hartung J, et al.: Hyperflexion and quadriplegia in the seated position. Anesthesiol Rev 5:34, 1985.
7. Gray H: The vertebral column. *In* Lewis WH (ed.): Anatomy of the Human Body, 24th ed. Philadelphia, Lea & Febiger, 1946.
8. Cailliet R: Neck and upper arm pain. *In* Cailliet R (ed.): Soft Tissue Pain and Disability. Philadelphia, FA Davis, 1977.
9. Dubuisson D: Nerve root damage and arachnoiditis. *In* Wall PD, Melzack R (eds.): Textbook of Pain, 2nd ed. New York, Churchill Livingstone, 1989.
10. Teng P: Spondylosis of the cervical spine with compression of the spinal cord and nerve roots. J Bone Joint Surg 42:392, 1960.
11. Murphy FL: Anaesthesia for orthopedic surgery. *In* Healy TEJ, Cohen PJ (eds.): Wylie and Churchill-Davidson's A Practice of Anaesthesia, 6th ed. London, Edward Arnold, 1995.
12. Saway PA, Blackburn WD, Halla JT, et al.: Clinical characteristics affecting survival in patients with rheumatoid arthritis undergoing cervical spine surgery. J Rheumatol 16:890, 1989.
13. Haynes RC Jr: Adrenocorticotropic hormone. *In* Gilman AG, Rall TW, Nies AS, Taylor (eds.): Goodman and Gilman's The Pharmacological Basis of Therapeutics, 8th ed. New York, Pergamon Press, 1990.
14. Hurd ER: Extra-articular manifestations of rheumatoid arthritis. Semin Arthritis Rheum 8:151, 1979.
15. Calin A, Porta J, Fries JF, et al.: Clinical history as a screening test for ankylosing spondylitis. JAMA 237:2613, 1977.
16. Ball J: The enthesopathy of ankylosis spondylitis. J Rheumatol 22:25, 1983.
17. Hunter T, Dubo HI: Spinal fractures complicating ankylosing spondylitis. Arthritis Rheum 26:751, 1983.
18. Adams RD, Petersdorf RG: Pyogenic infections of the central nervous system. *In* Thorn GW, Adams RD, Braunwald E, et al. (eds.): Harrison's Principles of Internal Medicine, 8th ed. New York, McGraw-Hill, 1977.
19. Beal JL, Lopin MC, Binnert M: Anesthesia for surgery of degenerative and abnormal cervical spine. Ann Fr Anesth Reanim 12:385, 1993.
20. Crosby ET, Lui A: The adult cervical spine: Implications for airway management. Can J Anaesth 37:77, 1990.
21. Lanza DC, Parnes SM, Koitni PJ, et al.: Early complications of airway management in head-injured patients. Laryngoscope 100:958, 1990.
22. Wells RM: Airway management in the blunt trauma patient: How important is the cervical spine? Can J Surg 35:27, 1992.
23. Lee C, Barnes A, Nagel EL: Neuroleptanalgesia for awake pronation of surgical patients. Anesth Analg 56:276, 1977.
24. Gordon EE: Natural history of the intervertebral disc. Arch Phys Med Rehabil 42:750, 1961.
25. Cloward RB: Lesions of the intervertebral disk and their treatment by interbody fusion method. Clin Orthop Rel Res 27:51, 1963.
26. Clarke E, Little JH: Cervical myelopathy: A contribution to its pathogenesis. Neurology 5:861, 1955.
27. Odom GL, Finney W, Woodhall B: Cervical disk lesions. JAMA 166:23, 1958.
28. Payne EE, Spillane JD: The cervical spine. Brain 80:571, 1957.
29. Perlow S, Markle P, Katz LN: Factors involved in the production of skeletal muscle pain. Arch Intern Med 53:814, 1934.
30. Cloward RB: The clinical significance of the sinuvertebral nerve of the cervical spine in relation to the cervical disc syndrome. J Neurol Neurosurg Psychiatry 23:321, 1960.
31. Holt EP: Fallacy of cervical discography. JAMA 188:799, 1964.
32. Hitselberger WE, House WF: A warning regarding the sitting position for acoustic neuroma surgery. Arch Otolaryngol 106:69, 1980.
33. Wilder BL: The etiology of midcervical quadriplegia after operation with the patient in the sitting position. Neurosurgery 11:530, 1982.
34. McCallum JE, Bennett MH: Electrophysiologic monitoring of spinal cord function during intraspinal surgery. Surg Forum 26:469, 1975.
35. McPherson RW, Szymanski J, Rogers MC: Somatosensory evoked potential changes in position-related brain stem ischemia. Anesthesiology 61:88, 1984.
36. Cottrell JE, Hassan NF, Hartung J, et al.: Hyperflexion and quadriplegia in the seated position. Anesthesiol Rev 5:34, 1985.
37. Levy WJ, York OH, McCaffrey M, et al.: Motor evoked potentials from transcranial stimulation of the motor cortex in humans. Neurosurgery 15:287, 1984.

38. Wiles JC, Hansen RC: Postoperative (pressure) alopecia. J Am Acad Dermatol 12:195, 1985.

39. Goerz G, Ippen H: Hautschaden bei bewebtlosen Patienten. Med Klin 63:2047, 1968.

40. Lawson NW, Mills NL, Ochsner JL: Occipital alopecia following cardiopulmonary bypass. J Thorac Cardiovasc Surg 71:342, 1976.

41. Anderton JM: Trauma associated with patient transfer and the positioning process. *In* Healy TEJ, Cohen PJ (eds.): Wylie and Churchill-Davidson's A Practice of Anaesthesia, 6th ed. London, Edward Arnold, 1995.

42. Givner I, Jaffe N: Occlusion of the central retinal artery following anaesthesia. Arch Ophthalmol 43:197, 1950.

43. Walkup HE, Murphy JD, Oteen NC: Retinal ischaemia with unilateral blindness—complications during pulmonary resection in prone position: Two cases. J Thorac Surg 23:174, 1952.

44. Hollenhorst RW, Svien HJ, Benoit CF: Unilateral blindness occurring during anaesthesia for neurosurgical operations. Arch Ophthalmol 52:819, 1954.

45. Jampol LM, Goldbaum M, Rosenberg M, et al.: Ischaemia of ciliary arterial circulation from ocular compression. Arch Ophthalmol 93:1311, 1975.

46. Gage M, Parnell H: Scalenus anticus syndrome. Am J Surg 73:252, 1947.

47. Nachlas IW: Scalenus anticus syndrome or cervical foraminal compression? South Med J 35:663, 1942.

48. Falconer MA, Weddel G: Costoclavicular compression of the subclavian artery and vein: Relation to scalenus anticus syndrome. Lancet 2:539, 1943.

49. Faris AA, Poser CM, Wikmore DW, et al.: Radiologic visualization of neck vessels in healthy men. Neurology 13:386, 1963.

50. Krueger BR, Okazaki H: Vertebral-basilar distribution infarction following chiropractic cervical manipulation. Mayo Clin Proc 55:322, 1980.

51. Schmidley JW, Koch T: The noncerebrovascular complications of chiropractic manipulation. Neurology 34:684, 1984.

52. Sherman DD, Hart RG, Easton JD: Abrupt change in head position and cerebral infarction. Stroke 12:2, 1981.

53. McAllister RG: Macroglossia—a positional complication. Anesthesiology 40:199, 1974.

54. Tattersall MP: Massive swelling of the face and tongue: A complication of posterior fossa surgery in the sitting position. Anaesthesia 39:1015, 1984.

55. Munshi CA, Dhamee MS, Ghandi SK: Postoperative unilateral facial oedema: A complication of acute flexion of the neck. Can Anaesth Soc J 31:197, 1984.

56. Ellis SC, Bryan-Brown CW, Hyderally H: Massive swelling of the head and neck. Anesthesiology 42:102, 1975.

57. Sulek CA, Gravenstein N, Blackshear RH, et al.: Head rotation during internal jugular vein cannulation and the risk of carotid artery puncture. Anesth Analg 82:125, 1996.

Patient Categories

Chapter 13

Extracorporeal Shock Wave Lithotripsy

Vinod Malhotra

BACKGROUND

Extracorporeal shock wave lithotripsy (ESWL) was introduced into clinical practice in the United States in February 1984 when the first treatment occurred at the Methodist Hospital in Indianapolis, Indiana. The first clinical model of the lithotriptor (Dornier HM3) employed a water bath in a steel tub and a metal gantry chair that suspended the patient in a sitting position. This first-generation lithotriptor is still commonly used, but it presents complex challenges of positioning and immersion.

Second- and third-generation lithotriptors have been developed since. The newer machines have eliminated the cumbersome wa- terbath and in the process have also elimi- nated positioning problems related to the gantry chair.[1]

POSITIONING CONCERNS AND THE WATERBATH LITHOTRIPTOR

For treatment in the familiar waterbath litho- triptor (Dornier HM3), the patient is placed in a gantry chair in a semi-sitting position (Fig. 13–1). The gantry chair is essentially a metal frame with foam padding that provides support under the shoulders and the hips while the flanks are exposed for shock wave treatment. The thighs and legs are supported

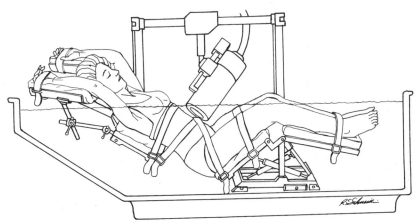

Figure 13–1

Patient in position in immersion tub ready for shock wave lithotripsy. (Modified from Riehle RA: Extracorporeal shock wave lithotripsy. Bull NY Acad Med 62:291, 1986.)

on metal plates with foam pads. These can be adjusted up or down, and the patient's lower limbs are secured with straps across mid-thighs and ankles. The head is supported in a U-shaped, firmly padded head rest that is detachable and slides in and out of the shoulder rest plate using a ratchet mechanism. The patient is positioned with a 15- to 30-degree side tilt toward the treatment side by using firm foam wedges under the contralateral shoulder. Finally, the patient is secured firmly in this position using a harness of straps straight across the lower chest and criss-crossed snugly across the abdomen (see Fig. 13–1). The gantry is then hoisted in the air and is pushed along the ceiling rails to be lowered hydraulically into the tub. This unique arrangement predisposes the patient to certain positioning risks (Table 13–1).

Mechanical Trauma

Even though the metal chair is padded, trauma can result from pressure or scraping metal edges. If general anesthesia is used, the anesthetized patient is lifted from the stretcher and transferred to the gantry chair. This arduous task predisposes personnel to lumbosacral strains and patients to impact injuries from hitting hard surfaces of the gantry chair.[2] The solution lies in using either sufficient numbers of personnel or a lifting device so that the patient is lifted gently and easily transferred to the gantry chair.[2] The head should be firmly supported during this transfer to avoid a whiplash injury to the neck. Until the patient is firmly secured to the gantry chair with appropriate restraining straps, attendants should stay on either side

of the patient to prevent a fall through the gap in the gantry chair. In many centers the attendants support the patient's weight by grasping towel slings passed under the lower back and buttocks until the restraining straps are secured.

The head rest should be adjusted to prevent extreme flexion or extension of the neck. The patient's head should also be adjusted for the body tilt to avoid neck strain due to excessive lateral flexion. With significant body tilt the patient's head may be unstable in the head rest. Therefore, a Velcro strap may be used across the forehead to safely retain the head in the support. The padding provided with the head rest is extremely firm, and an improperly adjusted head rest may cause pressure injuries to the greater occipital nerve as it passes over the nuchal ridge of the occipital bone. I have observed at least two such instances of occipital cephalgia lasting for 2 to 3 days. The pinna of the ear may also suffer pressure injury from the head support system.

The restraining straps should be taut but not too tight. Straps across the chest and abdomen that are excessively tightened may impair respiration in a spontaneously breathing patient during regional anesthesia or monitored anesthesia care. In spontaneously ventilating patients under regional anesthesia, Bromage and colleagues[3] described the development of a rapid, shallow pattern of respiration due to immersion and the restraining straps. If lower rib activity and abdominal wall motion are restricted by the restraining straps, the breathing becomes principally diaphragmatic. Sedation is likely to result in decreased ventilation and oxygenation. Restraining straps applied tightly across the thighs or ankles can impair regional circulation.

Table 13–1

Risks of Positioning During Lithotripsy

Cause	*Result*
Mechanical trauma	Pressure injury
	Scraping
	Hitting the metal frame
Outstretched arms	Brachial plexus injury
Sitting position, sympathetic block	Hypotension
	Incidence
	Spinal: 27%
	Epidural: 18%
	General: 13%
Position shift during procedure	Shock wave injury

Modified from Malhotra V: Extracorporeal shock wave lithotripsy. *In* Malhotra V (ed.): Anesthesia for Renal and Genitourinary Surgery. New York, McGraw-Hill, 1996. Reproduced with permission of The McGraw-Hill Companies.

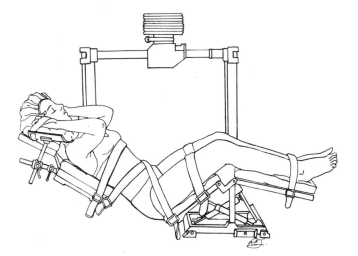

Figure 13–2

Patient is strapped into the support frame with the arms immobilized over the head. Brachial plexus stretch injuries can occur in this position. (Modified from Duval JO, Griffith DP: Epidural anesthesia for extracorporeal shock wave lithotripsy. Anesth Analg 64:544, 1985.)

Pressure injuries, when they occur, are commonly located in the gluteal region and over the coccyx. They usually result from thigh supports that are unevenly set, allowing the patient to tilt sideward and causing the metal edges to dig into the buttocks or the natal cleft.

In very obese patients, using biplanar fluoroscopy, bringing the kidney stone to lie in the focal zone of the lithotriptor is often very difficult. Consequently, it is not uncommon for the flank area of the patient to be wedged against the ellipse bowl at the bottom of the tub. Bruising or pressure necrosis may occur. Additionally, if the gantry is moved sideways when the flank is in contact with the bowl, serious scraping injuries to the back may occur. To avoid this complication, an assistant should frequently insert his or her hand between the patient's back and the ellipse during positioning to assure that the back and flank are free and clear of the ellipse. Sometimes, for the pathologically obese individual, there are no viable postural alternatives for successful lithotripsy, a procedure sufficiently less risky for them than is open renal surgery. Under these circumstances, minor complications that are easily treated are not sufficient reason to cancel the procedure.

Brachial Plexus Injuries

The Dornier HM3 lithotriptor provides arm supports that hold patients' arms above their heads using leather straps. Because arms are restrained overhead and the patient is in the sitting position, any downward movement of the torso may overstretch the arms and threaten the brachial plexus (Fig. 13–2).[4] There are anecdotal reports of brachial plexus injuries from many centers. In my experience, the patient in whom this is most likely to occur is young, lean, and female and undergoes general anesthesia. The use of muscle relaxants may further enhance the likelihood of such an injury. Protective measures include proper restraining of the patient, the use of regional anesthesia or monitored anesthesia care, and the use of alternative means of supporting the arms. I have found that applying inflatable flotation sleeves (water wings, arm floats) to the forearms allows the patient's arms to float by his or her sides and thereby reduces the likelihood of this injury (Fig. 13–3).

Postural Hypotension due to the Sitting Position

Sympathetic block and vasodilation with venous pooling during general, high epidural, or spinal anesthesia frequently result in postural hypotension as a supine patient is changed to the semi-sitting position. A 20% or greater decrease in blood pressure after repositioning is common.[5]

In my experience, the incidence of hypotension in patients undergoing general anesthesia is 13% as compared with 18% in patients undergoing epidural anesthesia and 27% in those undergoing spinal anesthesia.[5] Adequate hydration and prudent use of vasopressors help to minimize these changes. If hypotension occurs, one available solution is to immerse the patient in the bath up to the midthoracic level.

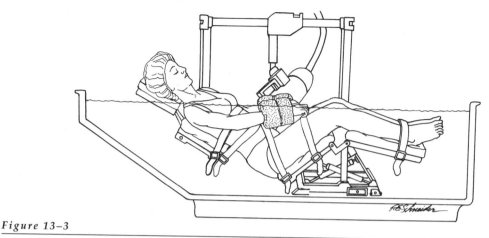

Figure 13–3

Inflatable flotation sleeves (arm floats, water-wings) around the forearms allow floating the patient's arms alongside the torso in the tub, thus avoiding stretch injuries to the brachial plexuses.

Shock Wave Injury due to Shift in Position

Although rare, this complication is likely if patients are incorrectly positioned in the gantry chair initially or if their positions change during the procedures. For example, pancreatic injury from misdirected shock waves has been reported.[6] This is usually accompanied by a significant increase in serum concentrations of amylase. Similarly, lower lung fields may be exposed to the shock wave if the patient is seated more vertically than normal in the gantry chair (Fig. 13–4).[7] To guard against these complications, the position of the patient should be monitored frequently during the procedure.

Physiologic Changes due to Positioning in Water

Cardiovascular Changes

Cardiovascular changes that occur as a result of immersion up to the clavicles increase central blood volume, central venous pressure

(CVP), and pulmonary artery pressures. Weber and co-workers[8] demonstrated that the increases in CVP and pulmonary artery pressure closely correlate with the level of immersion. With immersion to the clavicles, the CVP may increase by as much as 10 to 14 cm H_2O. Pulmonary artery pressures increase accordingly. In the semi-sitting position, CVP decreases slightly from its level in the supine position. Immersion to the umbilicus restores CVP to its level when the patient is supine. Immersion to the xiphoid process increases CVP level by only half as much as does immersion to the clavicles.[8]

In one study a decrease in cardiac output and an increase in mean arterial pressure and systemic vascular resistance were noted during ESWL performed with general anesthesia.[9] These and filling pressure changes are a source of serious concern for patients with advanced cardiovascular disease. Patients at risk for cardiac decompensation (i.e., those with congestive heart failure) are treated with minimal immersion so that only the shock

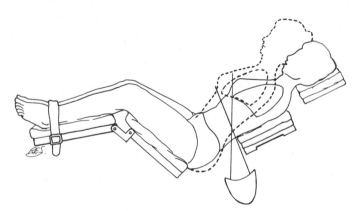

Figure 13–4

Patient positioned during lithotripsy in a Dornier HM3 lithotriptor. Solid lines depict a normal patient position in the gantry chair; the shock wave blast path is shown by the straight bold lines. The dashed line shows a more upright position of the patient, placing the lung field in the shock wave path. (From Malhotra V, Rosen RJ, Slepian RL: Life-threatening hypoxemia after lithotripsy in an adult due to shock wave–induced pulmonary contusion. Anesthesiology 75:529, 1991.)

Figure 13–5

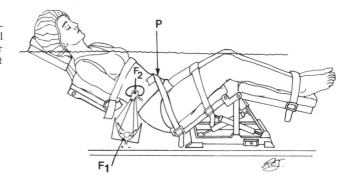

Diagram of the Dornier HM3 extracorporeal shock wave lithotriptor system. Underwater electromechanical shock waves generated at F_1 are concentrated on renal calculi positioned by remote control to lie at the point of secondary focus F_2. P indicates where hydrostatic measurements of surface abdominal pressure were made under the point of intersection of crossed restraining straps. (From Bromage PR, Bonsu AK, El-Fagih SR, Husain I: Influence of Dornier HM3 system on respiration during ESWL. Anesth Analg 68:363, 1989.)

wave entry site is covered by water. The exit site is left uncovered or is covered with a wet towel.

Pulmonary Changes

The harness tension before immersion has been shown to increase the abdominal surface pressure by approximately 15 cm H_2O (Fig. 13–5).[3] A study in healthy volunteers immersed in water up to their clavicles has shown that the hydrostatic pressure of water on the chest, estimated to be 20 cm H_2O with immersion to the clavicles, produces pulmonary changes that include decreases in expiratory reserve volume, expiratory lung volume, functional residual capacity, and vital capacity. The functional residual capacity may be decreased by 25% to 30%, and the vital capacity may be reduced by 20% to 30%.[10] In addition, because patients undergoing lithotripsy are strapped into the gantry chair and the straps across the abdomen are relatively

tight, they need to breathe with shallow, rapid respirations. Pulmonary blood flow increases. These contrasting changes promote a mismatch of ventilation and perfusion that, when combined with the altered breathing patterns, predisposes patients to hypoxemia if they are oversedated.

POSITIONING CONCERNS FOR NON-WATERBATH LITHOTRIPTORS

Patients are instructed to shift themselves onto the table for initial positioning. Frequently they may also be asked to turn prone. Hence, all sedatives should be avoided until the stone is focused to permit patient compliance.

Positioning extremely obese patients is a problem. Manufacturer guidelines for patient positioning in a Dornier model MFL 5000 lithotriptor are shown in Table 13–2. Extremely obese patients may have to be placed

Table 13–2

Positioning Hints*

Position	Suggestion
Supine	Upper third ureter
	Lower third ureter
	Renal
Prone	Middle third ureter
	L5 ureteral
	Obese patient with lower pole renal calculus
	Patient with nephrostomy tube in place
Extremely obese patient, prone	Place compression bank under patient to support abdomen
Kyphotic patient	Mild deformity: return to posteroanterior before going to lithotripsy
	Extreme deformity: position patient's head at opposite end of table
Thin patient, or lateral renal stone	Increase coupling pressure after fine tuning completed
	Use gel block

*Manufacturer's recommendations for Dornier MFL 5000.

Modified from Malhotra V: Extracorporeal shock wave lithotripsy. *In* Malhotra V (ed.): Anesthesia for Renal and Genitourinary Surgery. New York, McGraw-Hill, 1996. Reproduced with permission of The McGraw-Hill Companies.

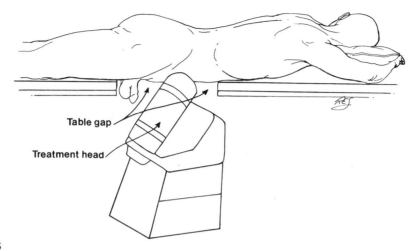

Figure 13–6

Patient lying prone on the table of a Dornier MFL 5000 lithotriptor. Note the large gap in the table that allows the treatment head to swivel into position to deliver shock waves. Pressure or pinching between table edges and the treatment head may result in damage to genitalia or the abdominal wall.

prone to permit the stone to be focused in the crosshairs of the biplanar fluoroscope. The prone position may cause respiratory distress for morbidly obese individuals, and some may not tolerate the posture at all. Simulation to focus the stone should be done before any anesthetic intervention. Occasionally, it may be impossible to bring the stone into focus in a person who is extremely obese.[11]

Because the gap in the table is fairly large and fixed, patients with a short torso are difficult to position because neither the shoulder nor hip find any support. Additionally, an injury can result from tissue getting caught in the gap between the table edges and the treatment head (Fig. 13–6). For example, in the prone position, the male genitalia may get squeezed, and in the very obese with a pendulous abdomen, the abdominal wall may get pinched. In the elderly the skin is very loose and sometimes, even in the supine position, skin folds may be pinched in this gap and contused.

REFERENCES

1. Rassweiler J, Henkel TO, Kohrmann KU, et al.: Lithotripter technology: Present and future. J Endourol 6:1, 1992.

2. Malhotra V: A modified stretcher-lifter device for safe transport of patients during lithotripsy. Anesth Analg 68:699, 1989.

3. Bromage PR, Bonsu AK, El-Fagih SR, Husain I: Influence of Dornier HM3 system on respiration during ESWL. Anesth Analg 68:363, 1989.

4. Duvall GO, Griffith DP: Epidural anesthesia for extracorporeal shock wave lithotripsy. Anesth Analg 64:544, 1985.

5. London RA, Kudlak T, Riehl RA: Immersion anesthesia for extracorporeal shock wave lithotripsy: Review of two hundred-twenty treatments. Urology 28:86, 1986.

6. Drach GW, Dretler S, Fair W, et al.: Report of the United States cooperative study of extracorporeal shock wave lithotripsy. J Urol 135:1127, 1986.

7. Malhotra V, Rosen RJ, Slepian RL: Life-threatening hypoxemia after lithotripsy in an adult due to shock wave–induced pulmonary contusion. Anesthesiology 75:529, 1991.

8. Weber W, Madler C, Kiel B, et al.: Cardiovascular effects of ESWL. *In* Gravenstein JS, Peter K (eds.): Extracorporeal Shock Wave Lithotripsy for Renal Stone Disease: Technical And Clinical Aspects. Boston, Butterworths, 1986, pp. 101–112.

9. Behnia R, Shanks, CA, Ovassapian A, et al.: Hemodynamic responses associated with lithotripsy. Anesth Analg 66:354, 1987.

10. Loellgen H, Von Neiding G, Howes R: Respiratory and hemodynamic adjustment during head out of water immersion. Int J Sports Med 1:25, 1980.

11. Malhotra V: Extracorporeal shock wave lithotripsy. *In* Malhotra V (ed.): Anesthesia for Renal and Genitourinary Surgery. New York, McGraw-Hill, 1996, pp. 111–149.

Chapter 14

Pathologic Obesity

Robert W. Vaughan
Marjorie Sue Vaughan

BACKGROUND

Anesthesiologists do not welcome enthusiastically the management of morbidly obese patients. Such reluctance is not without good reason. Despite thorough preparation, anesthetic care of this group of patients may be surprisingly difficult, even when a scheduled operative procedure seems minor. Frustrations frequently arise in the technical and mechanical aspects of management. Examples include transport to and from the operating room, placement of the intravenous and arterial catheters, problems in moving to and from the operating table as well as positioning on it, risks in control of the airway, and continuously securing a patent airway. The common presence of major organ system dysfunction makes the aforementioned problems even more complex. Thus, the challenges to safe and adept perioperative (preoperative, intraoperative, and postoperative) care include numerous difficulties and frustrations. To these problems, anesthesiologists must add concern regarding cardiopulmonary derangements that result from operative positioning (i.e., supine posture with retractors and intra-abdominal packs).[1]

In this chapter we review the definitions of obesity; enumerate the risks, independent of anesthesia and surgery, that this condition presents; review the physiologic consequences of severe obesity; and, finally, consider the anesthetic management related to specific positioning problems in this unique subset of the surgical population. Much has been learned during the hospitalization of obese patients that can be applied in the ambulatory surgical environment.

BASIC CONSIDERATIONS REGARDING MORBID OBESITY

With the advent of surgical procedures to treat morbid obesity (i.e., jejunoileal bypass and gastroplasty), anesthetic care has been customized for this specific subset of the adult obese population. Annually, 40,000 to 50,000 operations are performed in the United States for gynecologic, orthopedic, and intra-abdominal procedures in severely obese patients.

Defining and Measuring Obesity

Nutritionists, surgeons, internists, nurses, and anesthesiologists have suggested different ways to define obesity. Most indices of obesity are based on correlations between height and weight. Obesity exists by most definitions when an individual is 20% or more above the desirable weight designated by the Metropolitan Life Insurance Company's tables.[2] However, fat distribution may be more important than the total quantity of fat, as evidenced by an increased incidence of non–insulin-dependent diabetes mellitus and coronary heart disease in persons with elevated waist/hip ratios.[3] Moreover, a gradual rise in the percentage of fat develops as age increases.

Generally, measurement of fatness has employed indirect techniques (i.e., anthropometric, densitometric, dilutional), each with varying degrees of accuracy and reliability. Example measurements include waist/hip ratio, skin fold thickness, and water immersion. Densitometric and dilutional techniques now serve principally as tools for clinical research.

However, for the clinician who must measure degrees of fatness quickly and with time urgency (i.e., emergency operations), two easily calculated numbers are useful. One is the body mass index (BMI). BMI = weight (in kilograms) ÷ height^2 (in meters).[4] Ranges from BMI calculations in kilograms per square meter are defined as nonobese, less than 25; overweight, 26 to 29; and obese, greater than 30.[2] BMI correlates maximally with obesity and minimally with height. The second measurement, and the one that is the *most useful clinically*, is the Broca index to calculate ideal body weight. Patient height (in centimeters) − 100 = ideal body weight (in kilograms). For a typical morbidly obese patient with a weight of 327 pounds (147 kg) and height of 64 inches (162.5 cm), the calculated BMI would approximate 58 kg/m^2 whereas the ideal body weight would be 62.5 kg. The accepted definition for morbid (pathologic) obesity describes the individual who is twice the ideal weight for height. Therefore, in the above example, that 147-kg patient is definitely obese (BMI >30) and also morbidly obese (greater than twice the ideal weight of 62.5 kg).

Morbidly obese patients represent a specific subset of the total obese adult population; however, there are two categories of obesity within the morbid group. Subjects with normal levels of arterial carbon dioxide tension are referred to as having *simple obesity*. Those individuals with hypoventilation and resting hypercarbia are identified as having the *obesity-hypoventilation syndrome* (OHS).[5] Whereas this last group represents a fascinating syndrome (also referred to as pickwickian), such individuals are rare (5% to 10%) in the morbidly obese population. The importance of understanding the difference between the two groups lies in recognizing that the pickwickian syndrome, or OHS, is characterized by more severe biventricular cardiac enlargement, polycythemia, severe hypoxemia, hypercapnia, decreased vital capacity, and reduced maximum ventilatory ventilation.[6] Nevertheless, the principal ventilatory impairment in OHS remains alveolar hypoventilation completely independent of intrinsic (obstructive or restrictive) pulmonary disease. Further, simple obesity cannot be differentiated from OHS by observation alone. Associated circulatory abnormalities of OHS and simple obesity include pulmonary hypertension, right ventricular enlargement, and extreme hypervolemia.[6] All these findings are secondary to hypoventilation and can be exaggerated perioperatively by various position changes, especially the supine or head-down postures.

Risks

Studies have determined that a person who ranks above the 85th percentile in terms of body mass index (i.e., BMI of 38) has a significantly higher prevalence of hypertension, hypercholesterolemia, and non–insulin-dependent diabetes mellitus.[7] Mortality from cancers of the colon, rectum, and prostate gland in obese men and from cancers of the breast, uterus, ovaries, gallbladder, and biliary passages in obese women is greater than would normally be predicted in members of either sex who are not obese.[8, 9] Moreover, statistics from various studies indicate that the greater the degree of overweight, the higher the excess death rate, particularly in younger people and especially in males. Drenick and associates[10] analyzed survival of a group of 200 morbidly obese men (average weight of 143.5 kg and age range of 23 to 70 years) admitted to a Veterans Administration–sponsored weight control program between 1960 and 1970 (mean follow-up period 7.6 years). Techniques employing life expectancy tables were used to compare the mortality among these men with that among men in the general population; results demonstrated a 12-fold excess mortality rate for obese men 25 to 35 years of age (i.e., an exceptional risk in younger men). Additionally, a sixfold excess mortality was found in the group 35 to 44 years of age. Cardiovascular disease was the most common cause of death in the obese, with an almost 30% higher rate when all men in the United States were considered. These investigators concluded that the pathologically obese state causes the commonly occurring degenerative cardiovascular diseases to begin at an earlier age, to progress more rapidly, and to become life threatening more frequently.

Finally, obesity becomes a causal agent for a variety of chronic health problems, including cerebrovascular accidents, diabetes mellitus, atherosclerosis, cholelithiasis, cirrhosis, and cardiac disease.

RESPIRATORY AND CARDIOVASCULAR CONSEQUENCES OF OBESITY

Obesity increases resting alveolar ventilation commensurate with increased oxygen uptake

Effect Of Position On Lung Volumes

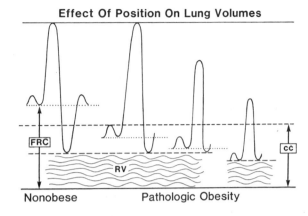

Nonobese   Pathologic Obesity

Figure 14–1

Effect of change in position on various lung volumes in a nonobese subject compared with a markedly obese subject. FRC = functional residual capacity; RV = residual volume; cc = closing capacity. (Redrawn from Vaughan RW: Pulmonary and cardiovascular derangements in the obese patient. *In* Anesthesia and the Obese Patient. Brown, PR Jr., ed.: *In* Contemporary Anesthesia Practice, vol. 5. Philadelphia, FA Davis, 1982.)

and carbon dioxide production. Because body surface area increases proportionally, obese subjects are not hypermetabolic. However, excessive fat produces additional deleterious effects on pulmonary mechanics, gas exchange, and circulatory function.

Severe obesity reduces respiratory system compliance. In this regard, obesity of the chest wall and abdomen can play a major detrimental role on gas exchange. Lung volumes are severely reduced in all but the erect posture (Fig. 14–1). Furthermore, the reduction in total respiratory system compliance results primarily from abnormal chest wall compliance. Because the energy cost of breathing is elevated and exceeds the increase in mechanical work, the calculated respiratory muscle efficiency decreases. Progressively, a severe preload (increased abdominal pressure) for inspiration must be added to the elevated afterload (abnormal respiratory system compliance).

Predictably, reduced compliance coupled with inspiratory muscle weakness profoundly affects certain lung volume measurements. Functional residual capacity (FRC), vital capacity, and total lung capacity can diminish as a consequence of the reduction in respiratory compliance. Reduction in both inspiratory capacity and expiratory reserve volume (ERV) decreases vital capacity. Although ERV decreases, residual volume either rises or remains unchanged. Consequently, from the previously described pulmonary changes one would predict abnormal pulmonary gas exchange. In those obese patients with minimal loss of ERV, ventilation to lower zones in the lung can be preserved. But in subjects with marked loss of ERV, what results is underventilation of the well-perfused lower regions of the lung with subsequent hypoxemia on

room air. Such severe hypoxemia from ventilation/perfusion mismatch occurs in awake obese patients with progressive loss of FRC.

Eucapnic, hypoxic obese subjects display shunting, probably through closed peripheral lung units, concomitant with low ventilation/perfusion ratios with increased venous admixture.[5] Coupled with these adverse pulmonary changes and the principal circulatory abnormalities of obesity, pulmonary gas exchange becomes severely deranged even with modest changes in positions. For example, in the obese person an increase exists in total, central, pulmonary, and cardiac blood volumes, with systemic and pulmonary blood volumes distributed as in the normal nonobese person. An increased cardiac output exists, and sometimes an elevated left ventricular end-diastolic pressure is noted as well. In addition, blood pressure, cardiac output, and blood volume combine to increase the actual work performed by the heart and to raise myocardial oxygen consumption.[11] Obesity, associated disturbances of lipid metabolism, and, perhaps, inactivity, may act through the common pathway of atherosclerosis to narrow coronary arteries supplying oxygen to an excessively worked, inadequately perfused myocardium. At the point where oxygen demand outstrips supply, clinical evidence of coronary artery disease (i.e., angina pectoris, myocardial infarction) can become manifest and even life threatening. Sudden death is a further possibility and has been documented in the pathologically obese.

ANESTHETIC MANAGEMENT

As previously suggested, even in the awake state, obese subjects manifest reduction in

FRC at the expense of ERV. When the supine position is assumed, a further decrease (10% to 40%) in FRC results in both nonobese and obese subjects. However, in the latter the reduced lung volume often places FRC below closing capacity so that airway closure occurs during tidal ventilation. Hypoxemia results from the increased venous admixture. If head-down tilt is added, further loss of FRC occurs so that more venous admixture results, accentuating the already severe arterial hypoxemia. Moreover, in the morbidly obese the blood volume, cardiac output, and oxygen consumption increase as excess body weight increases. A concomitant rise occurs in pulmonary artery pressure as well as in pulmonary artery wedge pressure. Sustained high levels of cardiac work seem to account for the ultimate development of left ventricular, and even biventricular, hypertrophy that has been observed at autopsy. In the pickwickian morbidly obese patients, severe hypoxemia and hypercapnia produce pulmonary hypertension. One could speculate that extravascular lung water can be expected to increase in a manner analogous to that in chronic obstructive lung disease with pulmonary hypertension. Lung compliance, already diminished, would be reduced still further. The distribution of ventilation would be even more abnormal, contributing to dangerous hypoxemia.

Paul and associates[12] studied the circulatory and respiratory effects of change in posture from sitting to supine in 11 morbidly obese patients scheduled for gastric bypass operations. In the supine position, further increases occurred in cardiac output, pulmonary artery pressure, and pulmonary artery wedge pressure. Oxygen consumption, contrary to observations in nonobese patients, also significantly increased in this position. No significant increase occurred in the alveolar to arterial oxygen tension gradient in the supine position, as compared with the sitting position. These investigators suggested that the principal factor in the tolerance to the supine position in these otherwise healthy obese individuals was the ability of the heart to respond to the greater preload and work of breathing by increasing cardiac output. This response minimizes the rise of filling pressure and the potential for pulmonary congestion. In addition, such cardiac compensation essentially masks the effects of increasing intrapulmonary shunting on arterial oxygenation. However, in those patients whose cardiac reserve is inadequate to meet the greater work of

breathing or the shift of blood to the central locations, appropriate increases in cardiac output might not occur. Clinical evidence of pulmonary congestion and hypoxemia would develop. Hypoxemia, in turn, would lead to reduced responsiveness of the central respiratory control mechanisms, leading to hypoventilation, hypercapnia, and acidosis. These changes would subsequently (1) increase pulmonary vascular resistance, (2) increase extravascular pulmonary water, (3) decrease compliance, and (4) further increase work of breathing, resulting in a vicious cycle.[13]

Such a syndrome in morbid obesity has been described by Tsueda and associates.[14] They reported an unusual complication that was observed in two morbidly obese subjects who were critically sensitive to position change. One patient died on assuming the supine position. The other, who was successfully resuscitated, was managed uneventfully during a minor emergency surgical procedure. Such a simple change to the supine position in severely obese subjects can precipitate disastrous consequences even before anesthesia and surgery.

The Intraoperative Period

In obese patients, the added effect of general anesthesia (i.e., reduced FRC) increases the likelihood of premature airway closure; gas trapping results as tidal ventilation moves within or below closing capacity. Such theoretical possibilities related to intraoperative oxygenation in the obese subject have been examined. Vaughan and Wise[1] studied 64 morbidly obese but otherwise healthy adults during intra-abdominal surgery to delineate patterns of pulmonary gas exchange. An inspired oxygen concentration of 40% did not uniformly produce adequate arterial oxygen (PaO_2). Furthermore, and without changes of the operative position, the placement of subdiaphragmatic abdominal laparotomy packs resulted in a consistent fall in PaO_2 in each patient (i.e., average PaO_2 of 65 mm Hg with a fraction of inspired oxygen [FIO_2] of 0.4). With a change of posture from horizontal supine to a 15-degree head-down position during operation and anesthesia, there was a significant reduction to a mean PaO_2 of 73 mm Hg; 75% of patients demonstrated PaO_2 values of less than 80 mm Hg.

In addition, Hedenstierna and colleagues[15] evaluated pulmonary variables in 10 morbidly obese subjects before and during general anesthesia and artificial ventilation. Airway closure, FRC, total efficiency of ventilation, and gas exchange (i.e., PaO_2 and $PaCO_2$) were measured. During spontaneous ventilation awake obese subjects demonstrated normal closing capacity and reduced FRC and airway closure within tidal ventilation, with resultant decrease in PaO_2. During anesthesia closing capacity was unaltered, but FRC was reduced further, causing marked hypoxemia. These investigators concluded that airway closure explains the severe increase in alveolar to arterial oxygen tension difference in obese subjects during anesthesia. Subsequently, Santesson[16] studied 8 morbidly obese patients to quantify venous admixture to ascertain whether improved oxygenation could be obtained by raising FRC with tidal ventilation of 5 to 7 mL/kg lean body weight. With two different levels of positive end-expiratory pressure (PEEP), 10 to 15 cm H_2O, he demonstrated that venous admixture can be reduced with the application of PEEP. However, because of a coincident fall in cardiac output, the oxygen availability (arterial oxygen content × cardiac output) falls, as PEEP is increased.

To corroborate Santesson's findings, Salem and co-workers[17] evaluated the influence of PEEP (10 to 12 cm H_2O) superimposed on intermittent large tidal volume (i.e., 1000 to 1200 mL) positive-pressure ventilation in 10 supine obese patients intraoperatively. Consonant with previous findings, a significant increase in arterial oxygen tension occurred when PEEP was discontinued. They concluded that under these conditions the use of PEEP superimposed on large tidal volume ventilation could not be assumed to produce any beneficial effect to improve arterial oxygenation. Oxygen tension and/or saturation must be measured to titrate PEEP during operations in morbidly obese patients.

The combined effects of obesity, anesthesia, and surgery on cardiorespiratory function could be expected to produce adverse oxygenation. Certainly, in those obese patients with reduced lung volumes, mismatches of ventilation and perfusion, increased pulmonary venous admixtures, and lower arterial oxygen tensions than predicted for age would be expected during any operative procedures. Superimposing the effects of the anesthetic induction on those of the supine operative posture would further reduce FRC, with additional alveolar units becoming overperfused in relation to ventilation and, thereby, augmenting pulmonary venous admixture. Moreover, potent inhalation anesthetics and certain fixed agents (e.g., sodium thiopental) reduce cardiac output both by vasodilatation and by a negative inotropic effect, thereby decreasing mixed venous oxygen tension further. As a result, PaO_2 could be dangerously reduced.

If, to this scenario of consequential hypoxemia, one adds the effects of surgical exposure and laparotomy packs, with retractors that can further reduce lung volume and restrict venous return, cardiac output could fall and further diminish oxygenation. For these valid reasons, when intra-abdominal surgery is planned in a morbidly obese patient, *continuous monitoring of arterial oxygenation* should be done from induction of anesthesia through emergence. Noninvasive pulse oximetry and capnography combined with intra-arterial monitoring have proved exceptionally useful in optimizing anesthetic care in morbidly obese patients.

POSTOPERATIVE CARE

Vaughan and associates[18] have demonstrated that some obese patients manifest significant reduction in arterial oxygen tension on postoperative days 1 and 2. At the reduced levels of PaO_2 that were demonstrated, hemoglobin/oxygen saturation functions on the more vertical portion of the oxyhemoglobin dissociation curve. Tissue hypoxia can easily occur. Not only do the patient's general physical status and the operative site affect postoperative oxygenation, but the surgical incision can contribute as well to postoperative hypoxemia.[19] For example, obese patients with vertical operative incisions have more prolonged periods of postoperative hypoxemia than do those with transverse incisions (Fig. 14–2).[19] Furthermore, Vaughan and Wise[20] studied the effect of position change on blood gas exchange both preoperatively and postoperatively in 22 morbidly obese but otherwise healthy nonsmoking young women who had no evidence of cardiorespiratory disease. There was a statistically significant decrease in arterial oxygen tension with assumption of the supine versus the semirecumbent position on postoperative days 1 and 2 (Fig. 14–3). However, no position difference was demonstrated in any variable by the third postoperative day.

Craig and colleagues[21] studied unanesthetized adults and related the effect of a change

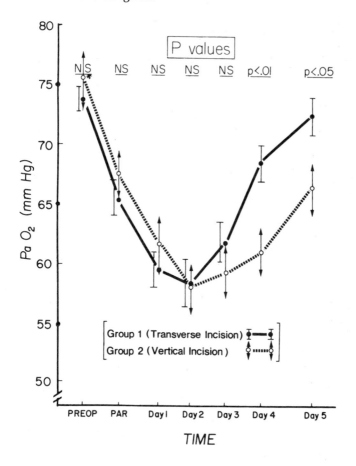

Figure 14–2

Graphic presentation of the fall in PaO_2 (mm Hg) with time postoperatively dependent on operative incision. Each point represents the mean of values for 23 patients in group 1 (solid line) or 25 patients in group 2 (interrupted line) with appropriate ± standard error of the mean (SE). (From Vaughan RW, Wise L: Choice of abdominal operative incision in the obese patient: A study using blood gas measurements. Ann Surg 181:829, 1975.)

Figure 14–3

Arterial oxygen tension (PaO_2, mm Hg) in 22 morbidly obese female subjects in the semirecumbent position (open bars) and the supine position (shaded bars) preoperatively and on postoperative days 1 through 3. All values were obtained with the patients at rest and breathing room air. NS = not significant. (From Vaughan RW, Wise L: Postoperative arterial blood gas measurement: Effect of position on gas exchange. Ann Surg 182:705, 1975.)

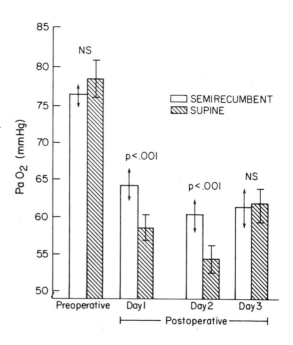

in posture to pulmonary gas exchange. In 22 normal subjects, they evaluated change in arterial oxygenation as well as change in the relationship of breathing level (FRC + tidal volume) to closing volume after change in position from seated to supine. They postulated that alterations of gas exchange from the seated to supine position would result from the interaction of three factors: (1) increased cardiac output in the supine position with its effects on mixed venous oxygen content; (2) increased uniformity of perfusion distribution and regional ventilation/perfusion relationships in the lung in the supine position; and (3) increased involvement of lung volume by airway closure in the supine position, tending to retard dependent zone ventilation and to lower dependent zone ventilation/perfusion relationships. Arterial oxygenation would be improved by the first two factors but impaired by the third. Because Craig's study involved adults who were not subjected to surgery, the results of Vaughan and Wise[20] that demonstrated a position difference for 48 hours postoperatively could be explained on the basis of adverse changes in the FRC minus closing capacity relationship.[19] A likely pathophysiologic explanation is that in an obese patient the additive effect of (1) reduced lung volume preoperatively, (2) the abdominal vertical incision with its attendant pain and splinting, and (3) the supine posture cause the increased involvement of the lung volume by airway closure for the first 48 hours after operation. As FRC returns toward preoperative levels by postoperative day 3, the overall effect of position change on arterial oxygenation can no longer be demonstrated. Our study indicates that maintaining severely obese subjects in the semirecumbent instead of the supine posture during the early postoperative period becomes a valuable, simple, noninvasive therapeutic tool to improve pulmonary gas exchange. The clinical implications for physicians and nurses concerned with postoperative recovery and intensive care show the need for heightened emphasis on the importance of positioning in obese patients.

In addition, the effect of lateral positioning on postoperative oxygenation in morbidly obese patients has been addressed as well. Our group studied 26 obese patients undergoing gastric partitioning operations to evaluate the effect on arterial blood gas levels of (1) lateral posture (left or right decubitus with the head elevated 30 degrees), (2) semirecum-

bent (45 degrees head-up angle), and (3) supine (left or right side with the head not elevated).[22] Patients were randomly assigned to either the right or left side-lying position for postoperative recovery room care. As previously demonstrated, the postoperative PaO_2 values were significantly lower than the preoperative values independent of any of the three positions. No significant difference between groups (right vs. left) occurred in either the semirecumbent (45-degree angle) or the supine postures. Therefore, considering postoperative oxygenation, the left or right lateral posture with head either level or elevated 30 degrees compares favorably with the semirecumbent position (45-degree head up, the "state of the art" postoperative posture) for morbidly obese patients.

No data exist that measure the pulmonary derangements and cardiovascular aberrations in the prone posture in morbidly obese patients. Nevertheless, it would be predicted from our previous studies that in the prone posture the morbidly obese patient would need careful continuous monitoring of oxygenation and arterial pressure. Moreover, extreme care should be exercised in using the prone position in the operative environment in such subjects. Continuous monitoring of airway management, cardiovascular stability, and pulmonary lung volume changes accompanied by controlled mechanical ventilation would indeed present challenges for any anesthesiologist.

Finally, an added caution should be offered for the postoperative transport of severely obese patients. We preferentially use a roller to facilitate transfer from operating room table to the patient's bed while maintaining continuous oxygen by face mask or endotracheal tube. Immediate attention is then directed at providing 30 degrees of head elevation during the patient's transport to the postanesthesia care unit. We routinely transport obese postoperative patients with supplemental oxygen by face mask or endotracheal tube. Such careful perioperative attention to the adverse effects of supine posture on oxygenation can now be expected to improve total perioperative care during induction of anesthesia, postanesthetic transport, and subsequent recovery.[23]

CONCLUSIONS

Anesthetic management should concentrate on the various aspects of preoperative, intraoperative, and postoperative care that are most likely to be abnormal in the morbidly obese patient. Because of the deranged cardiovascular and pulmonary dynamics associated with obesity, changes in position have predictably adverse consequences on lung volume, work of breathing, ventilation/perfusion ratios, and oxygenation. Certainly during the intraoperative period, whether electing regional or general anesthesia, the anesthesiologist must take into consideration the many variables that influence intraoperative oxygenation (e.g., regional distribution of blood flow with regional or general anesthesia, operative procedure, and surgical abdominal packing). Moreover, in a morbidly obese patient after any intra-abdominal procedure, a significant positional effect on oxygenation exists for 48 hours. Such a patient is optimally managed with the head elevated 30 to 45 degrees or in the lateral decubitus position with the head elevated or supine with supplemental oxygenation to improve gas exchange.

With knowledge of the deranged cardiorespiratory physiology unique to the morbidly obese, anesthetic management can be planned commensurate with care tailored by each member of the perioperative team (e.g., operating room nurses, anesthesiologists, surgeons, recovery room nurses, and intensive care nurses when necessary).[24] Attention to the important implications of positioning in such an unusual subset of obese patients could have a salutary effect on overall outcome. Such knowledge and understanding of the effects of posture on cardiorespiratory physiology will prove more conducive to safe care in these patients than in few others managed in the practice of anesthesiology.

A final admonition seems warranted. Lessons learned in the inpatient acute hospital environment apply just as importantly to the ambulatory surgical setting for all severely obese patients irrespective of operative procedure or surgical service.

REFERENCES

1. Vaughan RW, Wise L: Intraoperative arterial oxygenation in obese patients. Ann Surg 184:35, 1976.
2. Bray GA: Who are the obese? Obese Patient 9:5, 1976.
3. Krotkiewski M, Bjorntorp P, Sjostrom L, Smith U: Impact of obesity on metabolism in men and women: Importance of regional adipose tissue distribution. J Clin Invest 72:1150, 1983.
4. Keys A, Fidanza F, Karvonen MJ: Indices of relative weight and obesity. J Chronic Dis 25:329, 1972.
5. Rochester DF, Enson Y: Current concepts in the pathogenesis of obesity-hypoventilation syndrome: Mechanical and circulatory factors. Am J Med 57:402, 1974.
6. Burwell CS, Robin ED, Whaley RD, Bickelmann AG: Extreme obesity associated with alveolar hypoventilation: A pickwickian syndrome. Am J Med 21:811, 1956.
7. Garrison RJ, Castelli WP: Weight and thirty year mortality of men in the Framingham Study. Ann Intern Med 103:1006, 1985.
8. Lavecchia C, Franceschi S, Gallus G: Prognostic features of endometrial cancer in estrogen users and obese women. Am J Obstet Gynecol 144:387, 1982.
9. Snowdon DA, Phillips RL, Choi W: Diet, obesity and risk of fatal prostatic cancer. Am J Epidemiol 120:244, 1984.
10. Drenick EJ, Bale GS, Seltzer F, Johnson DG: Excessive mortality and causes of death in morbidly obese men. JAMA 243:443, 1980.
11. Vaughan RW, Conahan TJ: Cardiopulmonary consequences of morbid obesity. Life Sci 26:2119, 1980.
12. Paul DR, Hoyt JL, Boutras AR: Cardiovascular and respiratory changes in response to change of posture in the very obese. Anesthesiology 45:73, 1976.
13. Sharp JT, Henry JP, Sweany SK: The total work of breathing in normal and obese men. J Clin Invest 43:728, 1964.
14. Tsueda K, Debrand M, Zeok SS, et al.: Obesity supine death syndrome: Report of two morbidly obese patients. Anesth Analg 58:345, 1979.
15. Hedenstierna G, Santesson L, Norlander O: Airway closure and distribution of inspired gas in the extremely obese, breathing spontaneously and during anesthesia with intermittent positive pressure ventilation. Acta Anaesth Scand 20:334, 1976.
16. Santesson J: Oxygen transport and venous admixture in the extremely obese: Influence of anaesthesia and artificial ventilation with and without positive end-expiratory pressure. Acta Anaesth Scand 20:387, 1976.
17. Salem MR, Dalal FY, Zygmunt MP: Does PEEP improve intraoperative arterial oxygenation in grossly obese patients? Anesthesiology 48:280, 1978.
18. Vaughan RW, Engelhardt RC, Wise L: Postoperative hypoxemia in obese patients. Ann Surg, 180:877, 1974.
19. Vaughan RW, Wise L: Choice of abdominal operative incision in the obese patient: A study using blood gas measurements. Ann Surg 81:829, 1975.
20. Vaughan RW, Wise L: Postoperative arterial blood gas measurement: Effect of position on gas exchange. Ann Surg 182:705, 1975.
21. Craig DB, Wahba WH, Don H, et al.: "Closing volume" and its relationship to gas exchange in seated and supine positions. J Appl Physiol 31:717, 1971.
22. Vaughan RW, Vaughan MS: Morbid obesity: Implications for anesthetic care. Semin Anesth 3:218, 1984.
23. Vaughan RW, Vaughan MS: Anaesthetic management of patients with massive obesity. In General Anaesthesia, 5th ed. London, Butterworths, 1989, p. 749.
24. Brown BR Jr: Anesthesia and the Obese Patient. In Contemporary Anesthesia Practice, vol. 5. Philadelphia, FA Davis, 1982.

Pediatrics

S c o t t   E .   L e B a r d

BACKGROUND

Positioning the pediatric patient for surgery, though in many ways similar to the processes used for adults, may present different and unique concerns for members of the anesthesia care team. Mainly related to physiologic differences between adult and child, these concerns also involve the dissimilarities in physical sizes with their resulting impact on equipment requirements. The intention of this chapter, therefore, is to (1) briefly mention some physiologic aspects that may influence positioning concerns, (2) review management issues for the positions most commonly used in pediatric surgical procedures, and (3) mention some special situations that might warrant additional considerations.

PHYSIOLOGIC DIFFERENCES: PEDIATRIC VERSUS ADULT

The pediatric patient differs physiologically from an adult patient in multiple ways. The most significant differences pertaining to problems of positioning relate to differences in aspects of normal growth and development, in temperature regulation, and in the cardiorespiratory systems.

Growth and Development

The head circumference of an average term newborn is approximately 35 cm. With normal growth and development it increases to approximately 47 cm by 2 years of age, slowly growing during the remainder of childhood to an average adult head size of 53 cm, ap-

proximately 50% greater than at birth.[1] In contrast, there is a 20- to 30-fold increase in weight from newborn to adulthood. The weight of an average term newborn is 3.2 kg.[2] With normal growth and development, the average 1-year-old weighs 10 kg, the 3-year-old, 15 kg, the 10-year-old, 32 kg, and the theoretical average adult, 70 kg. Accordingly, the infant and toddler have a proportionately increased anteroposterior diameter of the head in comparison to the body, much more so than for the adult.

These growth differences impact equipment considerations during positioning. Whereas by 2 to 3 years of age most of the head supports used with adults can be easily fashioned for use in children, for infants this may not be true. Because the body size is not always proportionate to an adult, special equipment is often required for certain positions in infants and toddlers, or modifications are made to available equipment to meet the patient needs. Examples of how these modifications affect positioning management for the lithotomy, sitting, and lateral positions are considered in subsequent sections.

Temperature Regulation

Maintenance of body temperature is influenced by the ability to produce heat, distribute it throughout the body, and control its loss to the environment. Most temperature autoregulation occurs within the hypothalamus, with feedback messages sent to control cutaneous circulation, body activity, and pulmonary ventilation. Owing to differences in body composition in the infant when compared with an adult, the infant has only a finite ability to autoregulate his or her temperature for the following reasons: First, an infant has limited ability to produce heat because shivering thermogenesis is essentially nonexistent before age 3 months.[3] When heat production is needed, an increase in brown fat metabolism is required. Brown fat, however, accounts for only 2% to 3% of the body weight in an infant. Hence, this aspect of temperature regulation is somewhat limited.

Second, the ability to distribute heat throughout the body may be limited in the infant by cardiac output. Due to characteristics of an infant's or toddler's myocardial muscle, cardiac output is more related to heart rate than stroke volume. When a relatively slow heart rate is present, then further increasing the heart rate may influence heat distribution. However, if the normal physiologic state of tachycardia is present in the infant, there will be less ability to further impact distribution by manipulating cardiac output.

Finally, because heat loss usually occurs either through the skin or through increased ventilation, the infant is more predisposed to becoming hypothermic than is the adult.

- The skin of an infant, especially a premature infant, contains less keratin than does adult skin. Thus there is more evaporative water loss with concomitant heat loss in the infant.[4] The infant head accounts for approximately 20% of the body surface area, may need to be exposed for the operation, and provides an additional site for surface heat loss.
- Minute ventilation is high relative to body weight in the infant, resulting in increased evaporative water loss in a standard open breathing circuit.[5]

Therefore, when positioning a child, especially if the procedure is anticipated to take an extended period of time, efforts should be made to maintain an appropriate temperature. This may be done by having the operating room warm until the child is in the desired position and draped. A heating mattress, overhead heating lamps, or a head cover (plastic bag or stockinette cap) may be useful during this time. After positioning, if the surgical procedure and position allows for it, a forced-air heating device may be placed so as to optimize temperature stability.

Cardiorespiratory Systems

Pertaining to the circulatory system, there are two main factors that may influence position-

ing management in anesthetized infants or toddlers.

First, as mentioned earlier, owing to characteristics in the infant's or toddler's myocardial muscle, cardiac output is more influenced by heart rate than stroke volume. Therefore, the ability to increase cardiac output by increasing contractility is limited in this age group.

Second, all halogenated inhalation agents have the ability to depress myocardial contractility (halothane > isoflurane) and may depress baroreceptor reflexes (halothane > isoflurane). Therefore, even if a younger child were able to increase cardiac output to a greater extent than an older child or adult by increasing myocardial contractility, volatile anesthetic agents might depress this ability.

Because of these factors, exaggerated hemodynamic compromise is possible during positioning of the young pediatric patient who may be unable to compensate for significant postural changes (e.g., being placed upright).

Considering the respiratory system, an infant is more likely than an older child or adult to experience malpositioning of the endotracheal tube because the trachea is anatomically shorter. Consequently, once the final desired patient position is attained, auscultation of the lung fields should be performed to assure continued proper placement of the endotracheal tube for adequate gas exchange throughout the procedure. If the endotracheal tube does become displaced during the procedure, the infant or toddler is then at increased risk for hypoxemia because the dynamic aspect of its functional residual capacity is smaller than an adult. If extremes of truncal flexion are required, as might occur with the lithotomy, sitting, and jackknife positions, additional attention should be directed to assuring adequate gas exchange. Significant compromise of respiratory mechanics has been documented to occur in infants and toddlers because of extremes of truncal flexion.[6]

SPECIFIC POSITIONS

The exact positioning needs of any patient are influenced by the type of surgical procedure that is being performed. Also important are the preferences of the surgical team, many of which are traditional to the institution where the procedure is performed. These factors influence the care choices of the anesthesia team.

The Supine Position

Although the basic position for most abdominal surgery, the supine position is also frequently used for many orthopedic, urologic, ophthalmologic, otorhinolaryngologic, plastic, and thoracic operations. Exact requirements for a given surgical subspecialty thus become extensions of basic considerations about the supine posture.

For all patients, regardless of age or operative position, assuring a patent airway is a primary concern. The pediatric head is positioned in a neutral state to avoid respiratory obstruction due to flexion of the neck. Although rarely a significant concern when intubated, certain pediatric patients are susceptible to partial airway obstruction, especially without airway adjuncts in place. Examples include the premature infant with his or her proportionately larger head, the infant or child with marked untreated hydrocephaly and concomitant macrocephaly, or the child with macrocephaly from other causes such as gigantism, acromegaly, achondroplastic syndromes, mucopolysaccharidosis syndromes, or the Beckwith-Weidemann syndrome. If this is a concern, then a roll may be placed underneath the shoulders as shown in Figure 15–1 to help augment airway patency. If either a mattress of soft plastic foam or a heating mattress is being used, the roll should be located underneath this surface to allow the mattress to maintain contact with the body surface.

When intubated, the head is positioned neutrally or, alternatively, is turned to the side. Regardless of the position chosen, the stability of the endotracheal tube and anesthesia circuit must be carefully maintained. Head turning should not cause undue tension on the neck muscles or associated nerves for an extended period of time. Because the ears of young pediatric patients are soft and contain little cartilage, adequate padding should be provided for auricular tissues. Foam padding with cutouts for the ears usually suffices.

For prolonged surgical procedures, adequate padding of the operating table should be assured before induction of anesthesia.[7] Foam padding can be placed under any potential pressure spots such as the heels, buttocks, elbows, and head. Reports of alopecia in children after cardiac surgery suggest the need to consider repositioning the head during the procedure.[8]

Arms may be positioned at the side of the patient (see Fig. 15–1) or, as is frequently done, may be abducted and externally rotated as shown in Figure 15–2. The brachial plexus and shoulder joint of the abducted arm should be free from tension. Additional padding of the elbow should be considered.[9] When the arms are placed at the side, concerns are the same as for the adult. Reports of ulnar neuropathy in the supine young pediatric patient are extremely rare.

The Lithotomy Position

The lithotomy position is primarily used by urologic surgeons for cystoscopic surgery or reconstruction of external genitalia, but it may be used by general surgeons for colorectal operations or occasional gynecologic procedures in older children. A variant of this position, known as the frogleg position (Fig. 15–3) is also used frequently by general surgeons for perirectal procedures such as the Soave or Duhamel procedure for Hirschsprung's disease, the Pena procedure for an imperforate anus, or an incision and drainage of a perirectal abscess.

For the traditional lithotomy procedure, considerations in adult and pediatric patients are similar. These have been described in Chapter 6. The legs are placed in stirrups or in leg holders, with availability of appropriately sized equipment being the deciding factor. Regardless of the leg supports used, the legs must rest in a relatively normal, neutral position without undue strain or pressure on any joint. In addition, adequate padding must be applied to potential pressure points, such as the lateral aspect of the knee where the peroneal nerves traverse. This precaution de-

Figure 15–1

Smooth towel roll or foam pad placed beneath the shoulders to extend the neck and improve the infant airway.

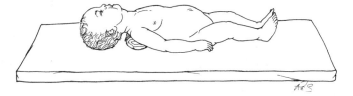

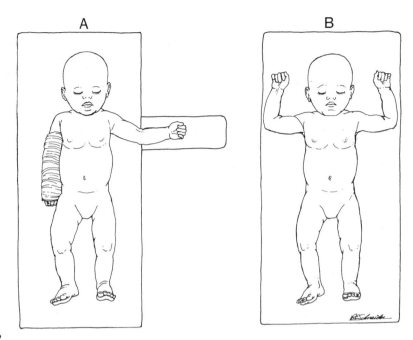

Figure 15–2

A. Either or both arms may be retained alongside the torso or abducted to approximately 90 degrees on boards.
B. Alternatively the elbow(s) of the abducted arm(s) may be flexed and the hand(s) placed in supination near the head. Padding is placed under the forearm or elbow as clinically indicated.

serves special attention in the younger child if the sizes of the leg supports are not proportionate to the size of the patient.

With the frogleg position the patient is traditionally moved to the end of the table where the legs are secured to the ether screen as portrayed in Figure 15–3. The soles of the

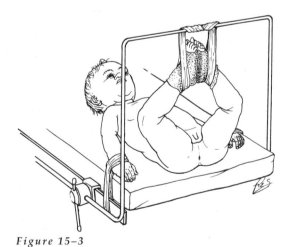

Figure 15–3

The "frogleg" lithotomy position in the small child utilizing an anesthesia screen as the support. The soles of the feet are placed together, wrapped securely but nonocclusively, and hung from the well-padded screen.

feet are placed together, padded as deemed necessary, wrapped securely with surgical draping, and finally hung from the horizontal portion of the well-padded bar. The trunk is concurrently positioned so that the buttocks are at, or very near, the distal edge of the surgical table. At this time, if it appears necessary, additional padding is placed under the buttocks to cushion potential pressure points or to elevate the hips enough to avoid inappropriate strain on the acetabular joints.

The other position used by some urologists that can have many of the same considerations is the split-leg position, portrayed in Figure 15–4. It provides the surgeon, sitting or standing between the legs of the patient, with excellent access to the perineum during reconstruction of external genitalia. In this position, the patient is moved to the end of the table with the buttocks placed at or very near the edge. The legs are placed either on individual extension boards or on a Y-shaped frame that serves the same purpose. The anesthesiologist must be sure that the leg extensions are firmly secured under the operating table mattress, that they extend outward an appropriate length to support the leg, and that they are adequately padded for the patient's protection. The weight of the leg(s) cannot be allowed to use the table edge as a

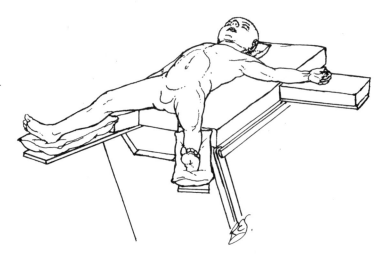

Figure 15-4

The "split-leg" position in the small child utilizing either individual leg extensions or a Y-shaped frame. The extremity support is secured firmly under the mattress of the operating table. Extra padding is applied to the extensions, and the legs are securely wrapped in position.

fulcrum and force the proximal end(s) of the leg extension board(s) through the mattress to place focal pressure on the lower back of the patient. On the extensions, additional foam padding is also placed under any potential pressure point, such as the heel, and the legs are secured with an elastic wrap or the equivalent.

Regardless of whether the frogleg or split-leg position is used, the patient is moved caudad toward the end of the table. Unless contraindicated, the anesthesia circuit should be disconnected from the endotracheal tube during this move to prevent unintentional extubation. In addition, invasive monitoring lines, intravenous tubing, or other attached monitors must be protected from being accidentally dislodged by the move. If either central venous lines or arterial lines are required for the procedure, they should be placed before repositioning the patient because normal accessibility of sites for vascular access will be limited subsequently.

The Head-Elevated Position

Variations of the head-elevated position are used by multiple surgical specialties. The sitting position, the most significant head-elevated position, is almost exclusively used by neurosurgeons for posterior craniectomies and procedures on the upper cervical spine. Milder degrees of head elevation are used by neurosurgeons, plastic surgeons, ophthalmologists, otorhinolaryngologists, urologists, or general surgeons for a variety of different procedures.

The sitting position, although infrequently used in children, especially if they are younger than 3 years old, is still occasionally used in some institutions. Most of the same preparations and precautions used for adults also apply to children, with size of the patient and equipment availability influencing much of the care. After induction and intubation of the child, all desired invasive monitors are routinely placed. This usually includes placement of an arterial line and central venous catheter and may include placement of a transesophageal echocardiographic probe. The arterial line is usually placed in a radial artery, but it may be placed anywhere at the discretion of the anesthesiologist. Depending on the size of the child, the adequacy of venous accessibility, and the technical equipment available in a given hospital, the central venous catheter may be placed in an internal jugular vein or an antecubital vein in the usual fashion. If the transesophageal echocardiographic probe is inserted before positioning upright, added attention must be directed to the endotracheal tube and airway so as to assure there is no unintentional extubation on moving to the sitting position. Before positioning the patient upright the lower extremities should be wrapped with elastic bandages to minimize the effects of venous pooling.

Specific aspects of establishing and using the sitting position in children warrant additional comment. First, as is true with the lithotomy position, the size of equipment available for establishing a sitting position may not be proportionate to the size of the child. For example, the back section of the operating room table may be longer than the torso of the child and, when elevated to support the sitting child, would obscure the operative site for the surgeon. Supports such as blankets

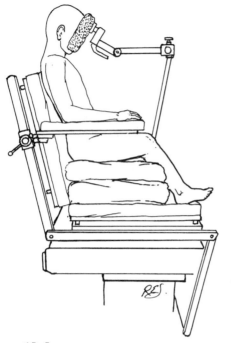

Figure 15–5

The sitting position in a smaller child. Supports are placed under the buttocks to raise the operative target above the cephalad edge of the table. Additional padding is placed under the popliteal region and under any potential pressure points.

under the patient's buttocks may be required to raise the operative target above the cephalad edge of the table top (Fig. 15–5).

Second, with a trachea that is shorter than that of the adult, the child is at higher risk for endobronchial intubation on flexion of the head. Ideally, after intubation the endotracheal tube is secured with its tip above the carina to allow it some safe caudad movement on positioning the child, yet assuring a stable airway in a neutral-to-mild neck extension position. Auscultation of both lung fields must be performed after positioning the child to assure that the endotracheal tube is properly placed, with adjustments made as indicated.

Third, because the cartilage of the tracheal rings is not as firm in the young child as in the adult, the use of a reinforced endotracheal tube should be considered. Not only does a reinforced tube help prevent kinking on neck flexion, it also helps prevent compression of the airway if a transesophageal echocardiographic probe is inserted.

Finally, although the incidence of venous air embolism in the sitting position is statistically similar with children and adults (33% vs. 45%), the incidence of hypotension has been noted to be significantly higher (69% vs. 36%) and the likelihood of successful aspiration of air through a central line significantly lower (38% vs. 68%).[10] Therefore, adequate venous access for resuscitation should be assured before surgical incision and a heightened surveillance for venous air embolism should be ongoing during the procedure with prompt intervention initiated as indicated.

Head-elevated positions of lesser degrees are primarily used by surgeons to facilitate better operative exposure and/or to decrease blood loss. Examples of these indications include sinus surgery, craniofacial reconstructions, and cervical resections. These positions are also used occasionally by neurosurgeons to control or manipulate intracranial pressure and by urologists for lithotripsy procedures. In general, the same concerns associated with the supine position are accorded to the head-elevated position. In addition, there are increased concerns regarding the chances of venous air entrainment in this position, the risk of which is proportionate to the degree of head elevation. Accordingly, appropriate monitoring and attention to this potential risk should be rendered as indicated for the procedure.

The Head-Down Position

The head-down position is rarely used for the pediatric patient. When requested, it is usually intended to facilitate surgical exposure during colorectal or genitourinary procedures.

In general, the same issues that are of concern for the adult patient in this position apply to the pediatric patient. When a person is placed head down, gravity-induced pressure exerted on the diaphragm by the abdominal contents can result in increased work of breathing during spontaneous ventilation. Functional residual capacity is decreased in this position, an issue that is rarely of any clinical significance for an older child. However, depending on the degree of head-down tilt, both the increased work of breathing and the decreased functional residual capacity can predispose to hypoxemia for the infant or toddler. Infants depend primarily on descent of the diaphragm instead of intercostal muscle action for lung expansion and inhalation of gases. Increased pressure against the diaphragm results in increased energy expenditure requirements for these muscles. The characteristics of the infant diaphragm are such that there is a lower content of type I (slow twitch, high oxidative capacity) muscle fibers when compared with the adult, thus predisposing the infant diaphragm to fatigue and subsequent impaired gas exchange.[11] Because oxygen consumption may be two to three times greater in infants and toddlers than in adults, a decrease in functional residual capacity and a sluggish diaphragm may rapidly lead to hypoxemia.

Two other considerations of the head-down position, intracranial pressure and myocardial performance due to induced volume loading, also warrant comment. As for the adult, this position should not be used if intracranial pressure is significantly elevated because it may induce cerebral ischemia. However, in contrast to the older adult, the additional preload effect on the myocardium does not usually predispose the child to compromised myocardial performance unless there is significant underlying dysfunction. Situations in which this might be an issue include the child with complex congenital heart disease or the child who has myocardial dysfunction from chemotherapeutic agents.

The Lateral Position

The lateral position is encountered in a variety of surgical procedures. General surgeons and cardiothoracic surgeons may use it for thoracic procedures, urologists for nephrectomies, and orthopedists for procedures on the hip or femur. Most of the considerations addressed in the adult patient (see Chapter 9) apply to the child, although there are dissimilar implications with some of these issues in different age groups.

When positioning the head, padding should be placed under the head to assure that the neck is in a neutral position to avoid undue strain on the neck muscles. This support may be constructed with blankets, with foam padding, or with a "donut." Because the small child's ear is relatively soft and contains little cartilage, creation of padding with a cutout for the ear ("donut") is recommended so as to avoid undue pressure on the auricle. Care should also be taken to assure there is no inappropriate pressure on the down-side eye.

In positioning the thorax in the lateral position, placement of an elevating pad (widely, and improperly, referred to as an "axillary roll") under the down-side chest wall just caudad to the axilla to prevent injury to the dependent brachial plexus region is warranted in the larger child. However, it is probably not needed in the very small child. With the tiny child, the patient weight is such that minimal forces are exerted on the down-side shoulder region, thus placing little strain or impingement on its brachial plexus. With the older child, forces exerted on the down-side shoulder region may be similar to that of the adult. Regardless of the size of the child, one should always check to assure that the down-side shoulder is not compressed. If a pad is deemed necessary under the down-side chest wall, then one that is appropriate for the size of the patient should be created and positioned so that it does not unduly flex the down-side thoracic wall. The chest pad must also allow the patient to be stabilized on the operating table, and an adequate radial pulse in the down-side extremity should be assured after positioning. For the up-side upper extremity, the arm is usually supported on a pillow or blanket, as shown in Figure 15–6. This prevents strain on the up-side shoulder joint and protects the ulnar nerve from potential pressure injury. In the larger child, an adjustable arm support is arranged so that the up-side arm is in a neutral position. Padding is added to prevent undue pressure against the ventral chest wall, in the axilla, or on the ulnar nerve.

When one is positioning the patient's trunk, supports are usually placed on both sides of the thorax and abdomen (see Fig. 15–6) to assure stability of the patient on the table during the procedure. For the larger child, the typical adult supports that attach to the operating table can be applied. Alternatively, "bean bags" are sometimes used. The bag, containing a huge number of tiny plastic pellets, is molded to the shape of the positioned patient and then stiffened to hold the body in place by evacuating the contained air. Some type of cloth covering should be placed over the bag to prevent direct contact between it and the skin. This cover absorbs moisture, helping to prevent irritation and possibly abrasion to skin that may be in contact with the plastic surface of the bag for prolonged periods. For the smaller child and infant, supports constructed of small sandbags or pads are useful. These supports are placed on each side of the trunk, and straps made of 3-inch rolled gauze or extended Kerlex dressings, which have been wrapped around the upper and lower part of the support, are brought

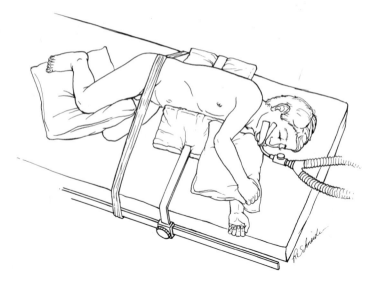

Figure 15-6

The lateral position in a larger child. Supports are placed to stabilize the trunk, and pillows are placed between the extremities for padding. Adhesive tape is applied across the up-side hip and shoulder as needed for stability.

underneath the patient. The supports are then snugged up against the trunk and the straps are tied to the rail on the opposite side of the table. Regardless of which support is used, care must be taken to assure that inappropriate pressure is not being exerted on the thorax or abdomen in a manner that impairs ventilation.

When positioning the lower extremities, a blanket or pillow should be placed between the legs (see Fig. 15–6) to help prevent potential pressure injury to the medial aspects of the knee and ankle that would be caused by the weight of the up-side extremity.

Once the lateral position is established, a few other aspects deserve comment. First, after achieving the desired position, tape is usually applied to both the shoulder and iliac crest regions and secured to the edges and undersurface of the operating table. These tapes help stabilize the child during the operation and should be applied firmly enough to immobilize the trunk without causing enough distortion of the skin to cause a traction injury. The tape across the up-side hip should be placed so as to avoid compressing the head of the up-side femur into its joint space, a situation that might compress nutrient vessels to the femoral head and lead to aseptic necrosis in that hip.

Second, for procedures that require optimal flank exposure, a kidney rest may be requested. The impact of this maneuver on the older child is similar to that of an adult. Ideally the child should be positioned such that the kidney rest elevates at the level of the down-side iliac crest, thus allowing optimal flank flexion with the least possible restriction of ventilation in the down-side hemithorax. When elevated, rarely is any hemodynamic or respiratory compromise noted in the pediatric patient. However, because this potential exists, when the kidney rest is raised attention should be directed toward the monitored cardiorespiratory variables to assure the child is not adversely impacted. For the very small child, the kidney rest may actually raise the entire trunk, resulting in suboptimal flank flexion. In this situation, the kidney rest may be replaced by a roll placed under the dependent flank before the skin preparation and draping.

Third, there is always the potential for movement of the endotracheal tube from added flexion or extension of the neck during positioning of the patient. Again, because the pediatric airway is proportionately shorter than the adult airway, there is a potential for displacement of the endotracheal tube caudally or rostrally. As in the adult, auscultation of both lung fields should be performed on final positioning to confirm appropriate placement of the endotracheal tube. If not already done at this time, the airway should be adequately taped or strapped to assure that draining salivary secretions do not result in loosening of the tape, with subsequent instability of the airway.

Some thoracic procedures may require either a double-lumen endotracheal tube or a standard endotracheal tube with a bronchial blocker to facilitate one-lung ventilation. In these situations, it is mandatory for the anesthesiologist to confirm continued placement of these devices in the desired location once the patient is finally positioned. This confirmation should be made with the aid of a fiberoptic bronchoscope, because migration of the endotracheal tube or bronchial blocking balloon has been documented to occur during positioning.[12] Not uncommonly, especially in the small child in which a bronchial blocker is used, the cuff to be inflated is dislodged. Failure to correct this before surgical incision can result in compromised ventilation or suboptimal surgical conditions, both of which only prolong the procedure and put the child at added risk.

The Prone Position

The prone position is used for a variety of procedures, the majority of these being performed by neurosurgeons and orthopedic surgeons, and a few by general surgeons and plastic surgeons. It is used for posterior craniotomies, spine-related procedures such as spinal fusions, resections of various masses such as lipomas, and repair of dermal defects. For this position, most of the same preparations and precautions considered for adults apply to children, with the weight of the child and equipment-related concerns influencing many of the management decisions.

An older (i.e., heavier) child usually has anesthesia induced on the transport cart before being moved to the operating table. That approach allows the patient to be rolled gently onto the table and its prepositioned ventral torso supports as opposed to the clumsier and more difficult maneuver of being lifted up, pronated, and having ventral supports added. In younger children anesthesia is commonly induced on the operating table, and then the child is turned to the prone position.

Regardless of which technique is chosen for turning a patient prone, two main concerns arise with the process:

1. The airway must be reliably secured after confirmation of proper placement of the endotracheal tube, with the breathing circuit disconnected just before turning. Failure to temporarily disconnect may result in the child being unintentionally extubated on being moved. Once the patient is turned prone and positioned on the table, the breathing circuit should be immediately reconnected and equal breath sounds confirmed bilaterally by auscultation.

2. Monitors must be initially placed in such a fashion that they ideally will not become tangled on turning. Because this is frequently easier said than done, consideration should be given to disconnecting all monitors except the pulse oximeter during positioning, with efficient reconnection to the patient at the earliest moment after the turn is completed. If invasive monitors are required for the procedure, these, as well as all required intravascular lines, should be placed before turning the child prone and carefully safeguarded during subsequent positioning changes.

Once in the prone position, padding and appropriate supports are positioned as displayed in Figure 15–7. In general, the supports that are used are influenced by the surgical procedure being planned and the size of the child.

For the small child, rolls may be placed in a variety of locations. In whatever manner they are placed, ultimately the rolls should permit the neck to be maintained in a neutral position and should assure that the thorax and abdomen are free from compression that would prevent relatively normal ventilation. The placement of the legs must not cause undue strain or pressure at the ankles or knees.

For the larger child, rolls may be placed in positions similar to an adult (see Chapter 10). They should reside parallel to the long axis of the body from just caudad of the clavicles to the anterior iliac crests, thus allowing for adequate chest excursion without pressing the clavicles dorsally to compress the retroclavicular space and its neurovascular structures. In the adolescent female, care should be taken during this process to assure there is no inappropriate pressure from the rolls on the breast tissue. A pillow or blanket may then be placed under the lower leg to avoid

Figure 15–7

The prone position in the larger infant or toddler with head rest. Note position of supporting rolls and the neutral position of the head.

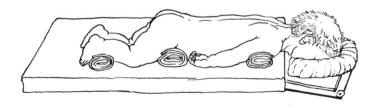

unnecessary pressure on the tibia or at the joints. Regardless of the patient's size, the arms may be either (1) placed alongside the torso in a neutral state, with forearms extended and either the palms or the thumbs facing the lateral surface of the thighs, or (2) placed with upper arms elevated alongside the head, elbows flexed, and hands either supinated or resting on the hypothenar edges. Forearms should be supported on arm extensions for the larger child or on the operating table for the smaller child. Padding placed underneath the elbows may distribute their compressive weight and protect the ulnar nerve.[9]

Depending on the surgical procedure, the head may be placed in a head rest or may rest on the table, turned to the side. If a head rest is to be used, as would occur in a posterior craniotomy, there are three main issues to be considered.

1. The size of the child influences the head rest that is chosen. Usually there will be an appropriately sized support, and the head can rest on the forehead and the mandible. However, occasionally an additional "donut" must be fashioned to create the necessary support (Fig. 15–8).

2. Regardless of what head rest is ultimately used, its padding must be adequate to cushion the head and protect the eyes from abrasive surface contact or global compression.

3. To secure the airway, a method must be used that will not fail in the presence of draining oral secretions and allow gravity and the weight of the airway appliances to dislodge the endotracheal tube. Reliable tape, or tape plus an adhesive compound, is traditional.

Alternatively, string ties may be fashioned to hold the endotracheal tube in place. The anesthesia circuit tubing should be supported, usually at the Y-connector (see Fig. 15–8) to minimize any outward traction that may exist on the endotracheal tube.

For posterior fossa surgery in hydrocephalic infants a unique position has been described.[13] Termed by its innovators a *bunny crouch*, it is a kneeling prone posture that arranges the infant rump-to-surgeon and offers a direct line of sight to the apex of the fourth ventricle with minimal loss of cerebrospinal fluid (Fig. 15–9). After a routine induction supine, the infant is turned prone and placed in a kneeling posture that frees the abdomen for effective ventilation. The neck is flexed and the head is situated on a foam pad, assuring adequate eye and face protection. The anesthesia circuit is carefully secured to prevent dislodgement of the endotracheal tube. Once appropriate padding is placed under the thorax and buttocks, restraining tapes are applied to prevent extension of the lower extremities and loss of the kneeling posture during the procedure. The table chassis can then be tilted as needed to level the thoracocervical spine of the patient.

For posterior spinal procedures, such as scoliosis repair, the Relton-Hall table is frequently used. As displayed in Figure 15–10, this table results in the patient being suspended by four adjustable pillars, one placed at the outer limit of each quadrant of the ventral torso, rather than resting on a flat surface. The configuration of the table mandates that anesthesia be induced while the patient is on the transport cart with all the appropriate monitors and lines placed before

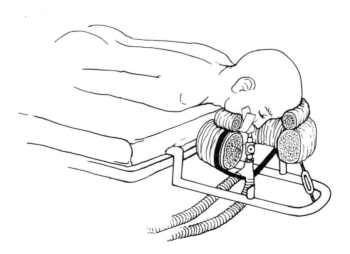

Figure 15–8

The prone position with head rest adapted to face size. Note the extra "donut" padding to support the head. The tape sling supports the endotracheal tube and breathing circuit. (Ring segments cut away for clarity.)

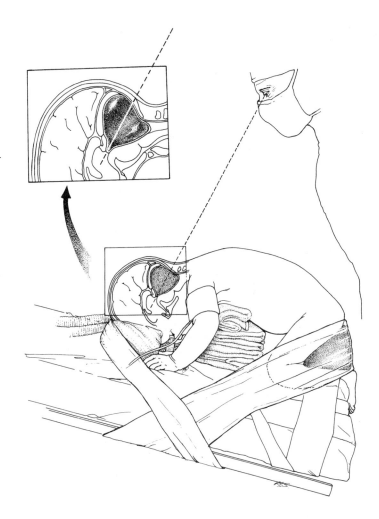

Figure 15–9

The kneeling "bunny-crouch" position provides line-of-sight access to the apex of the fourth ventricle for posterior fossa surgery in hydrocephalic infants. Pads under the buttocks and chest maintain the posture, relieve pressure on the abdomen, and provide optimum ventilation. Neck is flexed so that the forehead rests on a pad and frees the eyes, nose, and transoral appliances from compression. Once the patient is positioned, restraining tapes are applied to assure stability. (From Rayport M, Martin JT: New head-prone position for posterior fossa surgery in infants with severe hydrocephalus. Childs Nerv Syst 8:419, 1992. © Springer-Verlag.)

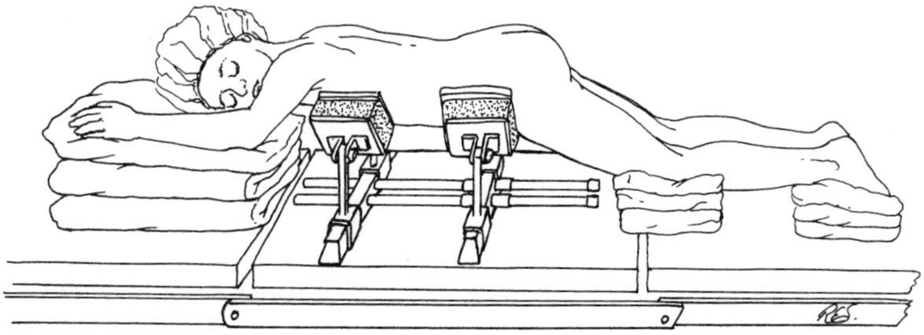

Figure 15–10

The Relton-Hall frame for posterior spinal operations. Padding is applied to potential pressure points as shown. Note the degree of body surface area exposed to room air and the points of contact from the four supports. Inguinal posts should not compress abdomen and axilla should be free of cephalad posts. (From Relton JES, Hall JE: An operation frame for spinal surgery. J Bone Joint Surg 49:327, 1967.)

positioning. Because the ventral surface of the patient is exposed to room air during the use of this table, the potential for heat loss is significantly increased. Hence, for the small child who may not be as able to maintain thermoneutrality, consideration should be given to using forced-air warming devices on the lower extremities because this has been shown to help maintain a desired temperature.[14] Because all the patient's weight is resting on the four supports, there must be adequate padding of these supports before positioning. It is not uncommon for an anesthesia team member to notice pressure-induced erythema at these points on completion of the procedure, underscoring the importance of appropriate padding.

The Jackknife Position

This position is used almost exclusively by pediatric surgeons for perirectal procedures, such as incision and drainage of a perirectal abscess. Many of the same considerations mentioned previously for the prone position, in terms of induction issues, monitors, extremity positioning, and securing of the airway, apply here. Otherwise, only minor variances exist in terms of positioning of the trunk and head.

For the larger child, induction of anesthesia takes place on the transport cart, monitors are placed, and the airway is secured; then the child is turned prone and positioned on the table (Fig. 15–11). As in the adult, the table top ultimately will be flexed, requiring the iliac crests to be situated over whatever table hinge will be used as the flexion point. Rolls are usually placed under the edges of the trunk parallel to its long axis, from just above the iliac crests to just below the clavicles, to minimize respiratory compromise. The head

is turned to the side with supports arranged to prevent undue strain on the neck muscles and padding applied to protect the downside ear. The arms are commonly raised to lie alongside the head and padding is placed under the elbows to prevent focal pressure on the ulnar nerve.[9] For the lower extremities, a pillow, blanket, or roll, is usually placed under the distal legs to provide support, thus minimizing exaggerated plantarflexion of the feet. Finally, as in all prone positions, once the patient is appropriately positioned, a repeat auscultation of the lung fields is performed to assure the endotracheal tube has not been inadvertently displaced.

For the smaller child, induction may be performed on the operating table, with monitors placed and the airway secured as previously noted. The child is then lifted up and turned prone, and an appropriately sized roll is placed under the hips to achieve the desired degree of flexion. Figure 15–12 portrays the usual position and padding required for the small child. Although additional rolls to support the trunk are usually not required, if a large roll for hip flexion is requested to help achieve optimal surgical exposure, ventilation may be impaired because it encroaches on the abdominal cavity. In this situation, additional support of the trunk should be provided, either with a roll underneath the clavicles or with rolls along the long axis of the trunk. Otherwise, all other considerations previously mentioned for the prone position in the smaller child apply.

SPECIAL SITUATIONS

Meningomyelocele

A patient with a meningomyelocele presents unique considerations. In the newborn with

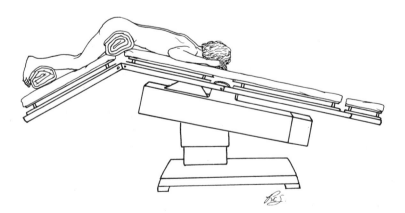

Figure 15–11

The jackknife position for the larger child, with hips flexed over the hinge between the thigh and leg sections of the operating table. (Additional padding omitted for clarity.)

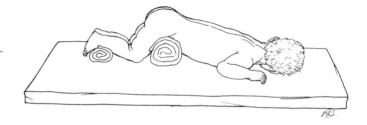

Figure 15–12

The jackknife position for the small child. Properly sized roll flexes the hips and reduces pressure on the abdomen.

an unrepaired defect, the meningomyelocele sac is frequently large and covered by a thin layer of tissue. Any significant pressure or physical trauma to the sac places it at risk for rupture, with the subsequent risk of acquired central nervous system infection. Therefore, in the newborn period, great care is taken to protect the sac from injury.

Because surgical repair is done under general anesthesia, and intubation is usually done in the supine position, the infant is usually placed supine on a "donut" large enough to surround and suspend the defect during induction. Figure 15–13 displays such a support, the "donut" frequently being fashioned out of surgical towels. It is also important to note that this support often partially suspends the trunk, requiring that an assistant should be present to stabilize the infant's trunk and thwart any potential for disruption of the sac during laryngoscopy and securing of the airway. Because the operation requires either the prone or lateral position until the defect is repaired, once the airway is secured, the infant is turned into the chosen position. Considerations noted in the previous sections

then apply. Alternatively, the intubation may be performed in the lateral position, thus obviating the concerns regarding the sac, but this option requires the participation of someone with experience and skill with intubation of infants.

In the older infant or child with meningomyelocele, there are additional concerns regarding the airway and the head position, as well as the extremities and buttocks. First, as pertains to the airway and head position, 85% to 90% of these children also have an Arnold-Chiari malformation with associated hydrocephalus.[15] Most commonly, ventriculoperitoneal shunts are placed in infancy before any potential development of elevated intracranial pressure, thus minimizing these potential concerns. However, because of the malformation, a few children may be at risk of herniation of the cerebellar tonsils[16] and consequent compromise of bulbar function and respiratory drive. Therefore, when caring for these children, the history should be searched for indications of nausea, vomiting, bulbar dysfunction, or an irregular respiratory drive. If there is potential for compromise, a conscien-

Figure 15–13

Newborn with a lumbar meningomyelocele supported on a "donut" that surrounds and protects the defect during induction and laryngoscopy. The remainder of the head and trunk may need to be supported manually during intubation to assure truncal stability and prevent accidental disruption of the sac.

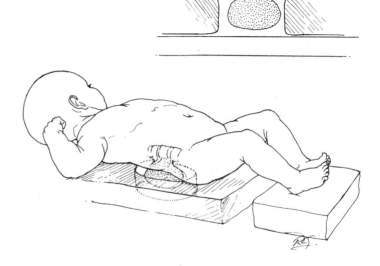

tious effort should be made to assure there is no undue neck extension during laryngoscopy or during the surgical procedure.

Second, as pertains to the extremities and buttocks, depending on the level of the defect, extremity contractures or pressure sores on the ischial spines may be present. When positioning, additional padding should be placed at any potential pressure points, and support should be placed under the extremities to minimize any undue strain on muscles or joints.

Down Syndrome

Trisomy 21 is mentioned here because of the issue regarding potential atlantoaxial instability in these patients. In 1983, the Special Olympics introduced a requirement for lateral neck radiographs in individuals with Down syndrome before participation in competitive activities. Later, the American Academy of Pediatrics published a position statement regarding screening for atlantoaxial instability.[17] Spurred by this controversy, further discussions took place among pediatric anesthesiologists and surgeons that led to some institutions developing screening policies that require lateral neck radiographs within at least 2 years before a planned procedure that might involve neck extension. The Academy recently revisited the issue, this time taking the stance that obtaining routine lateral neck radiographs is of potential but unproven value in detecting which of these patients is at risk for developing spinal cord injury during sports.[18] Because approximately 15% of pediatric aged individuals with Down syndrome have atlantoaxial instability by radiographic findings, and almost all of these individuals are asymptomatic, the routine practice of performing this diagnostic study preoperatively is certainly expensive and probably unnecessary. However, if the patient has symptoms of atlantoaxial instability, such as easy fatigability, difficulty in walking, abnormal gait, torticollis or head tilt, sensory deficits, or upper motor neuron and posterior column signs, consideration should be given to obtaining radiographic studies before performing a surgical procedure. If instability is documented radiographically and/or the child has symptoms, extra attention should be directed toward positioning of the head such that flexion or extension in any position is prevented or held to an absolute minimum and carefully monitored.[19]

Conjoined Twins

When confronted with the task of anesthetizing conjoined twins, the anesthesiologist has multiple concerns.[20-22] Depending on the location of attachment, there may be issues related to the integrity of the cardiovascular systems and potential shared circulations, the integrity of the thoracic cavities and the accessibility of the airways, and the integrity of the neurologic system. The impact of positioning on the cardiorespiratory systems warrants further discussion.

Because surgical procedures for separation most always require general anesthesia, management of the airways must be adequately planned. Depending on the location of conjoinment, the airway may be secured in the routine fashion after inhalational or intravenous induction, or consideration might need to be given to performing an awake intubation, an intubation from a lateral approach, or a fiberoptic intubation. Performing the intubation in a nonroutine position may result in temporary positioning concerns that need to be addressed at that time, perhaps the most significant of which is influenced by the impact of the integrity of the twins' respective cardiovascular systems. If there is a significantly shared circulation, then placing one of the twins above the other may result in shunting of blood to the dependent child, thus placing the nondependent child at risk for hypotension. Likewise, if there is a significantly shared circulation, when anesthetic agents are administered to one child to facilitate securing the airway, then the potential for depression of the cardiorespiratory systems in the other child exists and may need to be managed simultaneously.

Preterm Infants

Owing to the risk of postoperative apnea in preterm or former preterm infants who are younger than 44 to 60 weeks of postconceptual age,[23-25] spinal anesthesia has been advocated by some as the technique of choice for certain procedures.[26-28] If this technique is performed, it is important to note two aspects.

The first aspect relates to the positioning of the infant during placement of the spinal anesthetic. Because of an increased transcutaneous P_{CO_2} and decreased transcutaneous P_{O_2} that may occur in a lateral recumbent, fully flexed position, neck extension during placement of the spinal anesthetic has been advocated. Alternatively, the block may be performed in the sitting position with the head supported.[29]

The second aspect pertains to patient movement on successful placement of the spinal anesthetic. Because reports exist of high spinal blocks being produced when the legs are lifted for placement of the electrocautery grounding pad, the infant should be placed supine after successful injection of the local anesthetic, being rolled lateral for only a brief period if necessary for placement of the grounding pad.[30]

Musculoskeletal Disorders

A number of musculoskeletal disorders merit additional considerations regarding positioning.[31] These include the osteochondrodysplasias, the muscular dystrophies, and the connective tissue disorders. For example, as with Down syndrome, an increased incidence of atlantoaxial abnormalities occurs with achondroplasia and juvenile rheumatoid arthritis, mandating special consideration of the appropriate degree of neck extension and flexion allowable during positioning. With osteogenesis imperfecta, the bones are at significant risk for fracture, necessitating meticulous attention to gentle, nonstressful movement and appropriate padding of the patient during positioning efforts. The use of metal sleeves for protection of extremities during the procedure in a patient with this disorder should also be considered, especially if the posture of the surgeon could press on the child. Because myocardial dysfunction is often associated with muscular dystrophies, additional attention should be paid toward assuring hemodynamic stability during positioning, especially if the sitting position is planned. Finally, with many of these disorders, older children often have thoracic cavity deformities due to acquired scoliosis. These deformities may complicate the anesthetic care in certain positions because of abnormalities in ventilation/perfusion matching.

REFERENCES

1. Goudsouzian NG: Anatomy and physiology in relation to pediatric anesthesia. *In* Katz J, Steward DG (eds.): Anesthesia and Uncommon Pediatric Diseases, 2nd ed. Philadelphia, WB Saunders, 1993.
2. Developmental Pediatrics. *In* Behrman RE, Vaughan VC III (eds.): Nelson Textbook of Pediatrics, 12th ed. Philadelphia, WB Saunders, 1983.
3. Morgan J, Mumford P: Preliminary studies of energy expenditures in infants under six years of age. Acta Paediatr Scand 70:15, 1981.
4. Rutler N, Hull D: Water loss from the skin of term and preterm babies. Arch Dis Child 54:858, 1979.
5. Fonkalsrud EW, et al.: Reduction of evaporative heat loss and pulmonary secretions in neonates by use of heated and humidified gases. J Thorac Cardiovasc Surg 80:718, 1980.
6. Sly PD, Lanteri CJ, Kelly JH, et al.: Disturbance in respiratory mechanics with extreme truncal flexion during anaesthesia in children. Anaesth Intensive Care 19:220, 1991.
7. Webster CI: A pressure care survey in the operating theatres. Aust Clin Rev 13:29, 1993.
8. Ben-Amitai D, Garty BZ: Alopecia in children after cardiac surgery. Pediatr Dermatol 10:32, 1993.
9. Wadsworth TG: The external compression syndrome of the ulnar nerve at the cubital tunnel. Clin Orthop 124:189, 1977.
10. Cucchiara RF, Bowers B: Air embolism in children undergoing suboccipital craniotomy. Anesthesiology 57:338, 1982.
11. Keens TG, et al.: Developmental pattern of muscle fiber types in human ventilatory muscles. J Appl Physiol 44:909, 1978.
12. Bardoczky GI, et al.: Continuous spirometry for detection of double-lumen endobronchial tube displacement. Br J Anaesth 70:499, 1993.
13. Rayport M, Martin JT: New head-prone position for posterior fossa surgery in infants with severe hydrocephalus. Childs Nerv Syst 8:419, 1992.
14. Murat I, Berniere J, Constant I: Evaluation of the efficacy of a forced-air warmer (Bair Hugger) during spinal surgery in children. J Clin Anesth 6:425, 1994.
15. Stein SC, Schut L: Hydrocephalus in myelomeningocele. Childs Brain 5:413, 1979.
16. Holinger PC, et al.: Respiratory obstruction and apnea in infants with bilateral abductor vocal cord paralysis, meningomyelocele, hydrocephalus, and Arnold-Chiari malformation. J Pediatr 92:368, 1978.
17. American Academy of Pediatrics, Committee on Sports Medicine: Atlantoaxial instability in Down syndrome. Pediatrics 74:152, 1984.
18. American Academy of Pediatrics, Committee on Sports Medicine and Fitness: Atlantoaxial instability in Down syndrome: Subject review. Pediatrics 96:151, 1995.
19. Harley EH, Collins MD: Neurologic sequelae secondary to atlantoaxial instability in Down syndrome: Implications in otolaryngologic surgery. Arch Otolaryngol Head Neck Surg 120:159, 1994.
20. James PD, et al.: Anaesthetic considerations for separation of omphalo-ischiopagus tripus twins. Can Anaesth Soc J 32:402, 1985.
21. Diaz JH, Furman EB: Perioperative management of conjoined twins. Anesthesiology 67:965, 1987.
22. Hoshina H, et al.: Thoracopagus conjoined twins: Management of anesthetic induction and postoperative chest wall defect. Anesthesiology 66:424, 1987.
23. Steward DJ: Preterm infants are more prone to complications following minor surgery than are term infants. Anesthesiology 56:304, 1982.
24. Welborn LG, et al.: Postanesthetic apnea and periodic breathing in infants. Anesthesiology 65:658, 1986.
25. Kurth CD, et al.: Postoperative apnea in preterm infants. Anesthesiology 66:483, 1987.
26. Abajian JC, et al.: Spinal anesthesia for surgery in the high-risk infant. Anesth Analg 63:359, 1984.

27. Parkinson SK, et al.: Use of hyperbaric bupivacaine with epinephrine for spinal anesthesia in infants. Reg Anesth 15:86, 1990.
28. Webster AC, et al.: Spinal anaesthesia for inguinal hernia repair in high-risk neonates. Can J Anaesth 38:281, 1991.
29. Gleason CA, et al.: Optimal position for a spinal tap in preterm infants. Pediatrics 71:31, 1983.
30. Wright TE, et al.: Complications during spinal anesthesia in infants: High spinal blockade. Anesthesiology 73:1290, 1990.
31. Holtby HM, Relton JES: Orthopedic diseases. *In* Katz J, Steward DJ (eds.): Anesthesia and Uncommon Pediatric Diseases, 2nd ed. Philadelphia, WB Saunders, 1993.

Chapter 16

Obstetrics

Bradley E. Smith

BACKGROUND

Advancing pregnancy induces progressively more marked changes in maternal physiology. Inappropriate positioning during pregnancy, whether for normal sleep, for surgery, or for labor and delivery, can lead to hazards for both mother and fetus. Aortocaval compression by the pregnant uterus is the most well known of these conditions. The management of both general anesthesia and regional analgesia can interact with maternal positioning. Respiratory and circulatory functions are intimately related to positioning, as are regurgitation and aspiration of gastric contents and emergency care of the airway. The posture of a patient is important in tailoring the characteristics of some aspects of a regional block. Furthermore, nerve damage to the mother caused by faulty positioning is of concern, principally due to the frequent use of the lithotomy position (see also Chapter 6).

ALTERATIONS OF MATERNAL PHYSIOLOGY IN LATE PREGNANCY THAT ARE RELEVANT TO POSITIONING

The Respiratory System. Owing to an increase in tidal volume, respiratory minute volume progressively rises throughout pregnancy and eventually causes a mild compensatory respiratory alkalosis. Arterial Pco_2 of 32 mm Hg and pH of 7.44 are commonly encountered values.[1] Isolated lung compliance is relatively unaffected in pregnancy, but chest wall compliance (and thus total respiratory compliance) is significantly decreased nearing term.[2] Total compliance in the supine position, therefore, is reduced by about 20% from that of the nonpregnant state. Assumption of the lithotomy position by the pregnant patient further lowers total compliance to about half the prepartum value.[3]

Airway closure during tidal breathing may cause variable degrees of oxygen desaturation and significant depression of alveolar-arterial oxygen gradient. Closing volume (as estimated by closing volume/vital capacity) becomes progressively more impairing in many patients at term.[2, 4] Premature airway closure has been reported to occur in up to 50% of patients in the supine position, or in either lateral decubitus position, but disappears when the patient sits up.[1, 4] Therefore, the supine position should be avoided as often as possible or, at least, should be limited in duration.[1, 4]

The Cardiovascular System. Near term, cardiac output levels measured in the lateral recumbent position are as much as 40% greater than nonpregnant levels. However, assumption of the supine position reduces this elevated cardiac output by as much as 20% to 30% even without recognizable symptoms of aortocaval compression.[5] Cardiac output in pregnancy is higher in the sitting than in the supine position. In either the lithotomy position or in steep head-down tilt, cardiac output is 35% less than in the lateral recumbent position.[5] Again, we see reasons for limiting the use of the supine position, and even head-down tilt and lithotomy positions, as much as possible in pregnant patients who are near term.

Renal Function. The supine position decreases the ability of normotensive gravidas to excrete water, produces striking sodium retention, and reduces average glomerular filtration rate and renal plasma flow by up to 25%. These findings are now known to be associated with unrecognized aortocaval compression and must be guarded against during anesthesia and surgery for any purpose in late pregnancy.[6]

THE AORTOCAVAL COMPRESSION SYNDROME

Obstruction of the inferior vena cava and distal portion of the aorta, caused by the weight of the increasing mass of the uterus and its contents, leads to serious clinical pitfalls in late pregnancy (Fig. 16–1). Elective sleeping positions of healthy women have been found to be 64% 90-degree left lateral tilt, 10% 60-degree tilt, and 4% 30-degree tilt, whereas 20% elect right tilt and only 2% of the time is spent supine in sleep.[7] Presumably the body adjusts itself to avoid aortocaval compression. Aortic compression is more frequent in multiple pregnancies, with nonengagement of the fetal head, with the head in the occipitoposterior position, and before cervical dilatation reaches 6 cm. When pregnant patients at term are placed in left lateral tilt of less than 30 to 35 degrees, aortocaval compression occurs in 7% of patients not experiencing uterine contractions and in 40% of those having active uterine contractions.[8] Most authorities agree aortocaval obstruction is completely eliminated in the left lateral recumbent position.[8–16]

- If only the vena cava is obstructed in this manner (see Fig. 16–1C), a reflex tachycardia occurs that is followed by a profound drop in systolic pressure when the increased pulse rate can no longer compen-

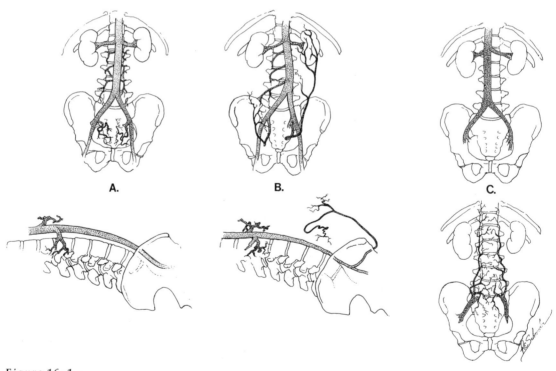

A.   B.   C.

Figure 16–1

Vascular compromise produced by an enlarged or a contracting uterus. *A.* Usual aortic relationships as shown in anteroposterior and lateral lumbar angiograms of a nongravid abdomen. *B.* Same patient at term. Angiogram shows the aorta deviated leftward and compressed against the ventral surface of the vertebral column by the uterine mass. Note the elongated left uterine artery. *C, top.* Angiogram of a normal inferior vena cava. *C, bottom.* Angiogram of caval obstruction in a gravid, supine patient with reduced venous return diverted into paravertebral plexuses. (Redrawn from Bieniarz J, Joshida T, Romero-Salinas G, et al.: Aortocaval compression by the uterus in late human pregnancy: IV. Am J Obstet Gynecol 103:19, 1969.)

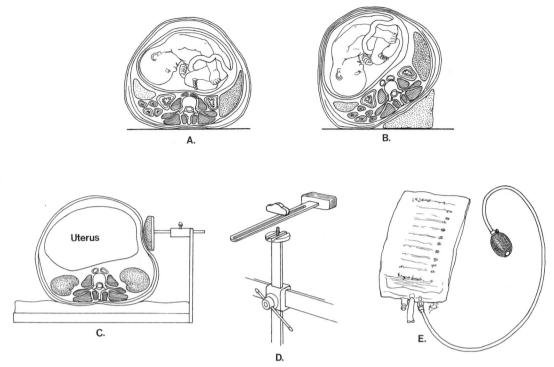

A.

B.

Uterus

C.

D.

E.

Figure 16–2

Methods of preventing the aortocaval compression syndrome. *A.* Compression of prevertebral vessels by uterus at term with mother supine provokes the syndrome. *B.* Wedge elevation of right hip moves uterine mass toward left hemiabdomen, relieving prevertebral vascular obstruction. *C.* Mechanical device for left uterine displacement in the supine position advocated by Colon-Morales. (Redrawn from Colon-Morales MA: A self-supporting device for continuous left uterine displacement during cesarean section. Anesth Analg 49:223, 1970.) *D.* Left uterine displacement device of Kennedy. (Redrawn from Kennedy RL, Friedman DL, Katchka DM, et al.: Hypotension during obstetrical anesthesia. Anesthesiology 20:153, 1959.) *E.* Inflatable container described by Redick for sustained elevation of right hip. (Redrawn from Redick LF: An inflatable wedge for prevention of aortocaval compression during pregnancy. Am J Obstet Gynecol 133:458, 1979.)

sate for the decreased venous return. During full vena cava compression, the parturient frequently perceives symptoms of dyspnea, faintness, and palpitations, but much evidence indicates that asymptomatic partial vena cava occlusion is quite frequent.[17]

• In a radiographic study, the right iliac vessels were compressed in up to 69% of pregnant patients at term who were placed in the supine position.[18] Obstruction of portions of the aorta and the common iliac vessels temporarily simulates an increase in peripheral resistance (see Fig. 16–1*B*), which may temporarily delay the systemic hypotension that would otherwise result from partial vena caval obstruction.[10, 15, 19]

• During compressive occlusion of the aorta by the uterus, brachial artery pressure is often normal or high despite a restricted cardiac output. Cardiac rate may be slowed owing to stimulation of the baroreceptors; however, perfusion of the lower extremities and placenta is poor.[19] This reduced placental perfusion can lead quickly to fetal heart rate signs of distress even without evident maternal changes (see Figs. 16–1*B* and *C*). Both fetal heart rate abnormalities and hypotension in the mother's legs are usually easily relieved by assuming the full left lateral decubitus position.[9, 11, 14, 20–22] Therefore, monitoring the onset of the aortocaval compression syndrome is aided by simultaneous leg and arm blood pressure monitoring.[14, 22]

Techniques to Minimize the Effects of the Aortocaval Syndrome. The compressive bulk of the gravid uterus can be shifted off the vessels of the lower abdomen in several ways (Fig. 16–2).

- A firm wedge[10, 23] (see Fig. 16–2E) or an inflatable bladder[24] can be placed under the right hip of a patient in the supine position to elevate the lateral pelvis enough to tilt the abdomen and shift the uterus to the left. The major vasculature is therefore decompressed (see Figs. 16–2A and B).[13]
- Manual force can be applied to the uterus to move it to the left flank.[10, 12, 25]
- A self-sustaining mechanical device can be attached to the operating table or added to the patient's bed to replace the manual displacing force (see Figs. 16–2C and D).[26, 27]
- The surface of the operating table or delivery table can be tilted to the left.[8, 15, 16, 28–30]
- The patient can be repositioned into a lateral decubitus position to free the major abdominal vessels from the uterine weight.[12, 13]

Kennedy and co-workers[25] reported that 18% of patients experiencing vaginal delivery in the lithotomy position under low subarachnoid anesthesia developed hypotension. However, manual displacement of the uterus to the left restored blood pressure in 93% of hypotensive parturients. Another group asserted that left lateral uterine displacement resulting from a self-supporting device that shifts the uterus was believed to provide better arterial oxygen saturation than did the displacement resulting from a 10- to 12-cm wedge placed under the right hip of the parturient.[23] Although earlier recommendations indicated that 15 degrees of left pelvic tilt is sufficient to avoid aortocaval compression syndrome,[21, 31] later reports indicate that 15 degrees is inadequate. Cardiac output and stroke volume during cesarean section were found by Secher and associates to be increased by manual left uterine displacement and by complete left lateral recumbency, but the 15-degree left lateral tilt position produced no significant change.[12] Eckstein and Marx[10] reported that left tilt was more effective than a right hip wedge, but thought that manual displacement of the uterus to the left was even more effective. In another study, intervillous blood flow was improved by approximately 30% when parturients moved from the supine position to the left lateral decubitus position.[32]

Newman and associates[30] compared cardiac output in supine position with that obtained first in the lateral decubitus position and then in the supine position with the table tilted left or right 15 degrees. Only the right table tilt position failed to improve cardiac output. Kinsella and colleagues[15] reported that decreased blood pressure in the leg was noted during contractions in 38% of women with left pelvic tilt of up to 20 degrees, but in 84% of these patients the obstruction was relieved by increasing the left pelvic tilt to 30 degrees. Of women studied in the right pelvic tilt position, 25% displayed aortocaval compression.[8] Most authorities believe that only 30 degrees or greater of left pelvic tilt is as safe as full left lateral decubitus.[16] Women in labor occasionally display aortic compression even in the semirecumbent position.[15] In advanced pregnancy, regional anesthesia has been reported to accentuate both the incidence and the severity of these aforementioned events because of the blockade of autonomic compensatory mechanisms.[33]

Datta and associates[34] reported that infants whose mothers had been in a supine semisitting position during epidural anesthesia displayed significantly lower pH values in cord blood than did infants whose mothers had been in the lateral position. In addition, infants whose mothers had been maintained with their backs elevated 30 to 45 degrees into a semisitting position were found to have higher concentrations of bupivacaine in their cord blood than was the case with infants whose mothers had been maintained in the lateral position. This finding may have been due to "ion trapping" caused by the slight acidosis found in the infants born from the supine position.

POSITIONING DURING GENERAL ANESTHESIA

Positioning and Aortocaval Compression

Left lateral positioning of parturients is mandatory even during general anesthesia.[13] Infants born by cesarean section when the mother received general anesthesia in the nontilt supine position demonstrated significantly lower Apgar scores[35] and greater degrees of acid-base derangements at birth than did newborns of supine patients who had been tilted.[31] Ansari and associates[36] found that the use of a 10-degree leftward tilt at cesarean section produced a significant improvement in oxygen saturation during general anesthesia but not during subarachnoid anesthesia. Right lateral tilt definitely does not substitute for left lateral tilt! During thiopental/succinylcholine/nitrous oxide anesthesia for cesarean section, Buley and co-workers[28] found that mothers who had been tilted toward the right were delivered of infants who had marked increases in metabolic acidosis at birth when compared with infants delivered of mothers who had been tilted toward the left.

Positioning and Pulmonary Aspiration

Radiographic evidence suggests that the fundus of the stomach can accommodate sizable volumes of fluid without reflux in the left lateral position, whereas in the supine or right lateral position reflux and regurgitation are anatomically more probable as regards to the gastric sphincter.[37] Although not widely accepted, some authorities advocate that routine induction of anesthesia and intubation of the trachea should be carried out with the patient in the left lateral recumbent position.[37, 38]

Positioning and the Complicated Airway

Unanticipated inability to intubate the trachea is a frequent cause of maternal mortality.[39] Some authorities have recommended that when tracheal intubation is impossible the parturient should be awakened before proceeding with the planned operative delivery.[40] Tunstall[41] has recommended, when anesthesia has just been induced and endotracheal intubation has proved impossible, that the parturient should be placed immediately head down on her left side. If partial respiratory obstruction persists, he advocates continuing the ventilation in this position with a face mask with the expectation of progressing to spontaneous breathing. He advocates passing a wide-bore stomach tube while the patient is still anesthetized in this position to suction away any recoverable gastric contents and to instill liquid antacid into the stomach.[41] If total respiratory obstruction develops, Tunstall[42] has advocated use of the esophageal obturator airway, or, it having failed, tracheostomy.

POSITIONING DURING REGIONAL ANESTHESIA: EPIDURAL ANALGESIA AND SUBARACHNOID ANESTHESIA

Positioning During Establishment of Epidural Block

Positioning, Comfort, and Aortocaval Compression

Vincent and Chestnut[43] have summarized studies that assessed the comfort of term parturients placed in either the left lateral decubitus position or the sitting position for the introduction of lumbar epidural catheters. No clear choice of position could be determined; therefore, if a parturient is uncomfortable in either of the positions, the other might be tried. Kinsella and co-workers[16] have suggested that the left lateral decubitus position with a pronounced and exaggerated flexion of the spine to facilitate epidural catheter placement frequently causes concealed aortocaval compression. They recommend that this position should be avoided throughout pregnancy to reduce the incidence of aortocaval compression. Another group demonstrated that 77% of parturients placed in the left lateral decubitus position during insertion of epidural catheters developed greater than 25% decreases in cardiac output during the procedure, whereas only 27% of parturients experienced similar decreases when the sitting position was used.[44]

Positioning and the Spread of Epidural Block

Although several earlier authors have reported lateralization of analgesia to the down side (decubitus side) of the patient,[45–48] a current consensus seems to deny the importance of gravity in the spread of drugs in the epidural space in the near-term pregnant patient. Hew and colleagues[47] reported that two thirds of the patients who remained in labor on the same side as the one on which they were placed for the introduction of the epidural anesthetic displayed a lower level of analgesia on the up side. They reported improvement in the equal spread of the block when the laboring woman was asked to lie on the side opposite to the position in which the block was started.[47] Without offering convincing evidence, Thorburn and Moir[49] advocated injecting epidural anesthetics for cesarean section with the patient in the sitting position and continuing in this position for at least 10 minutes before assumption of the supine left lateral tilt position. Park and co-workers[50] demonstrated no difference in either the sacral or the cephalad extent of the block when similar volumes of 1.5% lidocaine were injected epidurally in either the sitting or lateral decubitus position in men.

Hodgkinson and Husain[51] reported their surprise at being unable to demonstrate any gravity effects when the epidural space of parturients was injected with 20 mL of 0.75% bupivacaine in the sitting position and maintained thus for 5 minutes. They found limitation of cephalad spread only in obese parturients. Rolbin and associates[52] reported that maintenance of laboring women in the full left lateral decubitus position during epidural analgesia resulted in satisfactory analgesia. In contrast, Merry and colleagues[53] indicated an incidence of 30% asymmetrical cephalad spread of analgesia when patients were maintained in the left lateral decubitus position rather than supine. Nevertheless, sacral analgesia was unaffected by position. Merry's group[53] used small volumes of relatively more concentrated bupivacaine (0.5%) than did Rolbin and associates,[52] a difference in technique that might account for the conflicting findings. The total milligram dose (volume multiplied by concentration) seems to be a relative constant in obstetric epidural anesthetics of similar spread and duration, but lower concentration allows less motor block.

Other equally experienced authorities, such as Bonica,[54] Writer and associates,[55] and Rickford and Reynolds[56] have found no difference in the onset or the extent of sacral blockade of patients in the semi-upright position for injection of the epidural solution as compared with patients who remained supine. Ackerman and co-workers[57, 58] noted no difference in onset time or spread of block caudad or cephalad when similar volumes of 2% pH-adjusted 2-chloroprocaine were injected into the epidural space in the sitting versus supine position in either the first stage or second stage of labor.

Norris and Dewan[59] placed cesarean section patients either in 30 to 40 degrees of head-up tilt or in the supine position during injection of 23 mL of 3% 2-chloroprocaine into the epidural space. They found no difference in the rate of onset of equal blockade or the extent of blockade between the two groups, indicating little effect of head-up position in these pregnant patients. Norris and colleagues[60] also demonstrated convincingly that gravity does not cause lateralization of analgesia when 3% 2-chloroprocaine is injected into the epidural space of parturients remaining in the fully lateral recumbent position (either right or left) for 20 minutes. However, Pitkanen and associates established peridural block for cesarean section with 20 mL epidural 0.5% bupivacaine in the right lateral decubitus, then asked half of their patients to remain on the right side for 30 minutes while the other half turned to the left side for 30 minutes. There was no significant difference in lateralization, extent of the block, or plasma bupivacaine concentrations in their 40 patients.[61] Most observers do seem to agree, however, that doses of local anesthetic agents injected subsequent to the initial dose are not very likely to be influenced in their spread by gravity.[53, 62]

Positioning for the Management of Labor with Epidural Analgesia

Controversy over the best position in which to conduct labor with or without regional analgesia has spanned many years, many continents, and many cultures. Some physiologic facts that may be pertinent are available to us. Maintenance of the laboring parturient in the sitting position versus the supine position results in higher intrauterine pressure between contractions, greater bearing-down pressures (at least in nulliparas), and shorter durations of the second stage of labor.[63, 64] Berman and co-workers[65] suggested that the supine position during labor impaired not only uterine blood flow but also the umbilical circulation.

Huovinen and Teramo[66] reported that when epidural anesthesia used during labor was maintained in the continued left lateral positioning, only 10% of infants developed disturbing fetal heart rate patterns versus 56% abnormalities in similar patients laboring in the supine position. In the supine position, the occurrence of moderate arterial hypotension was associated in 50% of instances with disturbing fetal heart rate patterns. In patients who labored in the full left lateral decubitus position only 3% developed disturbing moderate blood pressure decreases; disturbing fetal heart rate patterns resulted in only 3% of those occurrences of reduced blood pressure.[66]

Preston and co-workers reported no difference in the satisfactory character of epidural analgesia between laboring patients who were maintained in the left semilateral position (with a wedge) versus similar women lying in the complete left lateral decubitus position.[67] There were no differences in pain scores, motor block scores, the incidence of uneven block, or the necessity to reposition the catheter or supplement the local anesthetic. However, 15% of their patients demonstrated evidence of severe fetal heart rate deceleration during maintenance in the wedge-tilt position versus none at all who were maintained in the full left lateral decubitus position.[67]

Fraser found transient hypotension in about 12% of parturients laboring under epidural anesthesia in both left lateral and supine positions, but severe hypotension occurred slightly more frequently in the supine patients.[68] Nonoperative, nonforceps deliveries were accomplished in only 34% of women in labor in the supine position versus 46% in patients who had labored in the lateral position. Forceps were required in 55% of patients who labored in the supine position but in only 38% of those who labored in the lateral position.[68]

Curtis and co-workers detected no significant changes in oxygen saturation in parturients who labored under epidural analgesia while in the supine, sitting, or left lateral posi-

tion.[69] However, in patients laboring without epidural analgesia, marked changes in transcutaneous oxygen tension were detected in all three positions. This was apparently caused by hyperventilation during the peak of contractions and hypoventilation between contractions. Maternal oxygen saturation was slightly higher in the sitting position than in supine. A finding unique to this study is that the lateral position was associated with the greatest falls in oxygen tension.[69]

Positioning During Subarachnoid Anesthesia

Positioning and the Comfort of Patient and Anesthesiologist

Stein and associates[70] studied the "Finster" position[71] with the patient straddling the table versus the standard sitting position with both legs off the same side of the table (Fig. 16–3). They found patients slightly more comfortable in the Finster position, perhaps because they can support themselves more easily and do not have the fear of falling. A few anesthesiologists complained of personal discomfort when patients were in the Finster position, perhaps because they must bend awkwardly over the side of the table to establish the block. However, there were no differences in the spread or evenness of the blocks.

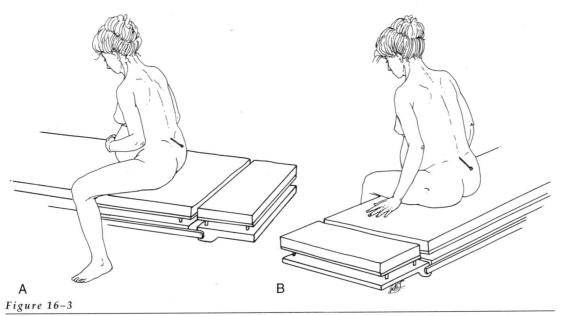

Figure 16–3

Sitting position for establishment of regional anesthesia in the gravid patient. *A.* The table-straddling position advocated by Finster. *B.* The classic position with patient's legs over side of table.

Position and the Spread and Lateralization of Subarachnoid Block

Historically, the baricity of intrathecal solutions has been deemed useful in controlling the character of subarachnoid block in nonpregnant and pregnant patients alike. However, the degree to which position can be used effectively for this purpose is now less clear. Several authors have demonstrated in nonpregnant patients that with 0.5% hyperbaric bupivacaine, position does affect spread and localization, but much less dramatically than might be expected.[72–74]

Sprague advocated that subarachnoid block in the parturient should be routinely established with the patient in the right lateral recumbent position.[75] Norris[76] injected hyperbaric bupivacaine to establish subarachnoid anesthesia for cesarean section with the patient always in the right lateral decubitus position, then immediately turned to the left lateral supine position with a left tilt of the surgical table, presumably to reduce lateralization of subarachnoid block that might result from the necessity of left body tilt to avoid aortocaval compression. However, Martin-Salvaj and co-workers[74] reiterated the conclusions of many older studies when they reported that, in nonpregnant patients, the subarachnoid injection of tetracaine, fentanyl, or epinephrine in the lateral position does not result in lateralization of either the motor or sensory block. The finding was true even in patients who remained in the lateral position as long as 18 minutes. However, after long duration of lateral position, the duration of both sensory and motor block was slightly longer on the down side of the body as compared with the up side.[74]

Patel and colleagues[77] studied the results of injecting 10 mg of hyperbaric bupivacaine (2 mL of 0.5% solution) in the lateral versus the sitting position at the L2–3 interspace before cesarean section. They found that the onset of sensory and motor block was about one third faster in the lateral position than it was in the sitting position. Thirty-eight percent of women whose subarachnoid drug was injected in the sitting position had insufficient analgesia, whereas in only 4% injected in the lateral position was anesthesia not satisfactory. Hypotension occurred in 48% of parturients injected in the lateral position, but only 13% of the sitting patients became hypotensive. Nausea was noted in 61% of lateral patients versus 22% in sitting patients.

Patel and colleagues[77] suggest that the faster onset of anesthesia while in the lateral position might relate to the anatomy of the lumbar curvature. They postulate that deposition of the solution at the L2–3 interspace relates to the cephalic end of the lumbar curvature, with pooling of the solution, which, on turning the patient supine, may account for a greater proportion gravitating cephalad.[77] In the sitting position, presumably all of the bupivacaine gravitates downward from the same injection site, with anesthesia in higher levels resulting from subsequent diffusion. Hirabayashi and associates[78] have offered radiographic studies suggesting this effect may be more prominent in pregnant women.

Bembridge and co-workers[79] reached similar conclusions after studying subarachnoid anesthesia for cesarean section established with hyperbaric 5% lidocaine in the lateral versus the sitting position. These findings were very similar in all respects to those of Inglis and associates,[80] who injected 2.5 mL of 0.5% hyperbaric bupivacaine in either the sitting or the right lateral decubitus position into the lumbar cerebrospinal fluid of patients who were to have cesarean sections. However, to complicate the consideration even further, Russell and co-workers[81] have reported that subarachnoid injection of drug while the patient is in the right lateral decubitus position enhances spread of the block to a greater extent than subarachnoid injection of drug while the patient is in the left lateral decubitus position.

Other Positioning Considerations in Subarachnoid Anesthesia

Barclay and colleagues[33] administered subarachnoid anesthesia with standardization of variables in nonpregnant patients, pregnant patients at term, and nonpregnant patients in whom inferior vena cava obstruction was artificially induced. In nonpregnant patients with induced vena cava compression, anesthetic levels rose higher than in the nonpregnant patients with unobstructed venae cavae and equaled levels attained in the pregnant patients, presumably indicating that aortocaval obstruction may result in higher block levels than might otherwise be anticipated. Santos and associates[71] have advocated use of a 10-degree head-down tilt of the surgical table immediately after injection of 2.0 mL of 0.5% bupivacaine before cesarean section to enhance the speed of onset and the height of sensory analgesia and to reduce the incidence of maternal hypotension.

PRECAUTIONS CONCERNING POTENTIAL NERVE DAMAGE DURING SURGERY OR OBSTETRIC DELIVERY IN PREGNANCY

Intrapelvic Nerve Damage

The sciatic, femoral, and obturator nerves may be damaged in their pelvic course by pressure from the fetal head or the obstetric forceps. Unilateral, or at times even bilateral, signs and symptoms may mimic nerve damage relating to some of the previously described position-associated hazards.[82] Early in this century the incidence of postpartum femoral neuropathy was an astonishing 4.7% (47/1000); now, 9 decades later, it has fallen to approximately 8/100,000 live births.[83] Vargo attributes that dramatic decrease to (1) labors that are currently less prolonged, (2) our very infrequent use of midforceps deliveries, and/or (3) the increased incidence of cesarean sections in modern obstetric practice.[83]

The Femoral Nerve

Use of the lithotomy position can lead to a femoral neuropathy. Extreme abduction of the thighs with external rotation at the hip is thought to be the cause.[84] The maneuver apparently results in ischemia of the femoral nerve as it is pulled on an angle beneath, and perhaps pinched against, the inguinal ligament (Fig. 16–4). In recorded cases, recovery has been complete within 10 weeks. This postural neuropathy can best be prevented by careful use of padded lateral thigh supports to limit the degree of abduction of the lower extremities.[84]

The Sciatic Nerve

Patients in the lithotomy position also can suffer sciatic nerve damage if the thighs and legs are externally rotated and the knees are extended. These maneuvers cause the nerve to be stretched between the sciatic notch and the neck of the fibula. Therefore, external rotation of the thighs and knees should be avoided, and the knees should remain flexed (Fig. 16–5).[85]

The Common Peroneal Nerve

Trauma to the common peroneal nerve can result in footdrop and anesthesia along the

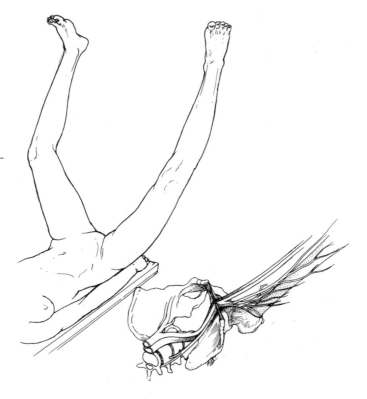

Figure 16–4

Femoral nerve damage due to excessive abduction and external rotation of the elevated lower extremities causing angulation and compression of the nerve under a tight inguinal ligament. (From McLeskey CH [ed.]: Geriatric Anesthesiology. Baltimore, Williams & Wilkins, 1996, in press.)

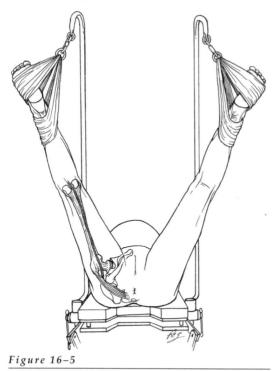

Figure 16–5

Sciatic nerve stretch damage due to extended leg in lithotomy position.

anterolateral surface of the leg and foot. In the lithotomy position the common peroneal nerve may be damaged by the pressure of the vertical supporting pole for the leg or by inadequately padded metal knee supports impacting the popliteal fossa. Compression, ischemia, and/or traction to the nerve have been said to be damaging factors.[86] This vulnerability has been thought to be due to the position of the nerve lateral and superficial to the proximal end of the fibula (Fig. 16–6A).[87] In addition, Dornette[88] stated that the common peroneal nerve can be damaged by pressure against an unpadded table while in the lateral recumbent position or by poorly positioned rolls under the knees (see also Chapter 6).

In surgical patients, Warner's group[89] identified extra risk factors to be (1) remaining in the lithotomy position for 4 hours or longer; (2) a lean body habitus; and (3) a history of smoking within 30 days of the procedure.[89] However, the use of regional anesthesia was not found to be associated with an identifiable risk of neuropathy. Approximately one half of Warner's patients with common peroneal neuropathy regained motor function within the first year, but none of the eight patients with sciatic neuropathy regained complete motor function within the first year.[89]

The Saphenous Nerve

In the lithotomy position, damage to the saphenous nerve can occur when the medial aspect of the lower leg is suspended outside an unpadded upright support. The nerve is compressed between the medial aspect of the tibia and the vertical metal brace (see Fig. 16–6B). Paresthesias may occur along the medial and anteromedial side of the calf.[87]

POSITIONING PREGNANT PATIENTS FOR SURGICAL PROCEDURES OTHER THAN THOSE RELATED TO THE DELIVERY OF THE FETUS

Very little original work has appeared in the literature concerning this subject. However, considerations derived from the previous sections of this chapter give some indications regarding necessary precautions.

- Respiratory function, in particular avoidance of alveolar-arterial oxygen deficiency, is more favorable in the semisitting position than in the supine, lateral, and lithotomy positions during late pregnancy.
- Cardiovascular function, in particular stroke volume, cardiac output, and blood pressure, is most acceptable in the left lateral decubitus position, slightly less acceptable in the 15-degree left tilt position, and least acceptable in the supine position.
- The lithotomy position is particularly detrimental to both respiratory and cardiovascular functions.

Therefore, some compromises among these various requirements should be sought that are also compatible with the positioning necessary for exposure of the surgical field. In any position that is less than full left lateral recumbency, deliberate efforts must be made to ensure that the gravid uterus is not impinging on the inferior vena cava, aorta, or iliac vessels. Blood pressures simultaneously recorded from the femoral and brachial vessels can be used to estimate whether these precautions have been successful. During some in-

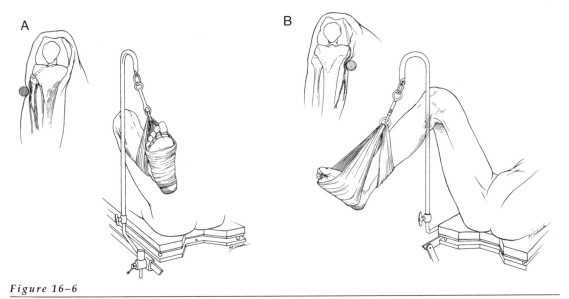

Figure 16-6

Compressive damage to the common peroneal nerve (*A*) or to the saphenous nerve (*B*) from an unpadded vertical post of the lithotomy leg holder pressing firmly against the extremity just distal to the knee joint.

tra-abdominal procedures, it may be possible for the surgeon to directly see the relationship of the uterus to the vena cava and aorta and even to use intraperitoneal packs to relieve compression. A prudent admonition is that the surgical procedure should be accomplished as swiftly as possible consistent with an acceptable outcome.

Whenever feasible, external fetal heart rate monitoring may be helpful to indicate the continued well-being of the fetus during the surgical procedure.[90] However, one must recognize that interpretation of the fetal heart rate tracing is an imprecise art in these circumstances. In addition, the effects of sedatives and anesthetics used for the procedure disturb the normal patterns and may give false indications of fetal compromise to obstetricians who are unfamiliar with these effects.[91]

REFERENCES

1. Awe RJ, Nicotra MB, Newsom TD, Viles R: Arterial oxygenation and alveolar-arterial gradients in term pregnancy. Obstet Gynecol 53:182, 1979.
2. Baldwin GR, Moorthi DS, Whelton JA, MacDonald KF: New lung functions and pregnancy. Am J Obstet Gynecol 127:235, 1977.
3. Marx GF, Murthy PK, Orkin LR: Static compliance before and after vaginal delivery. Br J Anaesth 42:1100, 1970.
4. Russell IF, Chambers WA: Closing volume in normal pregnancy. Br J Anaesth 53:1043, 1981.
5. Ueland K, Hansen JM: Maternal cardiovascular dynamics: II. Posture and uterine contractions. Am J Obstet Gynecol 103:1, 1969.
6. Lindheimer MD, Ehrlich EN: Postural effects on renal function and volume homeostasis during pregnancy. J Reprod Med 23:135–151, 1979.
7. Mills GH, Chaffe AG: Sleeping positions adopted by pregnant women of more than 30 weeks' gestation. Anaesthesia 49:249–250, 1994.
8. Kinsella SM, Whitwam JG, Spencer JAD: Aortic compression by the uterus: Identification with the Finapres digital arterial pressure instrument. Br J Obstet Gynaecol 97:700, 1990.
9. Goodlin RC: Importance of the lateral position during labor. Obstet Gynecol 37:698, 1971.
10. Eckstein KL, Marx GF: Aortocaval compression and uterine displacement. Anesthesiology 40:92, 1974.
11. Abitbol MM: Aortic compression and uterine blood flow during pregnancy. Obstet Gynecol 50:562, 1977.
12. Secher NJ, Arnsbo P, Heslet Andersen L, Thomsen A: Measurements of cardiac stroke volume in various body positions in pregnancy and during Cesarean section: A comparison between thermodilution and impedance cardiography. Scand J Clin Lab Invest 39:569, 1979.
13. Clark RB: Prevention and treatment of aortocaval compression in the pregnant patient. Anesth Rev 7:13, 1980.
14. Abitbol MM: Supine position in labor and associated fetal heart rate changes. Obstet Gynecol 65:481, 1985.
15. Kinsella SM, Spencer JA, Whitwam JG: Use of digital arterial pressure to detect aortic compression during labour. Lancet 2:714, 1989.
16. Kinsella SM, Whitwam JG, Spencer JAD: Reducing aortocaval compression: How much tilt is enough? BMJ 305:539, 1992.
17. Howard BK, Goodson JH, Mengert WF: Supine hypotensive syndrome in late pregnancy. Obstet Gynecol 1:371, 1953.
18. Ohlson L: Effects of the pregnant uterus on the ab-

dominal aorta and its branches. Acta Radiol Diagn 19:369, 1978.

19. Lees MM, Scott DB, Kerr MG: Haemodynamic changes associated with labor. J Obstet Gynaecol Br Commonwlth 77:29, 1970.

20. Bieniarz J, Joshida T, Romero-Salinas G, et al.: Aortocaval compression by the uterus in late human pregnancy: IV. Am J Obstet Gynecol 103:19, 1969.

21. Drummond GB, Scott SEM, Lees MM, Scott DB: Effects of posture on limb blood flow in late pregnancy. BMJ 4:587, 1974.

22. Marx GF, Husain FJ, Shiau HF: Brachial and femoral blood pressures during the prenatal period. Am J Obstet Gynecol 136:11, 1980.

23. Jassir C, Yu KC, Marx GF: Alveolar-arterial oxygen difference in parturient women with two types of uterine displacement. Anesth Analg 52:43, 1973.

24. Redick LF: An inflatable wedge for prevention of aortocaval compression during pregnancy. Am J Obstet Gynecol 133:458, 1979.

25. Kennedy RL, Friedman DL, Katchka DM, et al.: Hypotension during obstetrical anesthesia. Anesthesiology 20:153, 1959.

26. Colon-Morales MA: A self supporting device for continuous left uterine displacement during cesarean section. Anesth Analg 49:223, 1970.

27. Kennedy RL: An instrument to relieve inferior vena cava occlusion. Am J Obstet Gynecol 107:331, 1970.

28. Buley RJR, Downing JW, Brock-Utne JG, Cuerdin C: Right versus left lateral tilt for cesarean section. Br J Anesth 49:1009, 1977.

29. Crawford JS, Burton M, Davies P: Time and lateral tilt at cesarean section. Br J Anaesth 44:477, 1972.

30. Newman B, Derrington C, Dore C: Cardiac output and the recumbent position in late pregnancy. Anaesthesia 38:332, 1983.

31. Crawford JS: Principles and Practice of Obstetric Anaesthesia, 5th ed. Oxford, Blackwell, 1985, p. 286.

32. Kauppila A, Koskinen M, Puolakka J, et al.: Decreased intervillous and unchanged myometrial blood flow in supine recumbency. Obstet Gynecol 55:203, 1980.

33. Barclay DL, Renegar OJ, Nelson EW: The influence of inferior vena cava compression on the level of spinal anesthesia. Am J Obstet Gynecol 101:792, 1968.

34. Datta S, Alper MH, Ostheimer GW, et al.: Effects of maternal position on epidural anesthesia for cesarean section, acid-base status, and bupivacaine concentrations at delivery. Anesthesiology 50:205, 1979.

35. Apgar V: A proposal for a new method of evaluation of the newborn infant. Anesth Analg 32:260, 1953.

36. Ansari I, Wallace G, Clemetson CAB, et al.: Tilt cesarean section. J Obstet Gynaecol Br Commonwlth 77:713, 1970.

37. Pearce AJ: Intubation in the left lateral position: The logical choice for obstetric patients. Presented before the XVI meeting of the Society of Obstetrical Anesthesiologists and Perinatologists. San Antonio, 1984, p. 37 (abstract).

38. Zych A: Maternal position during induction of anesthesia for cesarean section. Anesthesia 38:1006, 1983.

39. Tomkinson J: Report on confidential enquiries into maternal deaths in England and Wales, 1976–1978. London, Department of Health and Social Security, 1982, vol. XV, p. 52.

40. American College of Obstetricians and Gynecologists: Technical Bulletin, No. 65. Washington, DC, American College of Obstetricians and Gynecologists, May 1982.

41. Tunstall ME: Anaesthesia for obstetric operations. Clin Obstet Gynaecol 7:665, 1980.

42. Tunstall ME: Failed intubation in obstetric anaesthesia: An indication for use of the esophageal gastric tube airway. Br J Anaesth 56:659, 1984.

43. Vincent RD, Chestnut DH: Which position is more comfortable for the parturient during identification of the epidural space? Int J Obstet Anaesth 1:9, 1991.

44. Andrews PJD, Ackerman WE, Juneja MM: Aortocaval compression in the sitting and lateral decubitus positions during extradural catheter placement in the parturient. Can J Anaesth 40:320, 1993.

45. Bromage PR: Spread of analgesic solutions in the epidural space and their site of action: A statistical study. Br J Anesth 34:161, 1962.

46. Grundy EM, Rao LN, Winnie AP: Epidural anesthesia and the lateral position. Anesth Analg 57:95, 1978.

47. Hew EM, Cole AFD, Rolbin SH, Virgint SJ: The effect of lateral position and volume on the spread of epidural anesthesia in the parturient. Anesthesiology 51:S300, 1979 (abstract).

48. Husemeyer R, White DC: Lumbar extradural injection pressures in pregnant women. Br J Anaesth 52:55, 1980.

49. Thorburn J, Moir DD: Epidural analgesia for elective cesarean section. Anaesthesia 35:3, 1980.

50. Park WY, Hagins FM, Massengale MD, Macnamara TE: The sitting position and anesthetic spread in the epidural space. Anesth Analg 63:863, 1984.

51. Hodgkinson R, Husain FJ: Obesity, gravity and spread of epidural anesthesia. Anesth Analg 60:421, 1981.

52. Rolbin SH, Cole AFD, Hew EM, Virgint S: Effect of lateral position and volume on the spread of epidural anesthesia in the parturient. Can Anaesth Soc J 28:431, 1981.

53. Merry AF, Cross JA, Mayadeo SV, Wild CJ: Posture and the spread of extradural analgesia in labour. Br J Anaesth 55:303, 1983.

54. Bonica JJ: Obstetric Anesthesia and Analgesia. Amsterdam, World Federation of Anaesthesiologists, 1980, p. 1680.

55. Writer WDR, Dewan DM, James FM III: Three percent 2-chloroprocaine for cesarean: Appraisal of a standard dose technique. Can Anaesth Soc J 31:559, 1984.

56. Rickford WJK, Reynolds F: Epidural analgesia in labour and maternal posture. Anaesthesia 38:1169, 1983.

57. Ackerman WE, Juneja MM, Kaczorowski DM, et al.: The effect of pH-adjusted 2-chloroprocaine on the onset of peridural analgesia in pregnant patients in the lying and sitting position during the first stage of labor. J Clin Anesth 1:177, 1989.

58. Ackerman WE, Herold JA, Juneja MM, Sweeney NJ: Effect of position on the spread of buffered 2% chloroprocaine administered epidurally for the second stage of labor. South Med J 83:277, 1990.

59. Norris MC, Dewan DM: Effect of gravity on the spread of extradural anaesthesia for cesarean section. Br J Anaesth 59:338, 1987.

60. Norris MC, Leighton BL, DeSimone CA, Larijani GE: Lateral position and epidural anaesthesia for cesarean section. Anesth Analg 67:788, 1988.

61. Pitkanen MT, Paatero H, Rosenberg PH: The effect of maternal lateral position or position change on epidural anesthesia and plasma bupivacaine concentrations. Reg Anesth 13:157, 1988.

62. Bromage PR: Epidural Analgesia. Philadelphia, WB Saunders, 1978, pp. 149, 150, 565.

63. Chen SZ, Aisaka K, Mori H, Kigawa T: Effects of sitting position on uterine activity during labor. Obstet Gynecol 69:67, 1987.

64. Caldeyro-Barcia R: The influence of maternal position during the second stage of labor. ICEA Rev 2:31, 1978.

65. Berman JA, Patel S, Marx GF, et al.: Umbilical velocity waveforms in different maternal positions before and after epidural anesthesia. Presented before the XVI meeting of the Society of Obstetrical Anesthesiologists and Perinatologists. San Antonio, 1984, p. 16 (abstract).

66. Huovinen K, Teramo K: The effect of maternal position on fetal heart rate during extradural analgesia. Br J Anaesth 51:767, 1979.

67. Preston R, Crosby ET, Kotarba D, et al.: Maternal positioning affects fetal heart rate changes after epidural analgesia for labour. Can J Anaesth 40:1136, 1993.

68. Fraser RA: Some aspects of management during lumbar epidural analgesia in active labor. Presented before the XVI meeting of the Society of Obstetrical Anesthesiologists and Perinatologists. San Antonio, 1984, p. 58 (abstract).

69. Curtis J, Shnider SM, Saitto C, et al.: The effects of painful uterine contractions, position, and epidural anesthesia on maternal transcutaneous oxygen tension. Presented before the XII meeting of the Society of Obstetrical Anesthesiologists and Perinatologists. Boston, 1980, p. 69 (abstract).

70. Stein DJ, Birnbach DJ, Bourlier RA, et al.: Comparison of two sitting positions for placement of spinal anesthesia in the patient for cesarean section. In press.

71. Santos A, Pedersen H, Finster M, Edström M: Hyperbaric bupivacaine for spinal anesthesia in cesarean section. Anesth Analg 63:1009, 1984.

72. Povey HMR, Albrecht Olsen P, Pihl H: Spinal analgesia with hyperbaric 0.5% bupivacaine: Effects of different patient positions. Acta Anaesthesiol Scand 31:616, 1987.

73. Wildsmith J: Baricity and spinal anesthesia: What solution when? Anesthesiol Clin North Am 10:31, 1992.

74. Martin-Salvaj G, van Gessel E, Forster A, et al.: Influence of duration of lateral decubitus on the spread of hyperbaric tetracaine during spinal anesthesia: A prospective time-response study. Anesth Analg 79:1107, 1994.

75. Sprague DYH: Effects of position and uterine displacement on spinal anesthesia for cesarean section. Anesthesiology 44:164, 1976.

76. Norris MC: Height, weight, and the spread of subarachnoid hyperbaric bupivacaine in the term parturient. Anesth Analg 67:555, 1988.

77. Patel M, Samsoon G, Swami A, Morgan B: Posture and the spread of hyperbaric bupivacaine in parturients using the combined spinal epidural technique. Can J Anaesth 40:943, 1993.

78. Hirabayashi Y, Shimizu R, Fukuda H, et al.: Anatomical configuration of the spinal column in the supine position: II. Comparison of pregnant and non-pregnant women. Br J Anaesth 75:6, 1995.

79. Bembridge M, MacDonald R, Lyons G: Spinal anesthesia with hyperbaric lignocaine for elective cesarean section. Anaesthesia 41:906, 1986.

80. Inglis A, Daniel M, McGrady E: Maternal position during induction of spinal anaesthesia for caesarean section: A comparison of right lateral and sitting positions. Anaesthesia 50:363, 1995.

81. Russell IF: Effect of posture during the induction of subarachnoid analgesia for cesarean section: Right v. left lateral. Br J Anaesth 59:342, 1987.

82. Bonica JJ: Obstetric Analgesia and Anesthesia. Philadelphia, FA Davis, 1967.

83. Vargo MM, Robinson LR, Nicholas JJ, Rulin MC: Postpartum femoral neuropathy: Relic of an earlier era? Arch Phys Med Rehabil 71:591, 1990.

84. Tondare AS, Nadkarni AV, Sathe CH, Dave VB: Femoral neuropathy: A complication of lithotomy position under spinal anesthesia. Can Anaesth Soc J 30:84, 1983.

85. Nicholson MJ, Eversole UH: Nerve injuries incident to anesthesia and operation. Anesth Analg 36:19, 1957.

86. Dawson DM, Krarup C: Perioperative nerve lesions. Arch Neurol 46:1355, 1989.

87. Britt BA, Gordon RA: Peripheral nerve injuries associated with anaesthesia. Can Anaesth Soc J 11:514, 1964.

88. Dornette WHL: Identifying, moving, and positioning the patient. In Dornette WHL (ed.): Legal Issues in Anesthesia Practice. Philadelphia, FA Davis, 1991, pp. 120–123.

89. Warner MA, Martin JT, Schroeder DR, et al.: Lower-extremity motor neuropathy associated with surgery performed on patients in a lithotomy position. Anesthesiology 81:6, 1994.

90. Liu PH, Warren TM, Ostheimer GW, et al.: Foetal monitoring in parturients undergoing surgery unrelated to pregnancy. Can Anaesth Soc J 32:525, 1985.

91. Boehm FH, Egilmez A, Smith BE: Physostigmine's effect on diminished fetal heart rate variability caused by scopolamine, meperidine and propiomazine. J Perinat Med 5:214, 1977.

Chapter 17

Geriatrics

John T. Martin

BACKGROUND

Positioning an elderly patient for a surgical procedure can pose difficult problems because of the presence of acquired infirmities. No minimum age can be placed on the term *geriatric*. Whereas an increasing number of senior citizens are now living to the century mark, and remain reasonably fit for the great majority of those years, some 60-year-olds will have dwindled to an extent not ordinarily present until several decades later. Most of the positioning problems of the aged are similar to those seen in younger patients and are presented generically elsewhere in this text. This discussion relates to those issues more common to the older population.

PROBLEMS OF AGING

Nutrition

Many geriatric patients have faced a serious change in lifestyle that accompanied either their retirement, retirement of their spouse, or the death of a loved one.

- Often, meal times assume a social significance not previously present and excessive nutrition combines with reduced general activity. Obesity commonly develops, frequently limiting activity even further.
- By contrast, the lonely, often hermit-like existence of some elders results in significant malnutrition, wasting, and limited physical activity. On occasion, and particularly in the presence of terminal disease, the result can be serious enough

to be compared with that of a cachectic survivor of a prisoner-of-war camp.

Both extremes of body habitus can cause physical stresses to be poorly tolerated. Positioning either an obese or a wasted patient presents problems of physical handling, extremity placement, bony prominence padding, and retraction of delicate skin.

The Vasculature

The effects of gravity on the vascular system of a normal patient are detailed in Chapter 6 regarding the lithotomy position. Although the values themselves are probably not altered with aging, the significance of deviations from normal is undoubtedly enhanced by sclerotic changes in the vascular tree. Segments of peripheral vessels may be partially obstructed by plaques, requiring a greater than normal perfusion pressure to provide flow.

Elevation of an extremity above the atrium in the presence of high-pressure flow segments may reduce postplaque flow more than would be anticipated from elevation alone in a normal circulation. Examples are the various lithotomy positions, the tilted lithotomy positions, and the hemilithotomy position. If a raised extremity of an elderly patient is compressed by a pneumatic device or an elastic wrap, or if driving pressure is reduced by the presence of regional or systemic hypotension, flow can be degraded to values that invite a compartment syndrome.[1]

Bruits may be present in the carotid vasculature, indicating the potential for compromised circulation if the patient's head is rotated to one side during positioning. Toole[2] found that a 60-degree lateral rotation of the head begins to reduce flow in the contralateral vertebral artery as it passes through the bony canals of the transverse processes of the sixth through the second cervical vertebrae. An 80-degree rotation obstructs flow. Were the vasculature normal, that flow restriction and eventual obstruction would be opposed by a simultaneous, proportional increase in the ipsilateral vessel. Caudad (retrograde) flow in a normal basilar artery might assist perfusion as cephalad flow in the vertebral arteries is diminished. In the presence of recognized arteriosclerotic vascular disease these compensatory mechanisms may not function adequately, and retaining the head in a sagittal alignment deserves strong consideration. Additional comments on head positioning are present elsewhere in this text.

The obvious message is that high-pressure perfusion segments must be assumed to exist in the vessels of aged patients. Therefore, vascular driving pressures must be carefully monitored so that postures required for a surgical procedure compromise regional blood flow to the least extent possible.

The Skeleton

In the aging skeleton, two major problems are present: (1) some form of arthritis is present in 50% of the population that is aged 75 or older,[3] and (2) bone reabsorption usually exceeds bone formation with subsequent skeletal calcium loss and diminished bone density. An increased vulnerability to fractures results. Poor nutrition, particularly regarding calcium and vitamin D intake, enhances the process.

Arthritis. Thirty percent of males and 53% of females in the free-living population older than age 55 have peripheral joint distress.[4] Twenty-five percent of men and 40% of women in that age group have frequent neck and low back complaints. Osteoarthritis is second only to obesity as a reason for an elderly patient to consult a family practitioner. Ranked as the most prevalent chronic health problem in a 1984 survey by the National Center for Health Statistics,[4] osteoarthritis was present in 49.5% of individuals aged 75 and older and caused an estimated 180,000 people to be confined to wheelchairs or beds. Michet[5] has published an extensive review of the subject.

Jenkinson and associates studied 100 patients admitted to an acute geriatric unit and found that about 40% of those who had some loss of function due to arthritis did not volunteer evidence of their joint disease.[6] Even with minimal involvement, major joints may have specific limitations of mobility to which the patient has gradually adapted. Flexion or extension deficits may dictate which arm carries heavy loads or how the individual navigates stairs. Neck motion awake may be restricted by pain, imposing significant limitations on the positions in which the individual can sleep comfortably. How these arthritic problems impact on a patient's ability to assume an intraoperative posture should be determined preoperatively. Severe postoperative pain can be caused during anesthesia by exceeding easily identifiable limits of skeletal mobility.

Osteomalacia. Osteomalacia, a disorder causing decreased bone mineralization, is associated with normal bone volume, bone deformities, bone pain, and fractures. It is caused by deficiencies of vitamin D or phosphates and may be associated with the use of drugs such as phenytoin, barbiturates, and aluminum-containing antacids.[7]

Osteoporosis. Osteoporosis, defined as "a state of inappropriately low bone volume for age, gender and race in association with normal mineralization processes and a normal ratio of unmineralized osteoid matrix to mineralized bone," is the most common metabolic bone disorder in the geriatric population. Involving about 20 million North Americans and costing up to $6 billion annually in medical care, its etiology is uncertain in 95% of its victims.[7]

Positioning Risks. Either osteoporosis or osteomalacia may impair fracture healing and predispose to refracture at a healed site during patient manipulation. Low bone mass increases the susceptibility for primary fractures[7] and renders perilous the mechanical manipulation of aged patients during positioning. Similar hazards may exist if bony metastases threaten skeletal continuity.

POTENTIAL COMPLICATIONS

Skin Damage and Decubiti

Loss of subcutaneous tissue and decreased elasticity of aged skin increases the likelihood of damage to superficial tissues when skin is stretched or compressed for long periods of time. Skin overlying bony prominences that support the weight of body parts, particularly the dorsal aspect of the calcaneus, may become relatively avascular with prolonged compression. Decubitus ulcers can result, with potentially significant systemic effects if secondary infection develops and is accompanied by septicemia. Careful padding of weight-bearing surfaces in cachectic patients is necessary, despite the fact that the precaution does not guarantee protection against compressive damage.[8] Tape that stretches elderly skin is potentially injurious, and alternative arrangements should be sought.

Hypoperfusion

Hypoperfusion due to positioning is usually regional rather than systemic. Sequestration of blood in lower extremities that are positioned below the level of the heart may occur in any elderly patient, but the presence of hypovolemia increases its potential for harm by reducing inferior vena caval return below the level needed to sustain an adequate cardiac output. Leg wraps that are tight enough to support venous channels against gravity pooling without themselves producing ischemia are the usual precautionary practice.

When one or both lower extremities are raised in a variant of the lithotomy position, hypoperfusion may occur either from a loss of driving pressure or from a serious increase in compartment pressures because of external compression associated with a leg holder, wrapped legs, or the weight of a surgical assistant leaning on the extremity (see discussion in Chapter 6).[1] Because it impairs driving pressure, controlled hypotension may be an undesirable addition to the vasculature of a geriatric patient. Ischemia that leads to a compartment syndrome is a serious and consequential complication for an otherwise uneventful anesthetic and surgical procedure.

Skeletal Distress

In the general interest of patient safety, the skeleton of every geriatric patient should be considered to be fragile and to have limited mobility. Preanesthetic evaluations should seek evidence of limited motion of major joints, inflexibility of the vertebral column, arthritic or disuse contractures, a history of fractures occurring with minimal stress, or the presence of known bony metastases. If extremes of rotation, flexion, or extension are known to be painful, the limits of comfortable

movement should be established before the induction of anesthesia. When the interview is conducted by persons other than those who are to administer the anesthetic, the findings must be carefully documented in a manner that is easily recognized by a subsequent chart reviewer. Having an awake patient assume a position intended for use during surgery is a helpful method for assessing the range of comfort of a distorted skeleton and evaluating alternative positioning.

Because of the presence of arthritis and abnormal bone metabolism, the most likely site of skeletal trauma during anesthesia and surgery can be assumed to be the neck of the elderly patient. Forced head extension needed for tracheal intubation can be replaced by introducing an endotracheal tube over a fiberoptic guide while the head remains in a neutral position. Keeping the cervical spine aligned with the thoracic vertebrae while the patient is being turned into either the lateral or the prone position is a basic concept, and maintaining that alignment in the lateral position is a recognized need. Retaining the pronated head in the sagittal plane of the torso rather than rotating it in either direction probably offers the least amount of trauma to geriatric cervical vertebrae and affects vertebral artery perfusion the least.

Stresses on individual joints should be minimized to the fullest extent possible during nursing maneuvers, patient transport, and surgical positioning. Soft padding can protect pressure points of positioned patients, although this fundamental practice is known not to guarantee the absence of compressive problems such as an ulnar neuropathy.[8] It may be sufficient, however, to diffuse the pressure of a weight-bearing bony prominence and prevent focal ischemia that produces a decubitus ulcer.

Because the geriatric population is increasing in numbers, and because the technology of joint replacement is increasing in both sophistication and availability, more elderly patients have prostheses now than was the case a decade ago. Although many of these joints may be quite supple, those that are not can complicate surgical positioning. Despite thoughtful handling, positioning stresses may fracture long bones in which the stems of prostheses are embedded or refracture a site that is only marginally stabilized by screws and plates that have been in situ for long periods. Detecting the presence of these devices in the preoperative interview, and modifying positioning techniques accordingly, may be key to the avoidance of reconstructive orthopedic procedures after the primary operation.

Primary or metastatic tumors may weaken bones sufficiently for pathologic fractures to be produced by the minimal stresses that occur during handling and positioning. Because indications of these events may be masked by the presence of general anesthesia or heavy sedation, a patient who reports peculiar sites of skeletal pain in the immediate postoperative period should receive a detailed evaluation to establish the need for rapid corrective treatment.

Neuropathies

Elderly patients with bony abnormalities such as osteoarthritis frequently have dysesthesias associated with specific body positions. Occipital pain from sustained neck rotation; an ulnar neuropathy from resting an arm on a flexed elbow; median nerve discomfort from long-term use of a mouse, a trackball, or a computer keyboard; and sciatic distress (either from hip flexion with an extended lower leg or from prolonged sitting on a wasted gluteal mass) are examples. Frequently the onset of symptoms occurs after only a few minutes in the offending posture. Changing position relieves the annoyance promptly; however, continuing the provocation can cause prolonged distress and may lead to a serious clinical neuropathy. These dysesthesias are well known to those so afflicted, and preoperative questioning can reveal their presence. Efforts can then be made to avoid stressful postures during the anesthetic and surgical procedure and to provide padding that may minimize compression. Similar prophylactic measures should be extended into the postoperative period because sustained postures in a convalescent bed can also be detrimental.

Other neuropathies may be disease related or provoked by posture, but these are rarely limited only to the elderly. They are discussed elsewhere in this text.

PREANESTHETIC EVALUATION

A careful inventory of skeletal distress should be a deliberate part of the preoperative interview of elderly patients. Positive information should be recorded in such a manner that it is inescapable for all who review the patient's chart before positioning. Knowing the posture intended for that particular procedure is mandatory. On occasion, a preanesthetic "dry run" of the intended position helps identify a need to choose a substitute arrangement for the operation. This concept is particularly useful for patients who have artificial joints, limited mobility of major joints, contractures of extremities, and painful portions of the spine. When potential problems exist with a position for which there is no suitable alternative, the recovery facility, whether the postanesthesia care unit or intensive care unit, should be alerted to specifically evaluate the state of the skeletal and peripheral nervous systems while the patient is subsequently in their care.

Postural neck distress identifies which positions to avoid during anesthesia and helps plan which head holders to use. Careful delineation of the limits of comfort should be established preoperatively and reviewed before induction of anesthesia or positioning.

A history of ulnar dysesthesias resulting from napping briefly in a chair with elbows resting on arm rails indicates that specific attention must be paid to padding elbows and distributing the weight of the extremity away from the cubital tunnel during anesthesia. As noted, however, padding is not always effective in preventing a neuropathy.[8]

Wrist and hand dysesthesias associated with pre-existing carpal tunnel syndromes, and those that appear while performing repetitive hand and wrist maneuvers (e.g., prolonged keyboarding), indicate the potential for postoperative carpal tunnel distress. Because the perioperative period may be associated with various degrees of peripheral edema, pre-existing or occult carpal tunnel syndromes may produce recurrent or new symptoms after an operation. These associations imply that the distal extremity should be returned to a neutral position after placement of catheters in appropriate vessels. Immobilizing such a hand dorsiflexed in a cock-up splint for a considerable time intraoperatively and postoperatively to preserve a radial artery catheter should be considered hazardous.

As noted previously, the presence of skeletal prostheses should be sought, and any limitations of mobility produced by the device(s) should be defined and documented in a way that is apparent when positioning of the patient on the operating table becomes necessary.

Frail physiques that have atrophic skin and unusually prominent bony landmarks merit the deliberately recorded use of carefully placed additional padding.

REFERENCES

1. Martin JT: Compartment syndromes: Concepts and perspectives for the anesthesiologist. Anesth Analg 75:275, 1992.
2. Toole JF: Effects of change of head, limb and body position on cephalic circulation. N Engl J Med 279:307, 1968.
3. Sorenson LB: Rheumatology. *In* Cassel CK, Riesenberg DE, Sorensen LB, Walsh JR (eds.): Geriatric Medicine, 2nd ed. New York, Springer-Verlag, 1990, p. 184.
4. Valkenburg HA: Epidemiologic considerations of the geriatric population. Gerontology 34(Suppl. 1):2, 1988.
5. Michet CJ: Osteoarthritis. Arthritis 20:815, 1993.
6. Jenkinson ML, Bliss MR, Brain AT, et al.: Peripheral arthritis in the elderly: A hospital study. Ann Rheum Dis 48:227, 1989.
7. Meier E: Disorders of skeletal aging. *In* Cassel CK, Riesenberg DF, Sorensen LB, Walsh JR (eds.): Geriatric Medicine, 2nd ed. New York, Springer-Verlag, 1990, pp. 165–177.
8. Kroll DA, Caplan RA, Posner K, et al.: Nerve injury associated with anesthesia. Anesthesiology 73:202, 1990.

Section VII

Potential Complications

Chapter 18

The Central Nervous System

Nikolaus Gravenstein/Betty L. Grundy
Emilio B. Lobato

BACKGROUND

An appreciation for the mechanisms and the consequences of injuries to the central nervous system (CNS) related to positioning the patient for surgery is the foundation on which their prevention is based. CNS injuries that result from positioning during anesthesia can be grouped into two categories: (1) those related to risk factors that can be detected preoperatively and (2) those with no recognizable risk factors. In this chapter specific problems in both categories of injuries are addressed and a few complications related to changes in position after certain operations are described. Injuries to peripheral nerves are discussed in chapters specific to the various positions and in Chapter 19.

RECOGNIZED RISK FACTORS

Increased Intracranial Pressure

Patients with increased intracranial pressure (ICP) or decreased intracranial compliance are at risk for exacerbation of intracranial hypertension during anesthesia. Increased ICP not accompanied by a corresponding increase in mean arterial pressure (MAP) decreases cerebral perfusion pressure (CPP). In the supine patient, CPP can be determined mathematically by using either ICP or central venous pressure (CVP), whichever is greater, as follows:

$$CPP = MAP - (ICP \text{ or } CVP)$$

As the ICP approaches MAP, CPP becomes insufficient and CNS ischemia results. Similarly, if MAP decreases while ICP is constant or increasing, again CPP decreases. The skull and spinal canal are rigid, almost-closed structures with little ability to compensate for volume changes (Fig. 18–1).[1] Once the rather limited compensatory mechanisms have been exhausted, even very small additions to intracranial volume, for example, by blood or cerebrospinal fluid (CSF), may dramatically affect ICP and, thus, CPP.

Both MAP and ICP are affected by positioning. Any posture in which the head is elevated may cause an orthostatic decrease in MAP because of peripheral and visceral venous pooling and subsequent decreases in preload and cardiac output. The result is diminishing CPP and cerebral blood flow.[2] Orthostatic changes in blood pressure can be lessened by assuring adequate hydration, by changing the patient's position slowly to allow cardiovascular compensation, and by wrapping the patient's legs to minimize venous pooling in the dependent lower extremities.

When the patient's position is changed from supine to one in which the head is higher than the heart, blood pressure measured at the level of the brachial or radial artery no longer equals ICP. In such cases, the zero reference point for the arterial blood pressure transducer should be at the level of

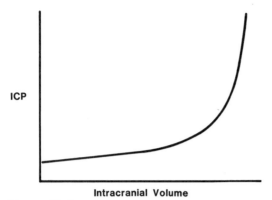

Intracranial Volume

Figure 18–1

Idealized intracranial pressure (ICP)–volume
compliance curve. (Adapted from Miller JD, Garibi J,
Pickard JD: The effects of induced changes of
cerebrospinal fluid volume during continuous
monitoring of ventricular pressure. Arch Neurol
28:265, 1973. Copyright 1973, American Medical
Association.)

the brain, that is, the external auditory meatus, not the wrist or heart. If blood pressure
is being monitored only by a sphygmoma-
nometer cuff, then the appropriate correction
should be made for estimating cerebral MAP.
The correction is based on the hydrostatic
pressure of the fluid column between the
brain and the point at which blood pressure
is being measured ($MAP_{systemic}$) (Fig. 18–2)*:

$$MAP_{cerebral} = MAP_{systemic}$$
$$- \frac{\text{height difference (cm)}}{1.3 \text{ cm/mm Hg}}$$

Thus, when the head is 30 cm above a brachial artery that is being used to measure
blood pressure, the actual $MAP_{cerebral}$ is 21 mm
Hg lower than $MAP_{systemic}$.

A head-elevated position may have a beneficial effect in a patient with increased ICP
(Table 18–1).[3–6] The decrease in ICP associated
with head elevation persists even when other
medical measures are taken to decrease ICP
and continues over time.[3] The opposite occurs
when the head is lowered. Therefore, a patient who arrives in the operating room with
the head elevated to help control ICP should
be kept in that position until anesthesia is
induced and ICP is being medically controlled. Typically, the decrease in intracranial
blood volume associated with improved cere-

bral venous drainage in the head-elevated position offsets the decrease in $MAP_{cerebral}$ so that
CPP is maintained or improved. If hydrostatic
and orthostatic decreases in $MAP_{cerebral}$ are
greater than the ICP decrease, then CPP will
actually decrease. CPP can be evaluated from
simultaneous measurements of ICP and MAP
referenced to the head.

Positions that increase CVP by interfering
with cerebral venous drainage and increasing
cerebral blood volume may increase ICP and
decrease CPP. In a rat model, a 3- to 7-mm Hg
rise in CVP increased cerebral blood volume
approximately the same amount as a 20-mm
Hg increase in arterial carbon dioxide partial
pressure ($PaCO_2$).[7, 8] Thus, position-induced
changes in cerebral venous pressure can have
an effect on cerebral blood volume of the
same magnitude as the consequences of a
clinically unacceptable increase (20 mm Hg)
in $PaCO_2$. Prone positions with the head
lower than the heart, and/or with the head
turned, inevitably result in some degree of
cerebral venous congestion. This is particularly true if a laminectomy frame is used and
the head is quite dependent. The higher mean
airway pressures required for mechanical
ventilation in prone patients may further impede cerebral venous drainage.[7] Careful padding of hips and shoulders, by reducing pressure on the chest and allowing the abdomen
to hang freely, improves thoracic compliance
and thereby decreases mean airway pressure.

Head turning and head-down tilt also
jeopardize cerebral venous drainage during

Table 18–1

**Position-Induced Changes in Intracranial
Pressure***

Intracranial Pressure (mm Hg)	
Supine Position	Head Elevated
1–5	7
6–10	10
11–15	8
16–20	12
21–25	13
26–30	12
32	9
61	7

*Changes in intracranial pressure recorded in 24 patients as
the head was elevated from 40 to 90 degrees.
Modified from Kenning JA, Touting SM, Saunders RL: Upright
patient positioning in the management of intracranial hypertension. Surg Neurol 15:148, 1981. Copyright 1981 by Elsevier Science, Inc.

---

*Equation modified for accuracy from Enderby GEH:
Postural ischaemia and blood pressure. Lancet 1:185,
1954.

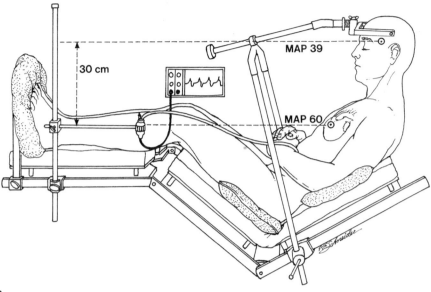

Figure 18–2

Relationship of transducer location to pressure to be measured. Transducer at heart level measures pressure at heart. Transducer moved to level of the ear, and zeroed there, measures intracranial pressure in sitting position independent of site of arterial cannulation. (MAP, mean arterial pressure.)

the placement of a central venous catheter. With increased ICP or abnormal intracranial compliance, the associated increase in cerebral blood volume may markedly decrease CPP.[9] When continuous clinical assessment of neurologic status is needed, the central venous catheter can either be placed by means of a long arm approach (basilic vein) or placed before general anesthesia is induced. The supraclavicular or infraclavicular subclavian approach does not require the head to be turned and may therefore be preferable to the internal jugular route. Occasionally, as in an uncooperative patient, such procedures can be done after induction of general anesthesia, and brain function can be monitored by electroencephalography (EEG), evoked potentials (EP), or transcranial Doppler studies.

During posterior fossa surgery, when the neck is flexed, epidural pressure increases in most patients (Fig. 18–3).[5] This is most likely a consequence of obstructed cerebral venous drainage in the neck. Even with neck flexion in sitting patients, when ICP would normally be expected to decrease, epidural pressure is increased. This is uniformly remedied by decreasing the amount of neck flexion.

In patients with normal intracranial compliance, excessive head turning can compress or obstruct the carotid or vertebral arteries and, thus, produce cerebral ischemia[10–13] or

embolic stroke despite normal systemic blood pressure. If a body position results in partial obstruction of a vessel in which flow is low, thrombosis may follow. Polycythemic patients are particularly vulnerable. Embolic stroke may occur in association with carotid artery atherosclerosis if pieces of atheromatous plaque are dislodged and flow into the intracranial circulation.

The simplest way to prevent position-induced stroke is to consider it a risk whenever a patient's head position is changed. To assess tolerance of an intended intraoperative position in patients with cerebrovascular disease, a trial of positioning should precede anesthetic induction. When the risk of brain ischemia is high, monitoring by EEG, EP, or transcranial Doppler may give warning early enough to allow intervention to prevent stroke and permanent sequelae. With cerebral ischemia, EEG shows a progressive loss of high-frequency electrical activity followed by an increase in power at the lower frequencies. Loss of EP is often preceded by increased latencies and decreased amplitudes of the relevant peaks. Such changes may herald compromise of blood flow to the nerve roots, the spinal cord, the subcortical structures of the brain, or the sensory cortex. With transcranial Doppler monitoring, a decrease in blood flow velocity in the middle cerebral artery may

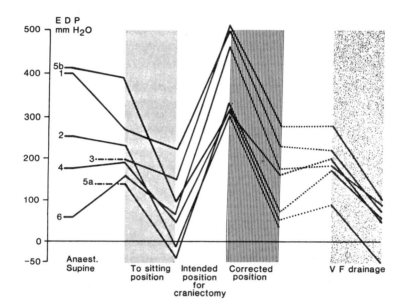

Figure 18–3

Epidural pressure (EDP) during positioning for posterior fossa surgery. Corrected position represents a decrease in patient's degree of neck flexion from the initial positioning by the surgeon. (VF = ventricular fluid.) (Adapted from Nornes H, Magnaes B: Supratentorial epidural pressure during posterior fossa surgery. J Neurosurg 35:541, 1971.)

indicate decreased cerebral blood flow.[14] If such a change is related to positioning, immediate adjustments should be made.

Although extracranial-to-intracranial arterial bypass procedures are now less common than in the recent past, positioning patients who have had this surgery requires special consideration. The superficial extracranial blood vessel, which now supplies the brain, is extremely vulnerable. Care must be taken to identify and protect this vessel, because its compression may produce an ischemic stroke. Whether congenital or acquired, ventriculoperitoneal shunts or a skull defect also present significant risks and must be identified before positioning so that the shunt or defect can be protected from pressure, skull pins, and injection of local anesthetics.

Cervical Instability

Instability of the cervical spine presents a particularly important challenge during positioning. Spinal injuries may be exacerbated during induction of anesthesia and again during positioning for the surgical procedure. While these patients are awake, neck pain and muscle spasm serve as alarms against additional cervical injury. The patient in cervical traction, a halo device, or a cervical collar realizes some protection from the external stabilization.

Induction of anesthesia and positioning should minimally disrupt physiologic and mechanical mechanisms of protection. Ideally,

the airway should be secured and the patient positioned and assessed to verify that the neurologic status does not vary from what it was before positioning. Because drug-induced, as opposed to position-induced, weakness mimicking a neurologic deficit has been described, some have suggested that, before anesthesia is induced, a neurologic examination follow sedation, both before and after endotracheal intubation.[15] The trachea may be intubated by using local anesthesia while the patient is awake. The tube can be placed orally or nasally and either blindly or under visual control with fiberoptic endoscopy. If the patient has extensive facial trauma or a possible basilar skull fracture, blind instrumentation of the nasopharynx is contraindicated; peroral fiberoptic endoscopy, or tracheostomy should be considered. An additional important benefit to awake intubation is that the patient can assist with the actual positioning before anesthesia is induced.[16] This strategy is especially useful for patients with posterior cervical instability who require cervical fusion in the prone position.

Once anesthesia is induced, evaluation of spinal cord function becomes more complex and requires either wake-up testing or somatosensory EP monitoring. Simply turning the patient to the prone position, even while in halo fixation, in cervical traction, or on a Stryker frame, may displace unstable cervical fractures.[17] Elderly patients with posteriorly displaced odontoid fractures are particularly at risk and may suffer respiratory arrest when turned prone.[18] The principles applied during positioning and induction of anesthesia remain applicable until the instability is repaired, external immobilization is accomplished, and the patient is again awake.

Patients with congenital craniocervical abnormalities represent another group that may suffer injury to the spinal cord or brain stem during intubation, positioning, or both, especially with atlanto-occipital assimilation, basilar invagination, or two block cervical fusions separated by an open interspace.[19] Patients with a congenital craniocervical lesion in association with Klippel-Feil syndrome,[19] Arnold-Chiari malformation, Morquio's syndrome,[20-22] Down syndrome,[23-26] or dwarfism[27, 28] should be carefully screened preoperatively.

UNRECOGNIZED RISK FACTORS

Air Embolism

Most spinal and intracranial neurosurgical procedures as well as many ear, nose, and throat procedures are done with the operative site elevated above the level of the heart to reduce venous bleeding. Any time a vein is open at a location above the heart, air embolism may occur when venous pressure is subatmospheric during some phase of the respiratory cycle. In addition to the embolic potential at the actual operative site, when pins on head holder devices puncture through the bony cortex into the marrow space they provide yet another place at which air entrainment may occur.[29] This is especially an issue if the head holder is repositioned and the original pin sites are left uncovered. Putting ointment around the occupied pin sites, as well as in newly vacated pin holes, may reduce the possibility of air entrainment at those locations.

Venous air embolism can cause CNS damage through two mechanisms: (1) decreased cardiac output or cardiovascular collapse and (2) paradoxical air embolism. By means of a patent foramen ovale, an atrial or ventricular septal defect, or an intrapulmonary shunt, venous air bubbles can migrate into the arterial circulation. Air may then accumulate in the cranial circulation and obstruct end arteries, producing ischemia.[30] At least one in five adult patients has a probe-patent foramen

ovale. When air embolism occurs, right atrial pressure rises while left atrial pressure falls, which, with a patent foramen ovale, leads to a right-to-left atrial intracardiac shunt. When the risk of venous air embolism is high, cardiac septa can be evaluated preoperatively with a flow-challenged echocardiogram. If right-to-left shunting is demonstrated, an alternative surgical posture should be strongly considered to minimize the possibility of paradoxical air embolism.[31]

Pneumocephalus

This complication, a function of both position and procedure, occurs most often in a craniotomy done while the patient is sitting (Table 18–2).[32, 33] Asymptomatic pneumocephalus, commonly seen whenever the dura is opened, is rarely troublesome. Tension pneumocephalus, however, is symptomatic and may be dangerous. In a series of 275 operations with patients sitting and the dura opened, a 3% incidence (8/275) of symptomatic pneumocephalus was reported.[34] Although there are many reports of symptomatic tension pneumocephalus, it remains an unusual complication. Because a pneumocephalus may require up to 3 weeks to disappear, at reoperation during that time interval nitrous oxide should probably be avoided until after the dura is opened to minimize the possibility of producing a tension pneumocephalus.[33] A preoperative computed tomographic scan can be obtained to rule out the presence of residual intracranial air. An asymptomatic pneumocephalus may complicate EP monitoring because intracranial air can insulate scalp electrodes and cause artifactual signals.[35] No way has been found to prevent this problem, but

Table 18–2

Incidence of Pneumocephalus with Different Positions for Neurosurgical Operations

Position	Incidence of Pneumocephalus	
	No. Patients	%
Sitting (n = 32)	32	100
Park bench (n = 40)	29 ·	73
Prone (n = 28)	16	57

Modified from Toung TJK, McPherson RW, Ahn H, et al.: Pneumocephalus: Effects of patient position on the incidence of aerocele after posterior fossa and upper cervical cord surgery. Anesth Analg 65:65, 1986.

it is expected that it will become less common as use of the sitting position progressively decreases.

Midcervical Tetraplegia

The devastating complication of midcervical tetraplegia is seen most often during neurosurgery with the patient sitting, the neck flexed, and the head rotated. The injury is attributed to stretching of the spinal cord with resultant compromise of the spinal vasculature, with or without local compression from an aggravated spondylosis or from a previously asymptomatic spondylitic bar.[36, 37] Because the neck is typically flexed after the induction of anesthesia, clinical assessment of neurologic function with the patient in the final position is impossible. Historically, the degree of neck flexion in any patient has been limited to that which is not at the extreme of the range of motion and is represented by two fingers placed between the chin and the sternum or clavicle. This method of limiting flexion appears adequate in most cases.

Although midcervical tetraplegia as a complication of body positioning remains rare, the literature contains reports of more than 25 cases of this complication.[34, 36, 37] An interesting case report from Zimbabwe supports the possibility of a stretched spinal cord as the cause of midcervical tetraplegia.[38] A 48-year-old man who was left tied up by bandits in a position of extreme cervical flexion for 12 hours had neurologic findings that included motor loss from C5 to T1 and a glove-type loss of sensation in both arms to the level of the elbow on the right and the C3 dermatome on the left. One case of midcervical tetraplegia has occurred in an infant who was supine intraoperatively with marked flexion of the neck, even though the chin was free of the sternum, the head was not rotated, and no hypotension occurred (Martin JT, personal communication, 1986).

Monitoring of somatosensory EPs elicited by stimulation of the median nerve may be helpful in identifying patients at risk for midcervical tetraplegia. Changes in somatosensory EP after neck flexion have been reported to return to normal upon repositioning.[39, 40] However, in anesthetized monkeys subjected to hyperflexion in the sitting position, somatosensory EPs were not always sufficiently sensitive to identify all individuals who were at risk: one of six monkeys was quadriplegic on awakening without a reported change in the somatosensory EP.[41] Motor evoked potentials may be helpful and are now being used clinically in some institutions.

Compromised function of the auditory nerve during positioning for a retromastoid craniectomy can be documented by monitoring brain stem auditory EP (Fig. 18–4).[42] In many cases the dysfunction is reversible, and hearing can be preserved.

UNCOMMON RISKS TO THE CENTRAL NERVOUS SYSTEM ATTRIBUTABLE TO POSITIONING

Excessive Loss of Cerebrospinal Fluid

During operations for CSF drainage (ventriculostomy, ventriculoperitoneal or ventriculoatrial shunt), ICP may increase before drainage, depending on positioning of the head and maneuvers that interfere with cerebral venous drainage. Once a cerebral ventricle has been entered, both during and after operation, excessive drainage of CSF may lead to pneumocephalus or formation of intracranial hematoma. With chronic hydrocephalus the risk is greatest because the often thin cerebral mantle collapses easily as CSF volume decreases and stretches small veins and arteries. Should these vessels tear, a subdural hematoma may result. For this reason patients should always initially be positioned in a flat recumbent position after CSF shunt placement, especially if a low pressure shunt valve has been used.[43]

When a ventriculostomy tube is connected to an external drainage bag, strict attention must be paid to the position of the drainage bag relative to the patient's head. This detail is easily overlooked when the patient or drainage bag mount is moved, and CSF may be accidentally infused or excessively drained.

Forced Head Rotation

Excessive head turning can compromise circulation to the spinal cord and brain stem even in unanesthetized patients (Fig. 18–5D). Perhaps the acute ischemic episodes associated with chiropractic manipulation have achieved greatest notoriety; injuries to the brain stem,[44] cervical spinal cord,[45] and cauda equina[46] have been reported. Either abrupt or

Figure 18-4

The lateral decubitus position for retromastoid craniectomy. The neck is stretched slightly and flexed. The head is rotated 15 to 20 degrees to the ipsilateral side. The up-side shoulder is distracted caudad by retaining tapes to improve access without compromising circulation to the extremity. (Redrawn from Grundy BL, Procpio PT, Janetta PJ, et al.: Evoked potential changes produced by positioning for retromastoid craniectomy. Neurosurgery 10:766, 1982.)

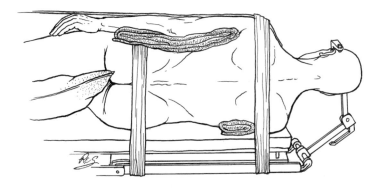

sustained spontaneous movements of the head can produce similar injuries. Neurologic injuries due to obstruction of the vertebral artery have been reported after calisthenics,[47] swimming,[48] ceiling painting,[49] yoga exercises,[50] and bow hunting.[51] A cadaver study provides insight as to why this occurs.[52] In 5 of 41 cadavers, extension and rotation of the head completely occluded the vertebral artery contralateral to the direction of head turning. When traction on the cervical spine was added to the extension and rotation of the head, the vertebral artery was completely occluded 32 times in 18 of the 41 cadavers. In 3, complete occlusion was bilateral. Similar changes have been demonstrated radiologically in healthy male volunteers[53] and in pa-tients with cervical spondylosis.[54] However, symptoms are likely only when contralateral vertebral flow is previously compromised.[55] Abrupt changes in head position, whether active or passive, may injure the intima of the vertebral artery at the atlantoaxial joint. Subsequent thrombosis with propagation or embolism of the clot may lead to progressive brain stem infarction.[56]

Anecdotal reports suggest that anesthetized patients are subject to similar position-related injuries. For example, a 61-year-old patient with pre-existing but undiagnosed severe spinal stenosis became paraplegic after hip surgery that was done with the lumbar spine extended and bent laterally.[57] In positioning anesthetized patients, care should be taken to

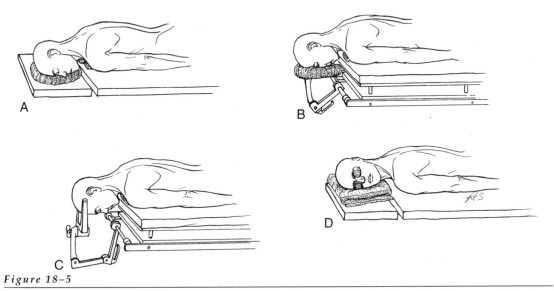

Figure 18-5

Methods of avoiding excessive head turning in the prone position. *A*, *B*, and *C* are acceptable. In *B* the neck is flexed only enough to support most of the weight of the head on the forehead without compressing the eyes. Extreme head rotation and extension, as shown in *D*, may be dangerous for some patients.

avoid extremes of head turning and spinal manipulation even when no specific risk factors for injury to the CNS are apparent. Positioning while patients are awake is preferable.

Central Cord Syndrome

The central cord syndrome consists of arm weakness, leg spasticity, and diminished perception of pain and temperature in the upper part of the body. It may occur after a decompressive cervical laminectomy, perhaps from either positioning or hypotension associated with an upright position. In one series of 300 patients, the incidence was 1.6%.[58] Orthostatic hypotension and inadequate neck immobilization, alone or combined, contributed to this complication.[58] Two simple measures may be preventive: (1) checking the blood pressure of these patients during their initial postoperative mobilization and (2) limiting their neck motion by fitting a firm cervical collar. Patients should be moved carefully after operations on the cervical spine.[58] After a cervical fusion or decompression, complete protection of the spinal canal may not follow immediately. Sustained postoperative immobilization such as that provided by a firm cervical collar is frequently required. Placing the collar securely before awakening, turning, or moving the patient is usually preferable.

Ischemic Optic Neuropathy

Ischemic optic neuropathy is a rare but serious affliction of the optic nerve that has been described in patients undergoing general anesthesia for various surgical procedures.[59, 60] It is usually manifested by a postoperative loss of vision that ranges from decreased light perception and/or narrowing of visual fields to blindness. The process can be unilateral or bilateral and may not become evident until several weeks after surgery. Funduscopic examination usually reveals a pale optic disc and various degrees of edema, findings consistent with an ischemic process involving the optic nerve.[60, 61] Perioperative factors associated with ischemic optic neuropathy include anemia, hypotension, blood loss, venous obstruction, and vascular abnormalities.[61, 62]

Ischemic optic neuropathy can be mistakenly attributed to improper positioning, but positioning is only considered causal if it provokes extreme local venous hypertension as a consequence of dependency or venous obstruction. A more common concern for the patient in the prone position for surgery is external pressure on the ocular globe, which can cause blindness by retinal vessel thrombosis. In contrast, ischemic optic neuropathy can occur without any evidence of direct pressure on the eye.

REFERENCES

1. Langfitt TW: Increased intracranial pressure. Clin Neurosurg 16:436, 1968.
2. Tindall GT, Craddock A, Greenfield JC: Effects of the sitting position on blood flow in the internal carotid artery of man during general anesthesia. J Neurosurg 26:383, 1967.
3. Kenning JA, Touting SM, Saunders RL: Upright patient positioning in the management of intracranial hypertension. Surg Neurol 15:148, 1981.
4. Miller JD, Garibi J, Pickard JD: Induced changes of cerebrospinal fluid volume: Effects during continuous monitoring of ventricular fluid pressure. Arch Neurol 28:265, 1973.
5. Nornes H, Magnaes B: Supratentorial epidural pressure during posterior fossa surgery. J Neurosurg 35:541, 1971.
6. Shapiro HM: Intracranial hypertension. Anesthesiology 43:445, 1975.
7. Todd MM, Weeks JB, Warner DS: The influence of intravascular volume expansion on cerebral blood flow and blood volume in normal rats. Anesthesiology 78:945, 1993.
8. Todd MM, Weeks JB, Warner DS: Microwave fixation for the determination of cerebral blood volume in rats. J Cereb Blood Flow Metab 13(2):328, 1993.
9. Lipe HP, Mitchess PH: Positioning the patient with intracranial hypertension: How turning and head rotation affect the internal jugular vein. Heart Lung 9:1031, 1980.
10. Sherman D, Hart RG, Easton J: Abrupt change in head position and cerebral infarction. Stroke 12:2, 1981.
11. Robertson JT: Neck manipulation as a cause of stroke. Stroke 12:1, 1981 (editorial).
12. Mehalic T, Farhat S: Vertebral artery injury from chiropractic manipulation of the neck. Surg Neurol 2:125, 1974.
13. Caplan LR, Zarins CK, Hemmati M: Spontaneous dissection of the extracranial vertebral arteries. Stroke 16:1030, 1985.
14. Chan KH, Miller JD, Dearden NM, et al.: The effect of changes in cerebral perfusion pressure upon middle cerebral artery blood flow velocity and jugular bulb venous oxygen saturation after severe brain injury. J Neurosurg 77:55, 1992.
15. Miller RA, Crosby G, Sundaram P: Exacerbated spinal neurologic defect during sedation of a patient with cervical spondylosis. Anesthesiology 67:844, 1987.
16. Lee C, Barnes A, Nagel EL: Neuroleptanalgesia for awake pronation of surgical patients. Anesth Analg 56:276, 1977.
17. Slabaugh PB, Nickel VL: Complications with use of the Stryker frame. J Bone Joint Surg 60:1111, 1978.
18. Lewallen RP, Morrey BF, Cabanela ME: Respiratory arrest following posteriorly displaced odontoid fractures. Clin Orthop 188:187, 1984.

19. Nagib MG, Maxwell RE, Chou SN: Anaesthetic considerations in Klippel-Feil Syndrome. Can Anaesth Soc J 33:66, 1986.
20. McCleod ME, Creighton RE: Anesthesia for pediatric neurological and neuromuscular disease. J Child Neurol 1:189, 1986.
21. Sjogren P, Pederson T, Steinmetz H: Mucopolysaccharidoses and anesthetic risks. Acta Anaesthesiol Scand 31:214, 1987.
22. Herrick IA, Rhine EJ: The mucopolysaccharidoses and anaesthesia: A report of clinical experience. Can J Anaesth 35:67, 1988.
23. Peuschel SM, Scola FH: Atlantoaxial instability in individuals with Down's syndrome: Epidemiology, radiographic and clinical studies. Pediatrics 80:555, 1987.
24. Kobel ME, Creighton RE, Steward DJ: Anaesthetic considerations in Down's syndrome: Experience with 100 patients and a review of the literature. Can Anaesth Soc J 29:593, 1982.
25. Williams JP, Somerville GM, Miner ME, et al.: Atlantoaxial subluxation and trisomy-21: Another perioperative complication. Anesthesiology 67:253, 1987.
26. Moore RA, McNicholas KW, Warran SP: Atlantoaxial subluxation with symptomatic spinal cord compression in a child with Down's syndrome. Anesth Analg 66:89, 1987.
27. Mayhew JF, Katz J, Miner M, et al.: Anesthesia for the achondroplastic dwarf. Can Anesth Soc J 33:216, 1986.
28. Waltz LF, Finerman G, Wyatt GM: Anesthesia for dwarfs and other patients of pathological small structure. Can Anaesth Soc J 22:703, 1975.
29. Grinberg F, Slaughter TF, McGrath BJ: Probable venous air embolism associated with removal of the Mayfield skull clamp. Anesthesiology 80:1049, 1995.
30. Gronert GA, Messick JM, Cucchiara RF, et al.: Paradoxical air embolism from a patent foramen ovale. Anesthesiology 50:548, 1979.
31. Cucchiara RF, Seward JB, Nishimura RA, et al.: Identification of patent foramen ovale during sitting position craniotomy by transesophageal echocardiography with positive airway pressure. Anesthesiology 63:107, 1985.
32. Toung TJK, McPherson RW, Ahn H, et al.: Pneumocephalus: Effects of patient position on the incidence of aerocele after posterior fossa and upper cervical cord surgery. Anesth Analg 65:65, 1986.
33. Reasoner DK, Todd MM, Scamman FL: The incidence of pneumocephalus after supratentorial craniotomy: Observations on the disappearance of air. Anesthesiology 80:1008, 1994.
34. Standefer M, Bay JW, Trusso R: The sitting position in neurosurgery: A retrospective analysis of 488 cases. Neurosurgery 14:649, 1984.
35. Schubert A, Zocnow MH, Drummond JC, et al.: Loss of cortical evoked responses due to intracranial gas during posterior fossa craniectomy in the seated position. Anesth Analg 65:203, 1986.
36. Hitselberger WE, House WF: A warning regarding the sitting position for acoustic tumor surgery. Arch Otolaryngol 106:69, 1980.
37. Wilder BL: Hypothesis: The etiology of midcervical quadriplegia after operation with the patient in the sitting position. Neurosurgery 11:530, 1982.
38. Levy LM: An unusual case of flexion injury of the cervical spine. Surg Neurol 17:255, 1982.
39. McCallum JE, Bennett MH: Electrophysiologic monitoring of spinal cord function during intraspinal surgery. Surg Forum 26:469, 1975.
40. McPherson RW, Szymanski J, Rogers MC: Somatosensory evoked potential changes in position-related brainstem ischemia. Anesthesiology 61:88, 1984.
41. Cottrell JF, Hassan NF, Hartung J, et al.: Hyperflexion and quadriplegia in the seated position. Anesthesiol Rev 12:34, 1985.
42. Grundy BL, Procpio PT, Janetta PJ, et al.: Evoked potential changes produced by positioning for retromastoid craniectomy. Neurosurgery 10:766, 1982.
43. Driesen W, Elies W: Epidural and subdural hematomas as a complication of internal drainage of cerebrospinal fluid in hydrocephalus. Acta Neurochir 30:85, 1974.
44. Krueger BR, Okazaki H: Vertebral-basilar distribution infarction following chiropractic cervical manipulation. Mayo Clin Proc 55:322, 1980.
45. Schmidley JW, Koch T: The noncerebrovascular complications of chiropractic manipulation. Neurology 34:684, 1984.
46. Dan NG, Saccasan PA: Serious complications of lumbar spinal manipulation. Med J Aust 24:673, 1983.
47. Nagler W: Vertebral artery obstruction by hyperextension of the neck: Report of three cases. Arch Phys Med Rehabil 54:237, 1973.
48. Tramo MJ, Hainline B, Petito F, et al.: Vertebral artery injury and cerebellar stroke while swimming: Case report. Stroke 16:1039, 1985.
49. Okawara S, Nibbelink D: Vertebral artery occlusion following hyperextension and rotation of the head. Stroke 5:640, 1974.
50. Hanus SH, Homer TD, Harter DH: Vertebral artery occlusion complicating yoga exercises. Arch Neurol 34:574, 1977.
51. Sorensen BF: Bow hunter's stroke: Case report. Neurosurgery 2:259, 1978.
52. Brown BSJ, Tatlow WFT: Radiographic studies of the vertebral arteries in cadavers: Effects of position and traction on the head. Radiology 81:80, 1963.
53. Faris AA, Poser CM, Wikmore DW, Agnew CH: Radiologic visualization of neck vessels in healthy men. Neurology 13:386, 1963.
54. Sheehan S, Bauer RB, Meyer JS: Vertebral artery compression in cervical spondylosis. Neurology 10:968, 1960.
55. Barton JW, Margolis MT: Rotational obstruction of the vertebral artery at the atlantoaxial joint. Neuroradiology 9:117, 1975.
56. Sherman DD, Hart RG, Easton JD: Abrupt change in head position and cerebral infarction. Stroke 12:2, 1981.
57. Wilkes LL: Paraplegia from operating position and spinal stenosis in non-spinal surgery: A case report. Clin Orthop 146:148, 1980.
58. Levy WJ, Dohn DF, Hardy RW: Central cord syndrome as a delayed complication of decompressive laminectomy. Neurosurgery 11:491, 1982.
59. Rizzo JF, Lessell S: Posterior ischemic optic neuropathy during general surgery. Am J Ophthalmol 103:808, 1987.
60. Williams EL, Hart WM, Tempelhoff R: Postoperative ischemic optic neuropathy. Anesth Analg 80:1018, 1995.
61. Brown RA, Schauble JF, Miller NR: Anemia and hypotension as contributors to perioperative loss of vision. Anesthesiology 80:222, 1994.
62. Johnson MW, Kincaid MC, Trobe JD: Bilateral retrobulbar optic nerve infarction after blood loss and hypotension. Ophthalmology 94:1577, 1987.

Peripheral Nervous System

William Dylewsky / Frederick S. McAlpine

BACKGROUND

As part of the typical perioperative routine, patients are sedated, anesthetized, and then positioned for their procedure. They represent a full spectrum of medical illnesses, and their positioning is as varied as the types of procedures that can be performed on them. What they all have in common is their vulnerability to injury during the perioperative period. Only continual awareness by medical personnel of the potential risks of peripheral nerve injury can offset this danger.

COMMON PERIPHERAL INJURIES INCIDENT TO ANESTHESIA AND POSITIONING

Peripheral nerve injury represents the most common serious perioperative anesthetic complication. Retrospective analyses of the overall incidence of nerve injuries have revealed little change in the past three decades. In 1973, Parks[1] reviewed 50,000 general surgical procedures and reported peripheral nerve injuries in 0.14%, whereas Blitt and co-workers[2] analyzed more than 81,000 anesthetic procedures between 1987 and 1993 and found an incidence of injury of 0.11%.

A simple presentation of the incidences of individual nerve injuries is, perhaps, not as useful as a detailed examination of the more common (and more troubling) perioperative complications. Particular attention in this chapter is paid to a discussion of the American Society of Anesthesiologists' (ASA) Closed Claims Study,[3, 4] an ongoing, structured evaluation of all types of anesthetic injuries obtained from completed claim files of professional liability insurance companies. As of January 1994, the database represented more than 3000 claims. Limitations of closed claims analyses have been well described[5] and include the retrospective nature of these studies as well as the time lag between event and evaluation. Closed claims analysis can never lead to incidence data because the population of anesthetics from which they are drawn is unknown. Nevertheless, these closed claims provide a useful collection of anesthetic events deemed serious enough to lead to allegations of malpractice. To include them in our discussion here is to provide a practical emphasis to this material. For example, although the overall incidence of peripheral nerve injuries in the surgical population is slightly over 0.1%, closed claims for nerve damage represented 16% of the total cases in the ASA study.

Brachial Plexus Injury

Peripheral nerves that are longer and more superficial have a greater possibility of being injured than do short and well-protected nerves. Figures 19–1 through 19–4 show the course in the upper extremity of the axillary, musculocutaneous, median, ulnar, and radial nerves together with the muscle groups they innervate.[6] Also shown are the sensory defi-

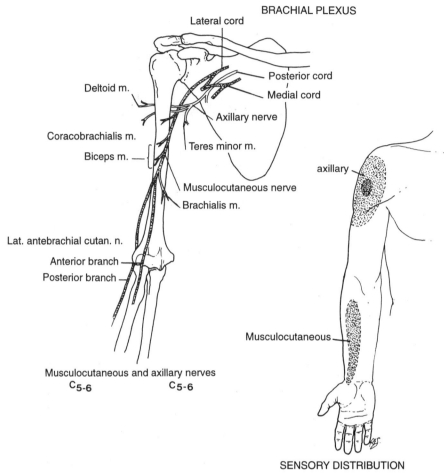

BRACHIAL PLEXUS

Lateral cord

Posterior cord

Medial cord

Deltoid m.

Axillary nerve

Coracobrachialis m.

Teres minor m.

Biceps m.

axillary

Musculocutaneous nerve

Brachialis m.

Lat. antebrachial cutan. n.

Anterior branch

Posterior branch

Musculocutaneous

Musculocutaneous and axillary nerves

C$_{5-6}$ C$_{5-6}$

SENSORY DISTRIBUTION

Figure 19–1

Musculocutaneous and axillary nerves. Motor branches and sensory loss from injury in area of shoulder joint. (Courtesy of Lahey Clinic, Burlington, MA; redrawn from Waxman SG, de Groot J [eds.]: Correlative Neuroanatomy, 22nd ed. East Norwalk, CT, Appleton & Lange, 1995.)

cits and motor deformities that may follow injury to these nerves.

The brachial plexus is probably the most susceptible of all nerve groups to injury. The clinical picture is usually that of a relatively painless motor deficit commonly affecting C5–7. The incidence of these lesions is cited as 0.02%.[7] Fifteen years earlier, Parks[1] reported the incidence as 0.06%. The brachial plexus was named as the site of injury in 23% of closed claims involving nerve injury—the second most common site.

Particular attention has been paid to brachial plexus injuries occurring coincident with a median sternotomy for cardiothoracic surgery. Several papers have documented that these injuries often occur bilaterally, principally to the lower segments of the plexus. Pain is a prominent postoperative feature,

and recovery is often protracted and incomplete. A large prospective study[8,9] of 531 patients undergoing open heart surgery at the Cleveland Clinic revealed an incidence of 4.9% who had sustained brachial plexus injury. The majority were injuries to the lower trunk of the plexus and most often involved the peripheral distribution of the ulnar nerve. In the Cleveland Clinic series, the majority of affected patients did *not* complain of pain and their deficits resolved over a 6- to 8-week period.

Ulnar Nerve Injuries

Ulnar nerve injuries are among the most common focal peripheral neuropathies reported during the perioperative period. For some patients, this represents the first evidence of ul-

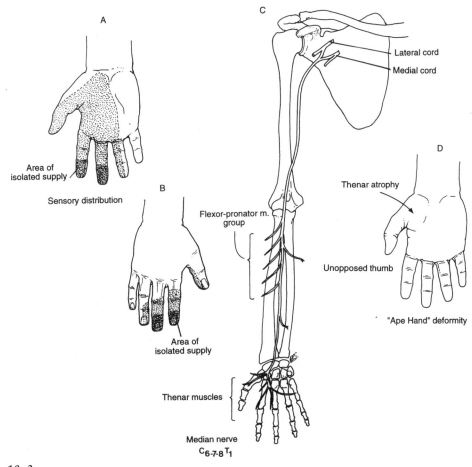

A

Area of
isolated supply

Sensory distribution

B

Area of
isolated supply

Thenar muscles

Median nerve
$C_{6-7-8}T_1$

C

Lateral cord

Medial cord

Flexor-pronator m.
group

D

Thenar atrophy

Unopposed thumb

"Ape Hand" deformity

Figure 19–2

Sensory and motor deficit associated with median nerve injury above the elbow. (Courtesy of Lahey Clinic, Burlington, MA; redrawn from Waxman SG, de Groot J [eds.]: Correlative Neuroanatomy, 22nd ed. East Norwalk, CT, Appleton & Lange, 1995.)

nar nerve injury; for others, previous symptoms had been mild and are now much more obvious and disabling. The importance of ulnar nerve difficulties is highlighted in the ASA closed claims study analysis by the fact that it represents over one third of all claims involving nerve injury.[3, 4]

Stoelting[10] described how the ulnar nerve is vulnerable to damage because of its superficial position, particularly in the cubital tunnel. Texts often point to the injury being caused by a hyperflexed elbow or to direct compression against a hard object, such as the edge of the operating table. In reality, the causes of perioperative ulnar nerve damage seem to be far more complex. Closed claims for ulnar neuropathies differed from those for other nerves in that the mechanism of injury was least often apparent and the injury was more likely to have occurred during general

anesthesia than during regional anesthesia.[4] Analysis of the closed claims data by Kroll and colleagues[3] revealed that of the 77 patients with ulnar nerve injury, 22 noted the time of onset of symptoms. Ulnar distress was first noted by 5 patients on awakening from anesthesia, by 3 others during the first postoperative day, by 10 during the first postoperative week, and by 4 at some time during 2 weeks to 1 month after anesthesia and surgery. That distribution suggests a postoperative cause in at least some patients. Support for the presumption is provided by a large retrospective study by Warner and colleagues in which 57% of patients with a new-onset perioperative ulnar neuropathy that lasted at least 3 months initially noted their symptoms more than 24 hours postoperatively.[11] Alvine and Schurrer[12] reported that patients whose ulnar nerve lesions develop in the periopera-

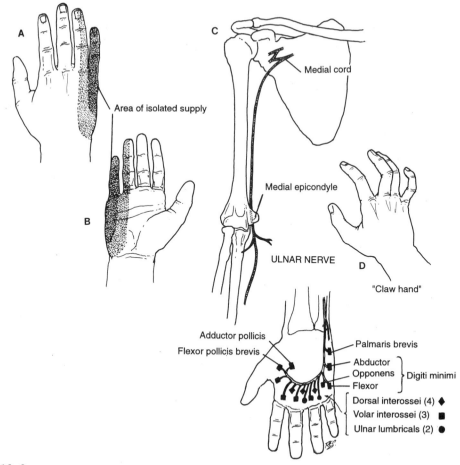

Figure 19–3

A through D. Sensory and motor deficit associated with ulnar nerve injury at the elbow. (Courtesy of Lahey Clinic, Burlington, MA; redrawn from Waxman SG, de Groot J [eds.]: Correlative Neuroanatomy, 22nd ed. East Norwalk, CT, Appleton & Lange, 1995.)

tive period uniformly have abnormalities on nerve conduction testing in both the affected and the contralateral arms. Given this variable onset of symptoms, coupled with a possible general predisposition to injury (the male/female ratio is approximately 4:1 in several studies),[11] it is not surprising that closed claims analysis revealed a mechanism of injury in only 5% of cases.[3]

Lower Extremity Nerve Injuries

Analysis of the anesthesia closed claims data for lower extremity injuries seems to be less broad and complete.[3] All lumbosacral nerve root injuries having an identifiable anesthetic cause (36%) were attributed to the administration of regional anesthesia. This, however, neglects to identify the vulnerability of the lower extremities to damage from position-

ing. Figures 19–5 through 19–7 demonstrate the distributions of the femoral, obturator, and sciatic nerves and their sometimes superficial courses. Stoelting[13] commented on how lower extremity neuropathies seem most likely to occur after surgical procedures performed on patients in the lithotomy position. Warner and associates[14] retrospectively reviewed operations performed with patients in the lithotomy position and found the incidence of persistent lower extremity motor neuropathies to be 0.03%.

ETIOLOGIC FACTORS IN PERIPHERAL NERVE LESIONS

The literature about perioperative peripheral nerve damage is filled with lists of specific

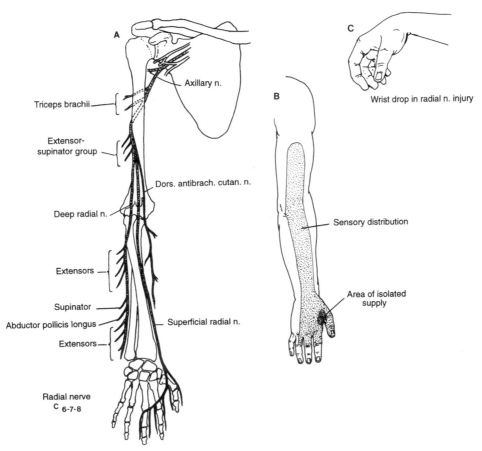

Figure 19-4

A through *C*. Sensory loss and wristdrop after radial nerve injury at the mid humerus. (Courtesy of Lahey Clinic, Burlington, MA; redrawn from Waxman SG, de Groot J [eds.]: Correlative Neuroanatomy, 22nd ed. East Norwalk, CT, Appleton & Lange, 1995.)

nerves or nerve groups and their specific potential mechanisms of injury. Perioperative neuropathies can be related to pre-existing conditions, anesthesia, intraoperative and postoperative positioning, or varied combinations of each. Because separating these causes is often impractical or impossible, this chapter will concentrate on the more important issue of common underlying pathways to nerve damage.

Neuroanatomy

The neuron is the key unit in the nervous system. It is made up of the cell body (perikaryon) and the cytoplasmic extension (axon). The axonal transport system is vital for neuron health and for supplying neurotransmitter precursors to the end plate. The life of the axon depends on its continuity with the cell body. Peripheral nerve fibers originate from sensory, motor, or autonomic cell bodies in the dorsal ganglia or ventral horn of the spinal cord. These fibers can be classified by size: larger myelinated A fibers, smaller preganglionic sympathetic myelinated B fibers, and small unmyelinated C fibers. Connective tissue surrounding the nerves is called perineurium. Tiny nutrient blood vessels, called vasa nervorum, run a longitudinal course with multiple anastomoses.

This histologic anatomy partly determines a nerve's susceptibility to injury. Nerve trunks containing numerous small fibers with abundant perineurium are less vulnerable than those composed of large fibers with little supporting connective tissue. An incomplete injury to nerves with small fibers is more functionally forgiving than the same injury to a nerve with a few large fibers. Anatomic location is another important factor. Some nerves (e.g., the sciatic and its branches)

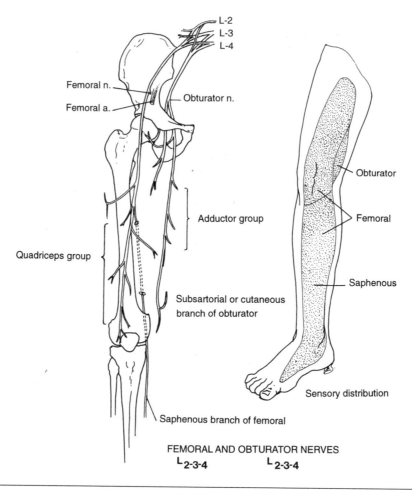

Figure 19–5

Muscles supplied by femoral and obturator nerves and sensory loss resulting from injury to the nerves at the groin. (Courtesy of Lahey Clinic, Burlington, MA; redrawn from Waxman SG, de Groot J [eds.]: Correlative Neuroanatomy, 22nd ed. East Norwalk, CT, Appleton & Lange, 1995.)

course for more than 1 meter in superficial planes or in direct contact with bone or fibrous tissue. Intraoperative manipulation, direct trauma resulting from the surgical procedure itself or from pulling of retractors, malpositioning of an extremity, or improper use of a tourniquet can compromise these vulnerable structures. The exact mechanism of injury varies from nerve to nerve, but the final common pathway to injury is reduction of blood supply from the intraneural vasa nervorum with resultant nerve damage.

Causes of Injury

The most likely causes of nerve injury include section, compression, traction, and ischemia. Identifying the cause, if possible, is important because the prognosis for recovery directly depends on the underlying nature of the neurologic deficit.

Section Injury. This may be due to an operation that specifically involves the nerve (e.g., carpal tunnel) or to inadvertent cutting of the axon directly with a knife or percutaneously with a needle.

Compression Injury. Usually caused by mechanical compression from external forces, this category includes tourniquet compression, crush injuries, tumors, healing fractures, edema, or hematoma. The pathologic condition induced by a compression injury depends on the magnitude, duration, and rate of application of the compressive force.[15] Intraneural injection injury would also fall into this category—the rise in intrafascicular pressure has been demonstrated to initiate a compression type of injury.[16] The

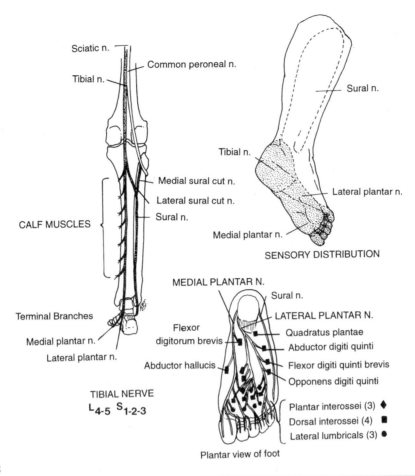

Sciatic n.
Common peroneal n.
Tibial n.
Sural n.
Tibial n.
Medial sural cut n.
Lateral sural cut n.
Sural n.
CALF MUSCLES
Lateral plantar n.
Medial plantar n.
SENSORY DISTRIBUTION

MEDIAL PLANTAR N.
Sural n.
Terminal Branches
LATERAL PLANTAR N.
Flexor
digitorum brevis
Quadratus plantae
Medial plantar n.
Abductor digiti quinti
Lateral plantar n.
Flexor digiti quinti brevis
Abductor hallucis
Opponens digiti quinti
Plantar interossei (3) ♦
Dorsal interossei (4) ■
Lateral lumbricals (3) ●

TIBIAL NERVE
L$_{4-5}$ S$_{1-2-3}$

Plantar view of foot

Figure 19–6

Tibial nerve. Sensory and motor deficit when nerve is injured at the knee. (Courtesy of Lahey Clinic, Burlington, MA; redrawn from Waxman SG, de Groot J [eds.]: Correlative Neuroanatomy, 22nd ed. East Norwalk, CT, Appleton & Lange, 1995.)

hypoxic axon may then be vulnerable even to agents with a low neurotoxicity profile.[17]

Traction Injury. Traction decreases the cross-sectional area of the nerve, raises its intraneural pressures, and compresses the vasa nervorum. Lundborg[18] demonstrated that as little as 8% elongation of a nerve will cause circulatory compromise, and complete ischemia will occur at 15% elongation. An example of traction injury occurs when the brachial plexus is stretched by having the neck extended and flexed to the opposite side or when the arm is in any extreme position, particularly when abducted and externally rotated.

Ischemic Injury. Femoral cannulation, a more frequent procedure since the advent of cardiac catheterization, has led to an increase in femoral nerve injury, usually at the level of the inguinal ligament where the artery is penetrated by instruments.[19] Other causes of inadequate blood flow to a peripheral nerve include placement of shunts for renal dialysis and arterial cannulation. These lesions frequently produce major degrees of axonal damage with resulting long-lasting and painful clinical effects.

In reality, the causes of perioperative neuropathies may be multifactorial. For example, the common brachial plexus injury seen with median sternotomy during heart surgery has been attributed to a variety of causes, including asymmetrical retraction of the sternum that stretches the plexus, fractured first rib stretching the plexus, cannulation of the internal jugular vein in the presence of anticoagulation causing local compression by means of hematoma formation, and internal mammary artery dissection causing excessive traction on the plexus.[8, 9, 13]

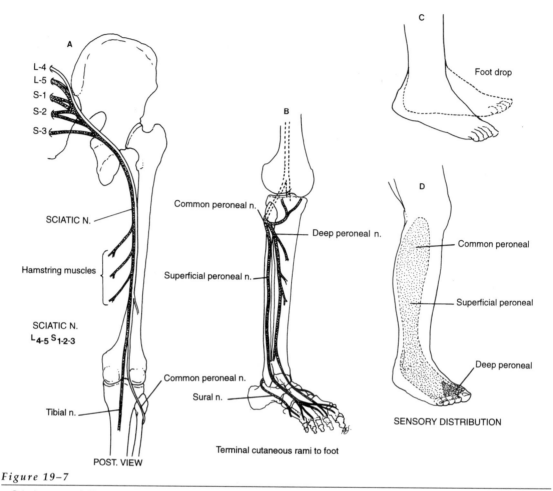

Figure 19–7

Sciatic nerve. *A.* Posterior view. *B.* Common peroneal nerve and its major branches. *C.* Footdrop from peroneal nerve injury. *D.* Sensory deficit associated with peroneal nerve injury. (Courtesy of Lahey Clinic, Burlington, MA.)

That there may be more than one factor involved in any of these injuries is not surprising. However, because the loss of blood supply to the nerve is what ultimately causes the injury, any additional pathophysiologic condition that further compromises perfusion of the vasa nervora may aggravate or increase the likelihood of a peripheral neuropathy. These include peripheral vascular disease, vasoconstriction with hypothermia or pressors, prolonged hypotension (either deliberate or not), and diabetes. For example, Warner and co-workers[14] found cigarette smoking (and presumably its vasoconstrictive effects) to be a major risk factor for lower extremity neuropathies after procedures performed on patients in lithotomy positions. The underlying function of the peripheral nerve itself may be hampered by disease. Table 19–1 lists some of the causes of peripheral nerve disease.

PERIPHERAL NERVE REACTION TO INJURY

Regardless of the mechanism of injury, paralysis or loss of sensation or both result from disruption of axonal function. The severity of the injury dictates the nerve's reaction to that injury, and that reaction dictates the clinical course. This reactive process must be well understood so that the physician can adequately estimate the severity of injury and the prognosis for recovery.

The mildest form of peripheral nerve injury is called *transient ischemic nerve block*. It commonly follows acute compression of a limb, can be duplicated with a blood pressure cuff, and is the result of ischemia of the entire limb rather than direct local mechanical forces on the nerve. No structural damage occurs after

Table 19–1

Etiology of Afflictions of Peripheral Nerves

Causes	Results
Trauma	Birth injury, fractures, stretch injury, cervical rib, herniated disk, bullet wounds, aneurysm, operation
Nutritional	Beriberi, pellagra, pernicious anemia, alcoholic neuritis
Metabolic	Diabetes, gout, porphyria
Heavy metal exposure	Lead, arsenic, mercury, bismuth, gold, silver
Vascular	Arteriosclerosis, arterial injury, emboli, tourniquet paralysis, Volkmann's ischemia, periarteritis nodosa
Infection and virus	Polio, diphtheria, leprosy
Tumors	Neuroma, Von Recklinghausen's disease, neurofibroma, malignancy

Courtesy of Lahey Clinic, Burlington, MA; from Nicholson MJ, Eversole UH: Nerve injuries incident to anesthesia and operation. Anesth Analg 36:19, 1957.

this type of injury, and recovery is complete after 20 minutes.

Seddon[20] proposed a classification of more severe localized nerve injuries. Figure 19–8 demonstrates his grades of nerve injury and the histologic events in their repair.

Neurapraxia. Seddon[20] used this term to describe a nerve injury that results in temporary paralysis or sensory loss. Pathologically, nerve fibers become demyelinated, especially those fibers near the periphery of the nerve trunk. The smaller and internal fibers are spared. However, continuity of the nerve trunk itself and the endoneural sheath is preserved. Although these palsies resolve, complete recovery takes nearly 4 to 6 weeks or longer. Remyelination tends to parallel clinical and electrical recovery, which is fastest in the fourth or fifth week.

Axonotmesis. Being a complete disruption of the axons within an intact sheath and connective tissue elements, axonotmesis usually occurs after a severe stretch injury.[20] This injury results in a degeneration of the nerve distally. The nerve usually regrows at 1 mm per day, and function gradually returns. However, complete recovery is much less likely than in injuries that do not disrupt axonal continuity. During this wallerian degeneration and subsequent regeneration, metabolic changes occur in the cell body at the level of the spinal cord that change metabolism from one geared for

synaptic transmission to one appropriate for the metabolic production of lipids and proteins for regeneration of the distal nerve stump (Fig. 19–9).

Neurotmesis. Seddon[20] reserved this term for the most severe of injuries: those with complete disruption of both axonal and connective tissue elements. These also result in degeneration of the nerve distal to the lesion, but, unlike axonotmesis, there is no opportunity for wallerian regeneration. These injuries do not heal normally and require surgical intervention to regain (at best) partial function.

DIAGNOSIS OF PERIPHERAL NERVE INJURY

When nerve injury is evident, a baseline neurologic examination should be documented and a comparison made to preoperative function. If the nerve deficit is still evident after 30 minutes, a neurapraxic or more severe lesion is likely. At this point, a review of the anesthetic, operative, and postoperative records is necessary to identify the following: unusual or extreme positioning; prolonged maintenance of one position; hemodynamic or metabolic extremes; coexisting medical problems, such as diabetes, alcohol abuse, vitamin deficiency, or coagulopathy; or evidence of equipment malfunction.

Initial presentation of the neuropathy may be subtle or dramatic and may go unrecognized in the midst of more dominating medical issues. Initial observations must be as objective as possible and documented carefully in the record. A neurologist should be contacted at an appropriately early moment to provide a baseline postoperative evaluation as well as to direct the patient's subsequent neurologic care. When the differential diagnosis includes a hematoma in the epidural space or elsewhere, emergency computed tomography or magnetic resonance imaging may become necessary.

Simplified Rapid Identification of Major Peripheral Nerve Injuries

A rapid method of identifying peripheral nerve injuries is presented in the hope that better statistical data will thereby be accumulated. During World War II, this method of examining large numbers of injured soldiers was devised and used at the Peripheral Nerve

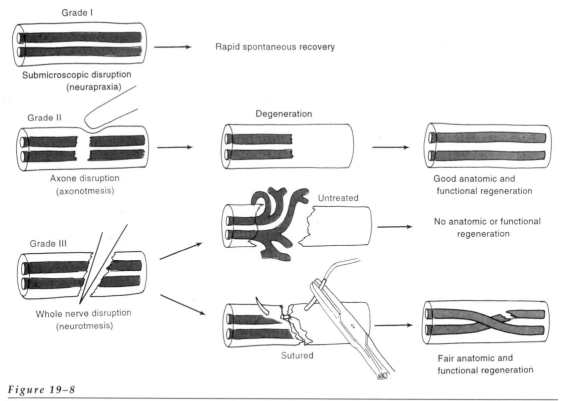

Grade I
Submicroscopic disruption
(neurapraxia)
→ Rapid spontaneous recovery

Grade II
Axone disruption
(axonotmesis)
Degeneration
Good anatomic and
functional regeneration

Grade III
Whole nerve disruption
(neurotmesis)
Untreated
No anatomic or functional
regeneration
Sutured
Fair anatomic and
functional regeneration

Figure 19–8

Grades of nerve injury and the histologic events in their repair. (Modified from Hicks SP, Warren S: Introduction to Neuropathology. New York, McGraw-Hill, 1950.)

Center, United States Naval Hospital, Oakland, California.[21]

Upper Extremity

The upper extremity may be tested rapidly for major nerve lesions in the following manner (Fig. 19–10)[21] :

Median nerve. When a pinprick over the palmar surface of the distal phalanx of the index finger is perceived normally, the median nerve is intact.

Ulnar nerve. When a pinprick can be felt over the palmar surface of the distal phalanx of the fifth finger, the ulnar nerve is intact.

Radial nerve. When the distal phalanx of the thumb can actively be extended, significant interruption of the radical nerve may be excluded.

Brachial plexus. Lesions of the brachial plexus can be identified as variable combinations of the median, ulnar, and radial nerves. Plexus injuries may involve two additional nerves of major clinical importance. These are the musculocutaneous nerve, injury to which produces loss of function of the bi-

ceps and inability to flex the forearm, and the axillary nerve, injury to which causes loss of deltoid function and inability to abduct the arm. Loss of these functions produces disabilities that are obvious and are usually not overlooked.

Palmar injuries. When injuries involve the palm of the hand, the sensation of each finger must be tested to avoid overlooking an interrupted digital branch of the median or ulnar nerve.

Lower Extremity

The lower extremity may be tested rapidly for major nerve lesions as follows (Fig. 19–11)[21]:

Femoral nerve. Ability to flex the thigh on the trunk indicates that the nerve supply to the iliopsoas muscle is intact. Ability to extend the leg and the presence of a knee jerk indicate that the extrapelvic portion of the femoral nerve is intact.

Obturator nerve. The obturator nerve is often injured along with the femoral nerve; an isolated lesion is rare. Ability to adduct the leg usually means that the nerve is intact.

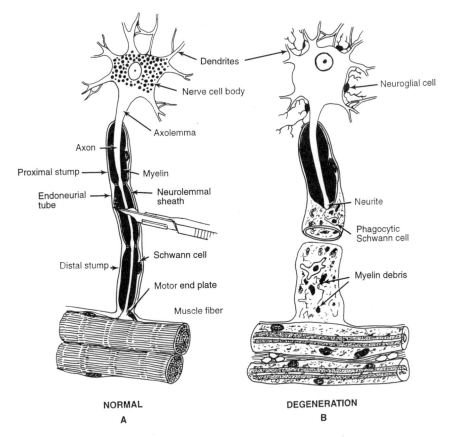

Dendrites

Nerve cell body

Axolemma

Axon

Proximal stump

Myelin

Endoneurial tube

Neurolemmal sheath

Schwann cell

Distal stump

Motor end plate

Muscle fiber

NORMAL
A

Neuroglial cell

Neurite

Phagocytic Schwann cell

Myelin debris

DEGENERATION
B

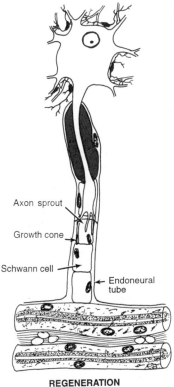

Axon sprout

Growth cone

Schwann cell

Endoneural tube

REGENERATION
C

Figure 19–9

Diagram of biologic events after transection of a peripheral nerve. *A.* Body of a central nerve cell within the spinal cord and its myelinated axon synapsing with a muscle in the periphery. Most nerves contain thousands of such fibers. *B.* Wallerian degeneration after transection. Schwann cells in the distal stump have transformed into phagocytic cells, which, most likely with participation by additional phagocytes derived from the blood, remove axonal and myelin debris. The body of the nerve cell is swollen, the nucleus is eccentric, the Nissl substance has lost its definition (chromatolysis), and neuroglial cells have interrupted some of the synapses of axons from other nerves on the cell body. This morphologic observation is interpreted as denoting a change in the metabolic state of the injured nerve cell from one geared to transmission of impulses to one appropriate for protein synthesis and repair. The distal muscle has lost its striations and is starting to atrophy. *C.* During successful regeneration, axon sprouts extend from the proximal axon, presumably attaching to the residual endoneural tube of the distal nerve stump through growth cones. The single line labeled *endoneural tube* represents schematically the residual basal membrane of the Schwann cell and nearby endoneural collagen strands, which together compose the endoneural tube. As the axon grows distally, it induces the remaining Schwann cells to form a myelin sheath around the axon. (Courtesy of Lahey Clinic, Burlington, MA; modified from Seckel BR, Chiu TH, Nyilas E, et al.: Nerve regeneration through synthetic biodegradable nerve guides: Regulation by the target organ. Plast Reconstr Surg 74:173, 1984.)

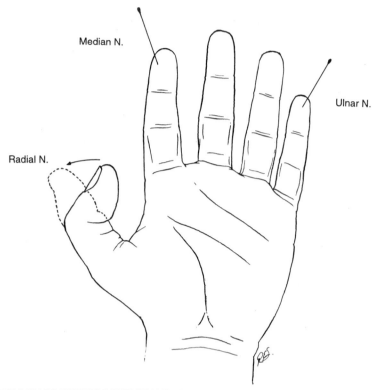

● INJURY TO MUSCULOCUTANEOUS NERVE =
LOSS BICEPS FUNCTION, INABILITY TO FLEX FOREARM
● INJURY TO AXILLARY NERVE =
LOSS DELTOID FUNCTION, INABILITY TO ABDUCT THE ARM

Figure 19–10

Method for rapid identification of major peripheral nerve injuries in the upper extremity. (Courtesy of Lahey Clinic, Burlington, MA.)

Sciatic nerve. This nerve gives off branches in the thigh to the hamstring muscles before it divides into the common peroneal and tibial nerves; therefore, ability to flex the leg at the knee indicates that the sciatic nerve is intact.

Common peroneal nerve. Ability to dorsiflex the great toe rules out injury to the peroneal nerve.

Tibial nerve. Ability to plantarflex the great toe rules out injury to the tibial nerve.

TREATMENT OF PERIPHERAL NERVE INJURIES

Immediate answers about the extent and outcome of nerve injuries may not be available for the patient and the concerned family. In general, more peripheral nerve injuries can be identified with greater precision than central lesions because simple tests or neurologic ex-

amination will provide sufficient evidence. More involved tests must be used to examine the spinal cord, nerve roots, or proximal plexus sites. These can take time, during which the anesthesiologist, surgeon, and the neurologist should remain in close, consistent communication with the patient.

Most position-related injuries are neurapraxic, and patients demonstrate substantial recovery soon after the onset of symptoms. Nonetheless, it is not prudent merely to ignore the patient's symptoms for the first few weeks in the hope that the injury is, indeed, neurapraxic. The timing of consultative support is a matter that is unresolved, but an argument can be made for early recognition of subclinical neural pathologic processes other than that of the patient's complaint. The differential diagnosis is based on careful sequential examinations, documenting the extent of injury as well as the degree and time course of recovery. If the neurologist docu-

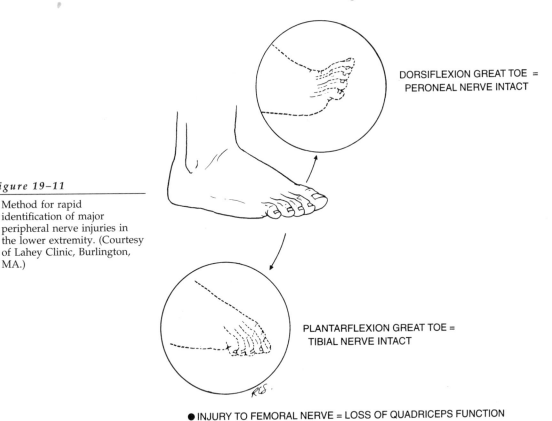

DORSIFLEXION GREAT TOE =
PERONEAL NERVE INTACT

PLANTARFLEXION GREAT TOE =
TIBIAL NERVE INTACT

● INJURY TO FEMORAL NERVE = LOSS OF QUADRICEPS FUNCTION

Figure 19–11

Method for rapid identification of major peripheral nerve injuries in the lower extremity. (Courtesy of Lahey Clinic, Burlington, MA.)

ments little progress, it is the responsibility of the electrophysiologist to deduce pathogenesis by deciding whether axonal loss has occurred or whether, instead, functional disturbances of fibers remain in continuity.

Detailing the steps that an electrophysiologist might take in evaluating the location of a particular nerve injury is beyond the scope of this chapter. No single test is specific for this evaluation, and several criteria are necessary to pinpoint the exact location and type of a lesion. Electromyography is performed to evaluate signs of denervation. Conduction studies are performed at several sites along the suspected nerve to determine which segment is affected and the functional integrity of its motor and sensory fibers.

Emphasis must be placed on the timing of the evaluation rather than on the specific tests employed. Many patients are referred for electrophysiologic evaluation only after spontaneous recovery is clearly delayed or absent. After a few weeks, the electrophysiologic changes of denervation are different from those seen in the acute stage. Reduction in amplitude of the evoked motor and sensory response is the most important sign of axonal loss.[19] The presence of even small responses indicates that the nerve is in continuity and that regeneration and reinnervation remain possible. In other words, prompt and consistent evaluation of these nerve injuries is imperative in establishing a prognosis.

In the earlier discussion of ulnar injuries, the question was raised about the contribution of pre-existing subclinical neuropathies to the postoperative clinical picture. An attempt to differentiate what represents acute perioperative injury from chronic neuropathy would seem to be useful to both patient and physician. Such a clarification is possible only when the patient receives a prompt and thorough neurologic evaluation.

For the majority of position-related injuries, time is the principal contributor to healing. For those injuries diagnosed as more serious and long lasting, a multidisciplinary approach may be warranted. When testing reveals that the injured nerve seems to be in continuity, a conservative approach, including follow-up studies, is indicated. Physical therapy can be provided to prevent disuse atrophy or contracture deformities until nerve function is restored. If no evoked motor or sensory response returns, complete denervation is likely, and surgical exploration may be indicated to ascertain whether the nerve trunk is in continuity or whether reconstructive repair is necessary. In the case of complete loss of function, occupational and physical therapists can advise patients about compensatory ways to accomplish basic tasks.

PREVENTION OF PERIPHERAL NERVE INJURIES

As is often true, prevention is the best form of therapy. Although never proven, most nerve injuries occurring in the perioperative period have been postulated to be the result of pressure from improper positioning or from inadvertent traction of the limb of a deeply anesthetized patient who may have a condition that predisposes to neuropathies. All personnel involved in caring for the patient, including the anesthesiologist, surgeon, nurses, and orderlies, must know the inherent potential hazards to which their patients will be subjected by undergoing the scheduled procedure. Although perioperative neuropathies appear to be a part of a complex, multifactorial process that often involves the exacerbation of pre-existing subclinical neuropathology, the care team must exercise continued vigilance to avoid errors in malpositioning and manipulation of the patient.

The first protective step is a careful preoperative examination and interview. Documentation must be made of concurrent illnesses or metabolic derangements. In addition, pre-existing neurologic deficits and limitations in motion should be discussed with the patient and described in the written record. If possible, the patient should be positioned on the operating room table before anesthesia is administered so that obviously uncomfortable or unphysiologic poses may be identified quickly and avoided. Throughout the operation, the anesthesiologist must continue to evaluate the nonoperative sites and rearrange cushions as necessary. The surgeon must likewise re-evaluate the duration and application of pressure applied to the surgical wound. Optimal metabolic control of the diabetic, alcoholic, or uremic patient is appropriate.

Perioperative diagnosis of neural function is difficult while the patient is often unable to report pain or paresthesias because of anesthesia and/or sedation. Because nerves and blood vessels are in close proximity, checking pulses and capillary refill distal to any possible site of nerve injury is advisable.[22] Placement of a pulse oximeter on the dependent limb in the lateral position is a qualitative measure of perfusion. Intact perfusion, however, is no guarantee of nerve preservation; somatosensory nerve stimulation has been demonstrated to be lost despite preservation of pulse.[22]

Supine Position

The brachial plexus and its peripheral branches can be safeguarded in the supine position by noting individual anatomic variations and restrictions of motion preoperatively; never abducting the arm beyond 90 degrees; keeping the hand and forearm in full supination when abducted to avoid ulnar compression at the elbow; if arms are above the head, keeping abduction and anterior flexion less than 90 degrees; avoiding prolonged extremes of flexion when the arm is flexed at the elbow; keeping the elbow padded when at risk; maintaining the arm level with the body; using a drawsheet extending above the elbow to keep the arm tight against the patient's body when at the patient's side to avoid contact between the table's side rail and the ulnar nerve at the elbow; employing the armboard with a locking mechanism to prevent hyperextension of the arm; avoiding extremes of plexus retraction or stretching; and preventing radial nerve compression by the vertical post unit of the body wall (Bookwalter) retractor against the upper arm or pressure caused by the vertical part of the ether screen against the upper arm. These points are shown in Figure 19–12.

Additional care must be taken when the supine patient is expected to be tilted head-down (see also Chapter 8). Figure 19–13 depicts the improper use of wristlets with the patient in the head-down position. The consequence is a stretch injury to the upper part of the brachial plexus (fifth and sixth cervical nerves), and that may lead to an Erb-Duchenne type of injury.

Figure 19–14A demonstrates the proper use of padded shoulder braces placed against the bony prominences of the acromioclavicular region to prevent the patient from sliding cephalad when the operating room table is tilted.

Figure 19–14B depicts a patient in a steep, head-down position with the arm on an arm-

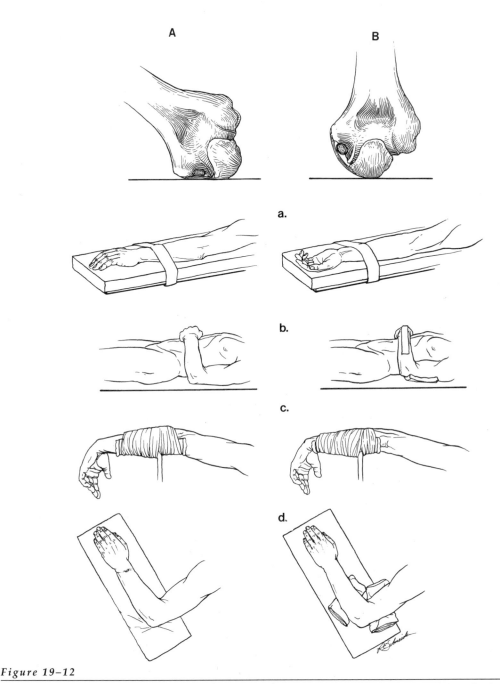

Figure 19–12

On the operating table, certain positions of the upper limb threaten external compression of the cubital tunnel (see column A, hazards), whereas judicious positioning of the extremity can minimize these hazards (see column B, protection). *a*. With the patient supine, pronation of the forearm places the cubital tunnel against the table surface, whereas full supination "lifts" the tunnel and the contained ulnar nerve away from compressive contact. *b*. A soft pad or a longitudinal adhesive strap or both attached to the dorsum of the forearm will prevent contact between the flexed elbow and the table surface. *c*. With the patient in the lateral decubitus position, the cubital tunnel can be freed effectively from external pressure of the arm rest by permitting the elbow to protrude from the support. *d*. With the arm placed alongside the head of a patient in the prone position, the medial epicondyle supports the flexed elbow and usually protects the cubital tunnel. However, a hypermobile ulnar nerve, dislocated from the tunnel, can be compressed externally and must be protected by properly placed soft pads. (Courtesy of Lahey Clinic, Burlington, MA; modified from Wadsworth TG: The cubital tunnel and the external compression syndrome. Anesth Analg 53:303, 1974.)

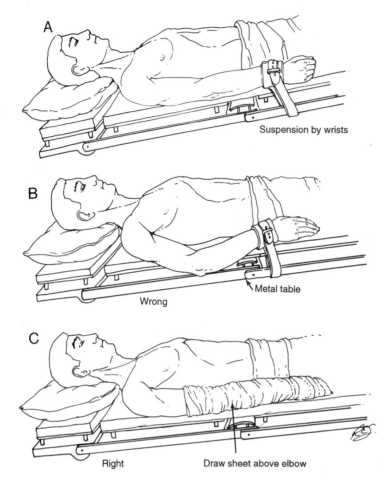

Figure 19–13

Dangers from improper use of wristlets. *A.* Patient suspended by wristlets when tilted head-down, threatening upper brachial plexus injury (Erb-Duchenne paralysis). *B.* Arm over side of table exposing ulnar nerve to potential injury. *C.* Correct use of drawsheet to restrain arm at side. (Courtesy of Lahey Clinic, Burlington, MA.)

board. The shoulder brace is against the shoulder opposite the outstretched arm and is all the support needed to keep the patient from sliding cephalad. When the extended arm is kept at an angle to the body of less than 90 degrees, the likelihood of injury to the brachial plexus is greatly minimized.

Figure 19–14C shows the incorrect use of the padded shoulder brace. The brace acts as a fulcrum when the arm is abducted beyond 90 degrees, leading to a lower brachial plexus injury at the level of C8–Tl. Abnormal stretching causes these lesions, which are also seen in the newborn after difficult breech delivery. The small muscles of the hand and wrist flexors are paralyzed. If the sympathetic rami of T1 have been injured, Horner's syndrome may be noted.[23] A claw hand deformity may result along with edema, cyanosis of the skin, and trophic nail changes (see Fig. 19–3D).

Figure 19–15 illustrates an armboard that can be locked at any desired angle. Pressure against it by a member of the surgical team will not cause it to move and result in an overly abducted arm.

Prone Position

The prone position for the anesthetized patient, correct and incorrect, is shown in Figure 19–16A. Arms placed above the head can cause stretch injury to the lower roots of the brachial plexus, resulting in tingling and numbness over the ulnar distribution. If the patient reports preoperatively symptoms of thoracic outlet syndrome (numbness or pain when hands are placed above the head), the arms should be placed next to the patient during operation. With proper support under the iliac crest and upper anterior thorax, the abdomen is unencumbered for abdominal breathing.

The edge of the table serves as a threat to the ulnar nerve in the prone position as well. In Figure 19–16B, the elbow is incorrectly placed over the edge of the table, permitting

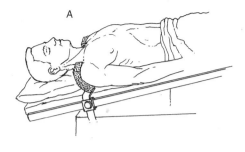

Figure 19–14

Shoulder braces. *A.* Correct application of padded shoulder braces. *B.* Arm out on board, no brace on that side, with angle of abduction 90 degrees or less. *C.* Incorrect use of brace with arm on board; angle of abduction greater than 90 degrees may result in lower brachial plexus injury. (Courtesy of Lahey Clinic, Burlington, MA.)

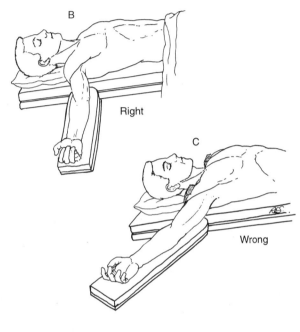

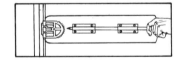

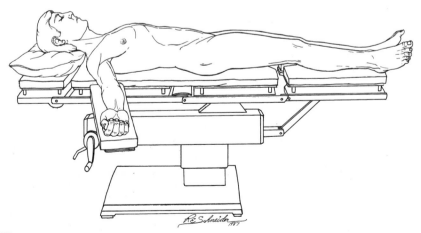

Figure 19–15

Armboard with locking mechanism to forestall hyperextension and brachial plexus injury.

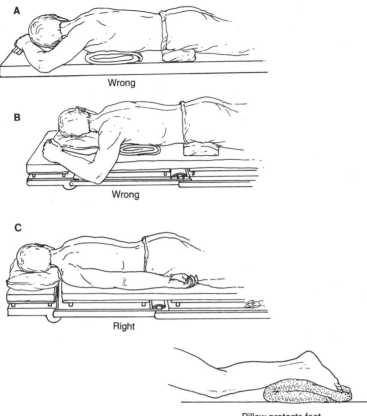

A

Wrong

B

Wrong

C

Right

Pillow protects foot

Figure 19–16

The prone position. *A.* Arm above head makes possible injury of lower brachial plexus. *B.* Arm over side of table may traumatize ulnar nerve in cubital tunnel or radial nerve as it moves around the humerus. *C.* Proper position of arm. Use of pillow to protect foot. (Courtesy of Lahey Clinic, Burlington, MA.)

nerve damage. The correct position is shown in Figure 19–16C, with the arms at the patient's side secured with a drawsheet. The feet are resting over a pillow to prevent plantar extension of the foot or the ankle and to shield the foot from contact with the end or edge of the operating table.

Lateral Decubitus Position

The posterior view of the lateral decubitus position is shown in Figure 19–17. The head, improperly supported in Figure 19–17A, compresses the dependent arm and may result in impairment of the neurovascular function of the arm. Figure 19–17B shows the head properly supported so that the head, neck, and spine are kept in the same horizontal plane. An instrument stand and screen are above the patient's head to keep the weight of drapes and surgical assistants off the patient's head and shoulders. Figure 19–17C shows the use of a pad near the axilla to distribute weight between the chest wall and the shoulder.

An anterior view of a patient in the lateral position is shown in Figure 19–18. To facilitate ventilation, the abdomen and chest are left free. A pillow is placed between the legs to distribute the weight of the upper leg on the lower leg. A metal "toboggan" (Wells Arm Protector, Mercury Enterprises, Inc., North Clearwater, FL) protects the arms and is properly padded.

Lithotomy Position

As mentioned earlier, the highest incidence of lower extremity position–related neuropathies occurs in the lithotomy position. Risk factors include duration of surgery of 4 hours or longer, a body mass index of 20 or less (thin body habitus), and a history of smoking within 30 days of the procedure.[14] Specific positioning recommendations for placing patients in the lithotomy position (see also Chapter 6) include the following:

- To protect the sciatic nerve, knees should be flexed whenever the hips are flexed, and external rotation of the hips should be minimized.
- To protect the tibial nerve, compression of the popliteal fossa should be avoided.

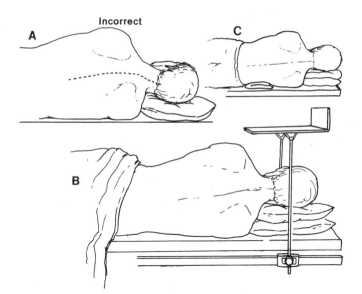

Figure 19–17

Lateral decubitus position, posterior view. *A.* Head improperly supported. *B.* Head properly supported, reducing compression of dependent arm. *C.* Use of pad to distribute weight between shoulder and chest wall. (Courtesy of Lahey Clinic, Burlington, MA.)

- To protect the saphenous nerve, equipment and personnel should not be permitted to press against the medial aspect of the upper third of the tibia.
- To protect the lateral femoral cutaneous nerve, the anterior-superior iliac spine should be well protected.
- To protect the superficial branch of the common peroneal nerve as it wraps around the head of the fibula, no pressure should be exerted against the lateral aspect of the lower leg just below the knee. This location is particularly at risk if it is permitted to rest against the poorly padded vertical pole of the leg brace used in the lithotomy position or if the crowding presence of team members working at the perineum forces the extremity laterally against the pole.

CONCLUSIONS

Despite the thousands of pages written in the past few decades about perioperative periph-

eral nerve injuries, the overall incidence of these injuries does not appear to have been substantially reduced. The answer may lie, in part, in the nature of the problem. Strategies to reduce nerve injury are well thought out, and one would be hard pressed to find a member of any operating room team who would not show respect for their principles. However, the daily maintenance of these strategies is difficult; they require tireless vigilance, constant communication between team members, and a sophisticated feedback system that will report and analyze complications discovered sometimes months later. The goal of reducing these injuries is further hampered by the frequent absence of an obvious explanation for the development of an injury and the occurrence of an injury despite acceptable positioning and monitoring.

Traditionally, texts have insisted that all perioperative nerve injuries are preventable if sufficient caution is consistently maintained by the operating room staff. Evidence exists,[3, 4, 11, 14] however, that nerve injury may occur despite routine application of accepted medi-

Figure 19–18

Lateral decubitus position, anterior view. Lower chest and abdomen are free. A pillow is placed between the legs, and a metal shield protects the arms. Up-side arm is placed on folded blanket. (Courtesy of Lahey Clinic, Burlington, MA.)

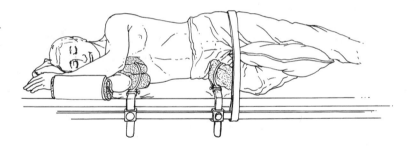

cal practices. Possibly, unavoidable events associated with anesthesia, surgery, and the postoperative period will produce additive effects on a previously damaged nerve and turn a subclinical neuropathy into an identifiable complaint or symptom (see Chapter 11).

Evidence is increasing to indicate that many perioperative neuropathies may occur during the postoperative period. Thus, increasing effort should be devoted to improving the education of postoperative surgical nursing staffs regarding the potential for position-related nerve damage, the means of recognizing causative factors, and the need for better preventive maneuvers.

Despite the scientific question of ability to avoid injuries, the legal implications for these injuries are clear. Nerve damage was the second most frequent complication reported in the ASA closed claims study.[3, 4] In these instances, medical care judgment was considered "standard" in 63% compared with 36% of instances not involving nerve damage. Nonetheless, the likelihood of payment for a claim of nerve damage was essentially the same regardless of whether the care was judged to have met the "standard." Future research designed to identify patients at risk for perioperative nerve injury and the development of monitoring procedures to evaluate nerve function during surgery could provide an early warning system for the physician. In the meantime, application of the basic, common sense techniques of safe patient positioning is part of the day-to-day responsibilities of all members of the operating room team.

REFERENCES

1. Parks BJ: Postoperative peripheral neuropathies. Surgery 74:348, 1973.
2. Blitt CD, Kaufer-Bratt C, Ashby J, Caillet JR: QA program reveals safety issues, promotes development of guidelines. Anesthesia Patient Safety Found Newsl 9:2:17, 1994.
3. Kroll DA, Caplan RA, Posner K, et al.: Nerve injury associated with anesthesia. Anesthesiology 73:202, 1990.
4. Cheney FW: The American Society of Anesthesiologists' closed claims project: Lessons learned. American Society of Anesthesiologists Regional Refresher Course. Park Ridge, IL, American Society of Anesthesiologists, 1994, pp. 1–7.
5. Keats AS: The Closed Claims Study. Anesthesiology 73:199, 1990.
6. McDonald JJ, Chusid JG, Lange J: Correlative Neuroanatomy, 4th ed. Palo Alto, CA, University Medical Publishers, 1947.
7. Cooper DE, Jenkins RS, Bready L, Rockwood CA Jr: The prevention of injuries of the brachial plexus secondary to malposition of the patient during surgery. Clin Orthop 228:33, 1988.
8. Lederman RJ, Breuer AC, Hanson MR, et al.: Peripheral nervous system complications of coronary artery bypass graft surgery. Ann Neurol 12:297, 1982.
9. Hanson MR, Breuer AC, Furlan AJ, et al.: Mechanism and frequency of brachial plexus injury in open-heart surgery: A prospective analysis. Ann Thorac Surg 36:675, 1983.
10. Stoelting RK: Postoperative ulnar nerve palsy—is it a preventable complication? Editorial. Anesth Analg 76:7, 1993.
11. Warner MA, Warner ME, Martin JT: Ulnar neuropathy: Incidence, outcome, and risk factors in sedated or anesthetized patients. Anesthesiology 81:1332, 1994.
12. Alvine FG, Schurrer ME: Postoperative ulnar-nerve palsy: Are there predisposing factors? J Bone Joint Surg Am 69:255, 1987.
13. Stoelting RK: Nerve injury during anesthesia. Am Soc Anesthesiol Newsl 58:6, 1994.
14. Warner MA, Martin JT, Schroeder DR, et al.: Lower-extremity motor neuropathy associated with surgery performed in patients in a lithotomy position. Anesthesiology 81:6, 1994.
15. Thompson GE, Lui ACP: Perioperative nerve injury. In Benumof JL, Saidman LJ (eds.): Anesthesia and Perioperative Complications. St. Louis, Mosby–Year Book, 1992, pp. 160–172.
16. Selander D, Sjostrand J: Longitudinal spread of intraneurally injected local anesthetics. Acta Anaesthesiol Scand 22:622, 1978.
17. Selander D, Brattsand R, Lundborg G, et al.: Local anesthetics: Importance of mode of application, concentration and adrenaline of the appearance of nerve lesions. Acta Anaesthesiol Scand 23:127, 1979.
18. Lundborg G: Structure and function of the intraneural microvessels as related to trauma, edema formation, and nerve function. J Bone Joint Surg Am 57:938, 1975.
19. Dawson DM, Krarup C: Perioperative nerve lesions. Arch Neurol 46:1355, 1989.
20. Seddon HJ: Three types of nerve injury. Brain 66:237, 1943.
21. Livingston KE: A simple method of rapid identification of major peripheral nerve injuries. Lahey Clin Bull 5:118, 1947.
22. Mahla ME: Nervous system. In Gravenstein N (ed.): Manual of Complications During Anesthesia. Philadelphia, JB Lippincott, 1990, pp. 383–419.
23. Clausen EG: Postoperative ("anesthetic") paralysis of the brachial plexus: Review of the literature and report of 9 cases. Surgery 12:933, 1942.

Chapter 20

Postanesthesia Care Unit Evaluation

Mary E. Warner

Concerns about the effects of patient positioning move with a patient from the operating room into the postanesthesia care unit (PACU) for several reasons. First, the same hemodynamic principles associated with positioning intraoperatively are present in the PACU. Second, patients in the PACU may not have regained all of their hemodynamic and autonomic protective reflexes, may not yet have complete control of their voluntary efforts, and may need to be protected by appropriate positioning and safety precautions. Finally, injuries may occur either during the intraoperative period or in the PACU and require early assessment to initiate promptly the appropriate diagnostic or therapeutic procedures.

Issues related to positioning of patients in the PACU include (1) protection of the awakening patient, (2) maintenance of appropriate hemodynamics, (3) assessment of neurologic function, and (4) evaluation of any apparent integumentary or peripheral injuries. Accurate assessment and documentation of the mental capacity, hemodynamic stability, and physical well-being of PACU patients are crucial. As noted by Aldrete,[1] interviews with the patient's family and friends may be needed to evaluate a postoperative condition against the preoperative status.

PATIENT ASSESSMENT IN THE PACU

For at least three decades, various scoring systems have been used as standardized as-

sessment tools in the PACU. In 1964, Carighan and colleagues[2] proposed a six-point postoperative recovery scoring system that evaluated the major physiologic systems. The intention was novel but was not universally accepted. Six years later, Aldrete introduced his version of a PACU scoring system.[3] This format uses a simple 0–2 point scale for five physiologic parameters (Table 20–1). Because it is easy to use and provides simple comparisons of scores over time, this method of assessment, now commonly known as the *Aldrete score,* has been adopted as the suggested criteria for discharge from the PACU by the Joint Commission of Accreditation of Health Care Organizations in the United States and by similar regulatory agencies in various other countries throughout the world. There has been one major criticism of the Aldrete score, namely, its use of skin color as a surrogate marker for oxygenation. Recently, Aldrete has modified his proposal to include quantitative assessment of oxygenation by pulse oximetry.[3] Variations of the Aldrete score (e.g., the Steward[4] and the Robertson[5] scores) are used in some PACUs.

Patients should be continuously monitored in the PACU as their awakening process is carefully supervised. On entry, the verbal report from the primary anesthesia provider should include information regarding the surgical/anesthetic course, pertinent preoperative conditions, and a suggested PACU treatment plan.[6] An initial assessment and scoring of the patient's physiologic and mental status should be made and documented. Thereafter,

Table 20–1

Major Components of the Aldrete PACU Recovery Scoring System

Component	Score	Requirement
Activity	0	Moves no extremity voluntarily or on command
	1	Moves two extremities voluntarily or on command
	2	Moves four extremities voluntarily or on command
Respiration	0	Apnea
	1	Dyspnea or limited breathing
	2	Able to breathe deeply and cough freely
Circulation	0	BP $\pm$ 50% of preanesthetic level
	1	BP $\pm$ 20%–50% of preanesthetic level
	2	BP $\pm$ 20% of preanesthetic level
Consciousness	0	Not responding
	1	Arousable on calling
	2	Fully awake
O_2 saturation	0	O_2 saturation <90% despite O_2 supplement
	1	Needs O_2 inhalation to keep O_2 saturation >90%
	2	Maintains O_2 saturation >90% on room air

Modified from Aldrete JA: The post-anesthesia recovery score revisited. J Clin Anesth 7:89, 1995. Copyright 1995 by Elsevier Science Inc.

interval PACU scores should be documented for comparison. A simple peripheral nerve function screen is a prudent addition to the documentation of the PACU score determined just before discharge from the unit.

PROTECTION OF THE AWAKENING PATIENT

Unconscious or semiconscious patients arriving in the PACU from surgery must be protected from injury. Tailoring the anesthetic to provide the most rapid return of protective reflexes and consciousness at its termination is the best method of providing this safeguard. The recent introduction and acceptance of short-acting intravenous and volatile anesthetics has increased the speed of awakening for many patients and increased the proportion of patients who are alert when first reaching the PACU.[7–10]

Despite these advances, however, some patients are semiconscious, confused, and thrashing about on admission to the PACU. They need quick protection from injury caused by flailing extremities and flopping heads. In some cases, padding of transport carts may be all that is necessary; in others, chemical or physical restraints may be appropriate. All of these patients should be rapidly evaluated for potential causes of their obtundation or semiconsciousness. Of a large number of possible causes, respiratory insufficiency and hypoxia would have the most

devastating effects and should be ruled out first. Fortunately, respiratory insufficiency and severe hypoxia are relatively rare events in the PACU. Rose and co-workers[11] noted severe hypoxia and hypoventilation to occur in less than 0.1% of their PACU patients. Metabolic derangements such as hyperglycemia or hypoglycemia and hyponatremia and associated neurologic impairment should also be considered early in the evaluation process.

If no apparent, potentially injurious etiologies are identified, and it appears that confusion and thrashing likely are associated with emergence from residual anesthetics, restraint may be needed. In these cases controversy arises, however, over whether to use chemical or physical restraints.[12, 13] Most physicians and nurses providing care in PACUs prefer to start with carefully titrated chemical (e.g., sedative or narcotic) restraint of a thrashing patient to prevent injury to the patient, care personnel, or the environment. Thereafter, physical restraints such as wrist or ankle bands are added as needed, according to institutional guidelines.[14] Lack of adequate guidelines for physical restraints has led to medicolegal and ethical limitations on their use.[15, 16] An example of written guidelines for the use of physical restraints in the PACU is found in Table 20–2.

MAINTENANCE OF APPROPRIATE HEMODYNAMICS

The most common hemodynamic problems encountered in PACUs are tachycardia and

Table 20-2

Potential Guidelines for Use of Restraints in Adults

Postulate: The use of physical restraints is appropriate only when less restrictive measures are insufficient, ineffective, or not feasible and when the restraint is necessary to protect the patient from injury to self or others.

1	Less restrictive interventions are to be evaluated and, whenever possible, tried before application of restraints. If such interventions are tried and found ineffective, insufficient, or not feasible, they will be identified and documented in the patient record.
2	An explanation will be given to the patient, family, or designated guardian about the process and rationale for the use of restraint. Some circumstances (e.g., short-term use of restraints in awakening PACU patients) may preclude or limit patient or family participation in the decision to use restraints.
3	Body holders, limb restraints, mitts, and bed enclosures qualify as restraints.
4	Nurse–physician collaboration is an essential component in the clinical assessment of a patient's need for restraint.
5	In a nonemergent situation, a physician will evaluate the patient as soon as feasible before writing the order for restraints.
6	In an emergency situation, the nurse can institute the restraint and will notify the physician immediately.
7	Restraints are prescriptive devices. All orders will be written for a limited period of time, not to exceed 24 hours. The order will specify the reason for restraint in behavioral terms. Verbal, telephone, and prn orders are not acceptable.
8	Collaboration between the nurse and physician will continue throughout the specified time that the patient is restrained. Evaluation of the continued need for restraint will include assessment of the patient's physical, emotional, and behavioral status related to the specific episode for which the order was written.
9	Communication of pertinent restraint care information will occur whenever a patient in restraint is moved from one patient care area to another.
10	Patients in restraint will be observed directly while in the PACU. Documentation on the PACU record will reflect the care provided during the period of restraint.
11	The neurovascular status of restrained extremities will be intermittently assessed and documented. Restraints will be intermittently removed to allow movement throughout the full range of motion, as appropriate.

Modified from the Adult Restraint Policy of Mayo Clinic Hospitals, 1995.

extremes of blood pressure.[17–20] Respiratory insufficiency and hypoxia first must be eliminated as causes.[21, 22] In general, tachycardia and hypertension are most often associated with high levels of pain perception by patients and should be treated appropriately.[23] In contrast, tachycardia and hypotension commonly result from intravascular fluid deficits and, less frequently, myocardial failure and sepsis. Before initiating treatment, it is important to distinguish between these possible causes because the treatments vary dramatically. The best treatment for hypovolemia is the rapid intravascular infusion of controlled volumes of fluid while carefully monitoring the responses. In the recent past, many physicians and nurses would also have tilted patients head down with the belief that this position would improve venous return and boost cardiac output and systemic blood pressure. In extreme cases of hypotension, pressure-filled constrictive devices (e.g., military antishock trousers) may have been tried. Today, these techniques for treating hypovolemia have been proven to be ineffective (see discussion in Chapter 8) and are seldom indicated. Myocardial failure requires careful hemodynamic assessment, inotropic support as

indicated, and, in some cases, respiratory assistance. Sepsis results in relative hypovolemia; intravascular volume expansion and sympathomimetic support often are needed.

A discussion of hemodynamic changes seen in the PACU, such as bradycardia and either hypertension or hypotension associated with bladder distention or myocardial ischemia, respectively, is beyond the scope of this text. There are many causes for hemodynamic aberrations, and each episode of hemodynamic instability requires careful and rapid evaluation by skilled clinicians.

ASSESSMENT OF NEUROLOGIC FUNCTION

A number of types of injuries may occur to patients during the perioperative period, but one category that requires particularly careful assessment and documentation is neurologic dysfunction. New neuropathies are not always apparent in the PACU, yet persistent routine searches for these afflictions provide prompt recognition and diagnosis plus the opportunities for early interventions that may improve the situation or prevent further exacerbation.

Alertness

A general assessment of alertness is part of most PACU scoring systems.[2-5] Unexpected delay in recovery of alertness mandates careful evaluation. In addition to confirmation of adequate oxygenation and ventilation, normal blood glucose and sodium levels, and appropriate acid-base status (if indicated), a neurologic examination should be performed to determine the presence or absence of intracranial pathology. Cerebral strokes from thromboembolism, ischemia, or hemorrhage may occur intraoperatively or in the PACU.[24, 25] If an intracranial pathologic process is suspected after physical examination, immediate neurologic consultation is needed and rapid diagnosis by using one of a variety of imaging techniques is often required.

Gross Nerve Function

During their stay in the recovery facility, all patients should be evaluated for dysfunction of major nerves. The initial evaluation often is performed by trained nursing staff with the subsequent involvement of responsible physicians or consultants added as needed. Proper nerve function should be documented, as should all evidence of dysfunction that might imply a new neuropathy. Assessment should include the function of major nerves such as the ulnar, median, and radial nerves of the upper extremities and the femoral, peroneal, and sciatic nerves of the lower extremities. Vision should be ascertained and compared with preoperative vision. Nerves at risk for dysfunction from certain surgical procedures (e.g., upper extremity nerves after cervical laminectomy) should be evaluated and their function documented. Specific nerves that may be injured in each intraoperative position are discussed in more detail in the chapters describing the positions.

Supine Position
(See Chapter 5)

Excluding nerve injuries of the upper extremities (see Chapter 11), various nerves of the face and neck can be injured during the intraoperative period. The same pressure phenomenon that may induce alopecia of the occiput after long cases performed on supine patients[26-28] may also affect the occipital nerve. Superficial nerves of the face such as the buccal and mandibular branches of the facial nerve may be stretched or compressed when work is performed around the face or when anesthetic techniques (e.g., taping airways) may place traction on the facial skin.[29, 30] The major nerves of the upper extremities can be traumatized or stretched in the process of placing an anesthetized patient in the supine position (see Chapter 11). Nerve injury may be procedure specific. For example, the lateral cutaneous femoral nerve may be injured during laparoscopic herniorrhaphy.[31] The ipsilateral facial nerve may be injured after acoustic neuroma surgery.[32]

Lithotomy Position
(See Chapter 6)

Perioperative neuropathies of nearly all lower extremity nerves have been reported. Of these, the most common motor neuropathies occur to the peroneal nerve. Warner and co-workers[33] found prolonged motor neuropathies in 55 of 198,461 (1:3608) adult patients who had procedures performed while in a lithotomy position; of these 55 neuropathies, 43 (78%) involved the peroneal nerve. Distal nerves in the lower extremities may also be damaged by high tissue pressures associated with compartment syndromes of the leg.[34] Renal failure and even cardiac arrest have been associated with the severe muscle destruction commonly associated with compartment syndromes.[34, 35] The reperfusion phenomenon that leads to this devastating problem may be manifest after the PACU stay. Distal pulses are often present in the legs of patients who subsequently develop a compartment syndrome. An early sign of compartment syndrome may be the onset of neurologic dysfunction of the peripheral nerves of the extremity.[35]

Head-Elevated Position
(See Chapter 7)

Some neurosurgical procedures that are performed in head-elevated positions will require assessment of specific neurologic functions. For example, the ability to hear and the function of the ipsilateral facial nerve should be determined in patients after removal of an acoustic neuroma.[32] Cervical spinal cord and brain stem nervous function may be compromised during and after posterior cervical surgery.[36–39] Specific attention should be given to swallowing mechanics and respiratory function. For patients who had their procedures performed with their heads turned, cervical radiculopathy and thoracic outlet syndrome may result.[40–42]

The Head-Low Positions
(See Chapter 8)

Steep head-down tilt may involve the use of restraints to stabilize the patient's position on the table. The brachial plexus may be stretched by caudally directed traction of the arms by wristlets or other arm restraints. It also may be stretched or injured by a shoulder brace if the patient shifts cephalad when in the head-low position.[43–46] If the upper roots (especially C5 and C6) of the brachial plexus are primarily involved (Erb-Duchenne type injury), the deltoid, brachialis, and brachioradialis muscles will be weak and sensation will be decreased over the deltoid area and radial surface of the forearm and hand. Injury to the lower roots of the plexus (e.g., C8–T1) is less common and may be associated with abduction of the arm on an armboard to more than 90 degrees, especially if an ipsilateral shoulder brace is used to prevent cephalad sliding of the patient.[44, 47]

The use of steep head-down tilt may also affect venous and lymphatic drainage of a variety of tissues. For example, scleral and conjunctival swelling and injection, nasal congestion, and facial edema are common after prolonged procedures performed in head-low positions, but these changes do not appear to cause prolonged problems. Edema of the glottis may, however, cause transient partial airway obstruction. This problem should be considered in any patient who has undergone a procedure in a head-low position when inspiratory stridor occurs after endotracheal extubation.

The Lateral Decubitus Positions
(See Chapter 9)

Patients who are operated on while in the lateral decubitus position without supportive pillows to prevent lateral tilt of the head may develop cervical radiculopathies,[47] a thoracic outlet syndrome, or even Horner's syndrome.[48] The down-side facial nerve may be compressed by unyielding lateral head supports (e.g., the fold of a blanket or towel) or stretched by a shift in position during a procedure. The up-side long thoracic nerve may be stretched in this position.[49] The major nerves of the upper extremities may be especially susceptible to injury or compression. The femoral nerve(s) may be pinched if the thighs are flexed too tightly.[50]

The Prone Positions
(See Chapter 10)

A variety of problems can arise in patients who have been placed in a prone position. Many of these potential problems may be associated with management of the head and neck during the establishment and maintenance of this position. For example, the head must be controlled during pronation of the patient; a flopping head can result in damaging impact and direct trauma or severe injury to the cervical vertebrae and spinal cord.[51] Cervical radiculopathy with neck and upper extremity pain and thoracic outlet syndrome are possible. Hyperextension of the head or cervical spine while in the prone position may entrap the greater occipital nerve and cause muscular spasms and headache in the postoperative period.[52] Superficial portions of facial nerves may be compressed if weight bearing is transmitted to them, especially if a hard surface (e.g., fold of a sheet or a wire cable) is directly in contact. Pressure on the orbits can increase intraocular pressure enough to cause retinal ischemia and blindness or may directly damage corneas, eyelids, or conjunctiva.[53–56] Hyperflexion of either the hips or knees may compromise blood flow during the operative period and cause ischemia and/or compartment syndrome of the lower extremities.

Evaluation of Gross Nerve Function

A limited neurologic evaluation early in the patient's PACU stay will detect most of the major neuropathies that may occur intraoperatively. Most neuropathies are identified initially in the PACU environment by assessing subjective symptoms such as tingling or pain in the distal extremities, although major neuropathies may be associated with distinct decreases in strength. An example of a simplified neurologic examination that may be useful in the PACU is shown in Table 20–3. Although an abbreviated examination adequately assesses nerve function in the distal extremities, further evaluation may be required to locate the level of specific nerve

Table 20-3

Simplified Neurologic Examination	
Nerve	*Test for Intact Function*
Median	Normal sensation on palmar surface of index finger
Ulnar	Normal sensation on palmar surface of fifth finger
Radial	Ability to abduct thumb
Sciatic	Ability to flex leg at the knee
Peroneal	Ability to dorsiflex great toe
Tibial	Ability to plantarflex great toe
Femoral	Ability to extend the leg at the knee
Anterior cutaneous	Normal sensation on the lateral surface of the thigh
Saphenous	Normal sensation on the medial surface of the leg

dysfunction. The presence or absence of symptoms or evident weakness of the following major nerve groups should be noted before discharge of patients from the PACU.

Upper Extremity Nerves

ULNAR NERVE

Sensory Evaluation. Ulnar paresthesias are localized to the volar surface of the medial half of the fourth digit and all of the fifth. The sensitivity of two-point discrimination testing to evaluate ulnar sensory changes within the PACU is probably no better than positive responses to questions that ask patients if they have any tingling or pain in their "ring" or "little" fingers.

Motor Evaluation. Ulnar nerve motor dysfunction can be readily determined if both grip and interosseous muscle weakness are found. Grip strength can be decreased by dysfunction of several nerves, including the ulnar nerve. However, decreased interosseous muscle strength, noted by asking patients to spread their fingers against resistance, is strongly suggestive of ulnar nerve dysfunction.

MEDIAN NERVE

Sensory Evaluation. Median paresthesias are localized to the volar surface of the first through third digits, plus the lateral half of the fourth digit. Although the median nerve also transmits sensation from the forearm, an abbreviated examination of sensation within the hand is reasonable.

Motor Evaluation. Median nerve motor dysfunction is present if there is weakness of wrist flexion and the lumbricales muscles. Decreased grip strength, wrist flexion, and "squeeze" or apposition of the fingers suggest median nerve dysfunction.

RADIAL NERVE

Sensory Evaluation. The dorsal surface of the hand, as well as the forearm, is innervated by the radial nerve or its branches. Because the median and ulnar nerves provide sensation to the volar surface and the radial nerve provides sensation to the posterior surface of the fingertips, patients may have varying degrees of crossover sensation in their fingertips. Some may note tingling of their fingertips, and further evaluation may be needed to determine which nerve group may be involved.

Motor Evaluation. Weakness of wrist extension and loss of ability to dorsiflex the distal phalanx first digit (thumb) suggest radial nerve dysfunction.

Lower Extremity Nerves

FEMORAL NERVE

Sensory Evaluation. Femoral paresthesias are found on the anterior surface of the thigh, extending below and medial to the knee. Paresthesias on the lateral thigh are associated with neuropathy of the lateral femoral cutaneous nerve.

Motor Evaluation. The quadriceps muscles of the thigh are innervated by the femoral nerve and its branches and cause extension of the leg at the knee. The rectus femoris muscle also assists with flexion of the hip; however, patients with femoral neuropathies often will be able to flex their ipsilateral hips because the iliopsoas muscle, innervated by nerves from L2–4, contributes to hip flexion.

SCIATIC NERVE

Sensory Evaluation. The sciatic nerve carries sensory input from the posterior thigh. In the popliteal fossa it splits into the common peroneal and tibial nerves. Paresthesias of the peroneal nerve are found on the lateral surface of the leg and foot. In addition, the deep branch of the peroneal nerve provides sensation between the first and second toes. The tibial nerve courses down the medial aspect of the leg and foot and carries sensory input from those areas.

Motor Evaluation. Proximally, the sciatic nerve innervates the hamstring muscle group, including the biceps femoris. These muscles extend the hip and flex the knee. Although the sciatic nerve may be injured before splitting into its distal branches, most motor deficits associated with this nerve occur after the branching. Distally, the tibial branch of the sciatic nerve provides motor innervation to the gastrocnemius and soleus muscles, among others, and permits active plantarflexion at the ankle. The peroneal nerve innervates the peroneal muscles on the anterior and lateral surfaces of the leg. These muscles dorsiflex the foot and toes at the ankle.

ASSESSMENT OF SOFT TISSUES AND OTHER STRUCTURES

Many soft tissues and other structures can be injured or altered in the perioperative period. In general, these structures are superficial and can be readily identified by careful visual examination in the PACU. Because many of the patients in the PACU will be cold and covered with blankets, care teams are often reluctant to incrementally remove these covers, expose their patients to the air-conditioned atmosphere, and completely inspect the body surfaces. It is essential that this visualization be performed and any unexpected alterations or injuries noted and treated.

Skin

Although the entire body surface should be inspected, certain areas are especially susceptible to injury. A large variety of forces can injure the skin, the most common being pressure on weight-bearing surfaces.[57] Chemical, thermal, and electric burns are usually found in distinct, well-circumscribed areas. Scratches, cuts, and bruises may occur anywhere but are particularly likely in the extremities because of their increased mobility and risk of exposure to traumatic forces.

Any weight-bearing surfaces should be inspected for pressure injuries to the overlying skin. These areas vary accordingly with the patient's position during the intraoperative period. For example, procedures done in the prone position may provoke pressure injuries to the skin of the face, shoulders, and knees. In contrast, injuries to the skin of these areas would be unlikely had the procedure required the supine position. Erythematous ar-

eas are common, but few cause any prolonged problems. Blisters or gross skin breakdown is unusual, but both must be noted and treated. Patients who receive corticosteroids and elderly patients who have lost much of their subcutaneous fat and integumentary support structure are especially susceptible to skin trauma.

Burns are usually distinguished by well-circumscribed borders that differentiate them from the more diffuse spread of skin lesions and rashes associated with cutaneous allergic reactions to various chemicals. For example, a povidone iodine (Betadine)–induced burn may occur if the solution is allowed to pool in contact with the skin for a prolonged period. In this example, only the skin in contact with the iodine solution is burned. In iodine-induced allergic reactions, the cutaneous response is generalized and less circumscribed. Thermal burns often result from improperly functioning heating equipment, especially units that transmit heat by direct contact of warm solids or liquids with the skin. Because of the reduced risk of skin injury from forced-air heating devices, as well as the superior heat transfer characteristics of warmed air compared with liquids and solids,[58] most active heating mechanisms now used are forced-air devices. In general, the use of heated water blankets and, in many hospitals, heated humidifiers for inhaled gases is being eliminated. Electrical burns still occur despite continual improvement in electronic grounding technologies. In general, electric burns are small and readily identifiable.

Oral Structures

Cut lips and tongues are often associated with the placement of rigid airways and endotracheal intubation. Many others occur during or after the anesthetic when patients may bite on airways and pinch their lips or tongues between their teeth and mechanical airways. Teeth may be chipped or broken by these same forces. Dental injuries have been reported to occur in approximately 0.3% (3/ 1000) of patients who receive a general anesthetic; most of these injuries occur to the upper incisors and involve chipping or partial dislodgement of these teeth.[59]

Eyes

In general, most eye injuries are superficial scratches or abrasions of the cornea.[60, 61] In these cases, pain and tearing are always present. Fortunately, superficial corneal abrasions rarely cause prolonged problems. Because superficial cells of the cornea replicate rapidly, patching the affected eye for 24 hours to prevent eye movement, plus reassurance to the patient, is often all the treatment needed.

More severe injuries to the cornea and other ocular problems require ophthalmologic assessment. Rarely, patients awaken blind in one or both eyes.[53, 54] Retinal artery ischemia may be due to external eye compression that elevates intraocular pressure.[54] Retinal artery ischemia and increased intraocular pressure also may occur from nitrous oxide diffusing into and expanding inert gas bubbles that have been introduced to stabilize detached retinas. These gases are absorbed from vitreous humor at rates that vary from 10 days for sulfur hexafluoride to 30 days for carbon octoflurine. Nitrous oxide is over 100 times more diffusible than these inert gases[62]; and its ability to expand the bubble, increase intraocular pressure, and occlude the retinal artery depends on the initial size of the bubble.

Post-Tonsillectomy Position

After removal of masses such as the tonsils from the upper airway, safe recovery from general anesthesia is best accomplished by arranging the patient either in the lateral position with the face turned slightly toward the mattress or in what has been informally referred to as the "post-tonsillectomy position" (Fig. 20–1).

The posture allows secretions to drain away from the hypopharynx while affording both a relatively unobstructed view of the face and an accessible, patent upper airway.

- Pillows are placed between the legs, and the down-side leg is kept straight while the up-side leg is flexed at the knee and hip.
- The up-side arm is flexed with the pronated hand near the head.
- Depending on the amount of ventral tilt involved, the down-side arm can be extended slightly behind the patient's torso to avoid compromising its axillary neurovascular bundle.
- Ventral circumduction of the down-side shoulder must not be sufficient to stretch its suprascapular nerve.
- Support for the ventral chest wall may be needed to prevent the patient from rolling fully prone.

Strict surveillance of an obtunded patient of this type is an obvious necessity because continued nasopharyngeal bleeding must be recognized promptly and treated. Reanesthetizing a child who is hypovolemic and whose stomach is full of swallowed blood and clots immediately after a tonsillectomy is a rare but legendary task that has historically been associated with a tragic outcome.

CONCLUSIONS

The level of alertness, hemodynamic stability, gross neurologic function, and integrity of su-

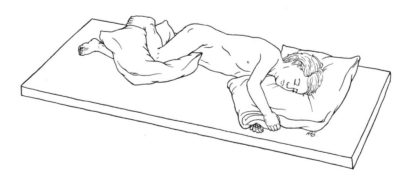

Figure 20–1

The post-tonsillectomy position. The patient is semi-prone with the down-side leg extended, pillows between the lower extremities, and the up-side leg flexed at the hip and knee to help stabilize the ventral tilt of the torso. The down-side arm is bent to a variable degree at the elbow and rests palm up in the general vicinity of the head while pillows separate the upper extremities. A relatively firm pad may be needed against the ventral chest wall to prevent inadvertent turning into the prone position that could circumduct the down-side arm across the chest and stretch the down-side supraclavicular nerve. Access to the face should be maintained to aid removal of oral drainage.

perficial structures of all patients in the PACU should be assessed to the extent possible on their admission to the unit, re-evaluated as indicated while there, and assessed finally before their discharge. Findings should be documented succinctly in the patient's permanent record in a location that can be easily found if the data are subsequently needed. These efforts are inexpensive, are well within the skill levels expected of the care team, and add little, if any, time to PACU stays. Early identification of abnormal parameters may allow physicians to recommend treatments that either improve outcomes or prevent further injury.

REFERENCES

1. Aldrete JA: Complications of positioning: Recovery room assessment. *In* Martin JT (ed.): Positioning in Anesthesia and Surgery, 2nd ed. Philadelphia, WB Saunders, 1987, p. 329.
2. Carighan G, Kerri-Szanto M, Lavelle J: Post-anesthetic scoring system. Anesthesiology 25:396, 1964.
3. Aldrete JA: The post-anesthesia recovery score revisited. J Clin Anesth 7:89, 1995.
4. Steward D: A simplified scoring system for the postoperative recovery room. Can Anaesth Soc J 22:111, 1975.
5. Robertson G, MacGregor D, Jones C: Evaluation of doxapram for arousal from general anesthesia in outpatients. Br J Anaesth 49:133, 1977.
6. Litwack K: Immediate postoperative care: A problem-oriented approach. In Vender JS, Spiess BD (eds.): Post Anesthesia Care. Philadelphia, WB Saunders, 1992, pp. 1–8.
7. Ding Y, Fredman B, White PF: Recovery following outpatient anesthesia: Use of enflurane versus propofol. J Clin Anesth 5:447, 1993.
8. Kalman SH, Jensen AG, Ekberg K, Eintrei C: Early and late recovery after major abdominal surgery: Comparison between propofol anaesthesia with and without nitrous oxide and isoflurane anaesthesia. Acta Anaesth Scand 37:730, 1993.
9. Schwender D, Muller A, Madler M, et al.: Recovery of psychomotor and cognitive functions following anesthesia: Propofol/alfentanil and thiopental/isoflurane/alfentanil. Anaesthetist 42:583, 1993.
10. Nightingale JJ, Lewis IH: Recovery from day-case anaesthesia: Comparison of total i.v. anaesthesia using propofol with an inhalation technique. Br J Anaesth 68:356, 1992.
11. Rose DK, Cohen MM, Wigglesworth DF, DeBoer DP: Critical respiratory events in the postanesthesia care unit: Patient, surgical, and anesthetic factors. Anesthesiology 81:410, 1994.
12. Tammelleo AD: Restraints: A legal catch-22? RN 55:71, 1992.
13. Stabler-Haas S, McHugh M: Patient restraints: A question of assault and battery. Crit Care Nurse 12:30, 1992.
14. Joint Commission on Accreditation of Health Care Organizations: Accreditation Manual for Hospitals, 1993, p. 235.
15. Fiesta J: Legal answers. Nurs Manage 23:20, 1992.
16. Anonymous: Montana state court establishes constitutional requirements for the use of seclusion and restraint. Hosp Community Psychiatry 42:1266, 1991.
17. Zelcer J, Wells DG: Anaesthetic-related recovery room complications. Anaesth Intens Care 15:168, 1987.
18. Cohen MM, Duncan PG, Pope WBD, Wolkenstein C: A survey of 112,000 anaesthetics at one teaching hospital (1975–1983). Can Anaesth Soc J 33:22, 1986.
19. Hines R, Barash PG, Watrous G, O'Connor T: Complications occurring in the postanesthesia care unit: A survey. Anesth Analg 74:503, 1992.
20. Shander A, Puri S: Recovery from anesthesia. Hemodynamic consequences of emergence. Int Anesthesiol Clin 29:13, 1991.
21. Parr SM, Robinson BJ, Glover PW, Galletly DC: Level of consciousness on arrival in the recovery room and the development of early respiratory morbidity. Anaesth Intens Care 19:369, 1991.
22. Russell GB, Graybeal JM: Hypoxemic episodes of patients in a postanesthesia care unit. Chest 104:899, 1993.
23. Marymont JH III, O'Connor BS: Postoperative cardiovascular complications. *In* Vender JS, Spiess BD (eds.): Post Anesthesia Care. Philadelphia, WB Saunders, 1992, p. 26.
24. Oliver SB, Cucchiara RF, Warner MA, Muir JJ: Unexpected focal neurologic deficit on emergence from anesthesia. Anesthesiology 67:823, 1987.
25. Sloan TB: Postoperative central nervous system dysfunction. *In* Vender JS, Spiess BD (eds.): Post Anesthesia Care. Philadelphia, WB Saunders, 1992, pp. 188–189.
26. Abel RR, Lewis GM: Postoperative alopecia. Arch Dermatol 81:72, 1960.
27. Patel KD, Henschel EU: Postoperative alopecia. Anesth Analg 59:311, 1980.
28. Wiles JC, Hansen RC: Postoperative (pressure) alopecia. J Am Acad Dermatol 12:195, 1985.
29. Glarber DT: Facial paralysis after general anesthesia. Anesthesiology 65:516, 1986.
30. Fuller JE, Thomas DV: Facial nerve paralysis after general anesthesia. JAMA 162:645, 1956.
31. Kraus MA: Nerve injury during laparoscopic inguinal hernia repair. Surg Laparosc Endosc 3:342, 1993.
32. Portmann M, Riemans V, Bebear JP: Facial nerve problems in acoustic neuroma surgery. Adv Otorhinolaryngol 22:207, 1977.
33. Warner MA, Martin JT, Schoeder DR, et al.: Lower-extremity motor neuropathy associated with surgery performed on patients in a lithotomy position. Anesthesiology 81:1332, 1994.
34. Martin JT: Compartment syndromes: Concepts and perspectives for the anesthesiologist. Anesth Analg 75:275, 1992.
35. Lampert R, Weih EH, Breuching E, et al.: Postoperative bilateral compartment syndrome resulting from prolonged urological surgery in lithotomy position. Anaesthetist 44:43, 1995.
36. Toole JF: Effects of change of head, limb and body position on cephalic circulation. N Engl J Med 279:307, 1968.
37. Sherman DD, Hart RG, Easton JD: Abrupt change in head position and cerebral infarction. Stroke 12:2, 1981.
38. McPherson RW, Szymanski J, Rogers MC: Somatosensory evoked potential changes in position-related brain stem ischemia. Anesthesiology 61:88, 1984.

39. Patel RI, Thein RMH, Epstein BS: Costoclavicular syndrome and the sitting position during anesthesia. Anesthesiology 53:341, 1980.
40. Kim BY, Ngeow JYF, Kitahata LM, Swift CA: EEG changes with lateral rotation of the head. Anesthesiol Rev 12:36, 1985.
41. Berwick JE, Lessin ME: Brachial plexus injury occurring during oral and maxillofacial surgery. J Oral Maxillofacial Surg 47:643, 1989.
42. Beal JL, Lopin MC, Binnert M: Anesthesia for surgery of degenerative and abnormal cervical spine. Ann Fr Anesth Reanim 12:385, 1993.
43. Sloan TB: Postoperative central nervous system dysfunction. *In* Vender JS, Spiess BD (eds.): Post Anesthesia Care. Philadelphia, WB Saunders, 1992, p. 192.
44. Clausen EG: Postoperative ("anesthetic") paralysis of the brachial plexus: A review of the literature and report of nine cases. Surgery 12:933, 1942.
45. Wood-Smith FG: Postoperative brachial plexus paralysis. BMJ 1:1115, 1952.
46. Mitterschiffthaler G, Theiner A, Posch G, et al.: Lesion of the brachial plexus caused by wrong positioning during surgery. Anasthesie Intens Notfallmedizin 22:177, 1987.
47. Britt BA, Gordon RA: Peripheral nerve injuries associated with anesthesia. Can Anaesth Soc J 11:514, 1964.
48. Jaffe TB, McLesky CH: Position induced Horner's syndrome. Anesthesiology 56:49, 1982.
49. Martin JT: Postoperative isolated dysfunction of the long thoracic nerve: A rare entity of uncertain etiology. Anesth Analg 69:614, 1989.
50. Raber G, Schneider HP: Femoral nerve paralysis after vaginal hysterectomy and its forensic importance. Zentralbl Gynakol 115:273, 1993.
51. Shellhas KP, et al.: Vertebrobasilar injuries following cervical manipulation. JAMA 244:1450, 1986.
52. Smith RH: The prone position. *In* Martin JT (ed.): Positioning in Anesthesia and Surgery. Philadelphia, WB Saunders, 1978, p. 42.
53. Wolfe SW, Lospinuso MF, Burke SW: Unilateral blindness as a complicaton of patient positioning for spinal surgery. Spine 17:600, 1992.
54. Morin Y, Renard-Charalabidis C, Haut J: Definitive transient monocular blindness caused by ocular compression during general anesthesia. J Fr Ophthalmol 16:680, 1993.
55. Cucchiara RF, Black S: Corneal abrasion during anesthesia and surgery. Anesthesiology 69:978, 1988.
56. Gild WM, Posner KL, Caplan RA, Cheney FW: Eye injuries associated with anesthesia: A closed claims analysis. Anesthesiology 76:204, 1992.
57. Little DM Jr: Posture and anaesthesia. Can Anaesth Soc J 7:2, 1960.
58. Sessler DI: Temperature monitoring. *In* Miller RD (ed.): Anesthesia, 4th ed. New York, Churchill Livingstone, 1994, pp. 1373–1375.
59. Warner MA, Muir JJ, Warner ME: Incidence and risk factors for dental injury. Anesthesiology 81:A1231, 1994.
60. Batra YK, Bali M: Corneal abrasions during general anesthesia. Anesth Analg 56:363, 1977.
61. Watson W, Moran R: Corneal abrasion during induction. Anesthesiology 66:440, 1987.
62. Wolf GL, Capuano C, Hartung J: Nitrous oxide increases IOP after intravitreal sulfur hexafluride injection. Anesthesiology 59:547, 1983.

Chapter 21

Medicolegal Considerations

Kenneth J. White

MEDICAL MALPRACTICE

Medical malpractice is generally defined as injury to a patient that was caused by the doing of, or failing to do, some particular thing or things that a physician or surgeon of ordinary skill, care, and diligence would have done, or refrained from doing, under like or similar circumstances, and that the injury complained of by the patient was the direct and proximate result of such action or inaction.[1]

The yardstick by which the physician's conduct is measured is referred to as *standard of care*. That term denotes the level of practice of a reasonable physician or specialist, if the defendant physician practices a medical specialty, in light of the then existing scientific knowledge concerning the procedure or diagnosis at issue. As a general rule, and although there are exceptions in certain states, the standard of care is defined as a national standard, not a provincial one indigenous to a local community.

Standard of care does not mean the highest or even the best level of practice. It refers to what would be considered reasonable practice under the circumstances. Likewise, a physician does not, by working his or her craft, guarantee a perfect or even good outcome absent a written or oral statement to the contrary. As a general proposition, the law recognizes that reasonable medical judgment often encompasses a wide range of acceptable approaches to a given medical condition or problem and that the practice of medicine is, in many instances, more art than science.

Thus, the incorrect exercise of reasonable judgment when viewed in retrospect, or the presence of undesired or even disastrous treatment results, does not necessarily render the physician liable for malpractice. The physician's conduct is to be viewed by the state of the practice at the time treatment was rendered, and by the facts known, or which should have been known by the physician at that time, not retrospectively with knowledge subsequently acquired.

In actions such as medical malpractice, the burden or obligation of proof is on the plaintiff, the person bringing the suit. In the context of a medical claim, that person is the patient or the patient's estate. The patient must prove the elements of the claim of medical malpractice by a preponderance of the evidence. The term *preponderance* generally translates to what is more likely than not, or, in other words, what has a 51% probability.

Before liability for medical malpractice can be established, the patient must prove four basic elements. If the plaintiff fails to prove any one of these elements, an action for medical malpractice will not be successful.

1. *There must be proof that the physician owed a duty to the patient.* This burden is usually met by establishing the physician–patient relationship. That is, the physician undertook to render medical care or treatment to the patient.

2. *The physician must be shown to have deviated from or breached the standard of care in rendering the treatment.* In most instances, this requires testimony by a competent expert wit-

ness who must render testimony critical of the defendant physician by stating that the accused physician's conduct fell below the standard of care required under the circumstance of the patient's treatment.

3. *The patient must prove that there was a direct and proximate cause between the physician's deviation from the standard of care and the patient's injury.* There must be proof, more likely than not, that the physician's breach of duty caused harm to the patient. A breach of duty, even if flagrant, does not give rise to a claim for medical malpractice if that breach did not result in harm to the patient. In other words, even if a physician breached the standard of care, and harm occurred to the patient, unless the patient can prove by a preponderance of evidence that the breach caused the harm, no claim for malpractice exists.

4. *The patient must prove the harm or damage that was caused by the deviation from the standard of care.* Traditional notions of harm include pain and suffering, loss of income, medical expenses, and wrongful death if a patient's death is brought about by the physician's wrongful action or inaction.

RES IPSA LOQUITUR

The phrase *res ipsa loquitur,* which means "the thing speaks for itself," is a rule of evidence that, in certain circumstances, allows a jury to draw an inference of negligence. This doctrine is applicable to a variety of circumstances outside medicolegal actions. However, because of the unique setting under which anesthesia is administered, res ipsa loquitur is frequently alleged in medical malpractice cases involving peripheral nerve injuries diagnosed after anesthesia.

Although the specific requirements vary from state to state, res ipsa loquitur may be applied where the evidence establishes that the instrumentality causing the injury to the patient was under the exclusive management and control of the defendant health care provider(s) and that the incident occurred under such circumstances that in the usual course of events it would not have happened if ordinary care had been observed.[2] When a patient undergoes general anesthesia for a surgical procedure unrelated to an extremity or the spine and, on awakening, manifests a neurologic problem in an extremity, the doctrine of res ipsa loquitur may be applicable. Under such circumstances, it is possible to argue that a peripheral neurologic injury should not

occur but for negligence that arguably occurred while the patient was unconscious and under the control of the operating room personnel, thus potentially rendering liable the anesthesiologist, surgeon, and nursing personnel involved in positioning the patient.

The apparent ease of applicability of this doctrine, however, has probably caused a considerable amount of confusion, if not unwarranted concern, to health care professionals over their potential liability for untoward results after surgery.

The doctrine of res ipsa loquitur is merely a rule of evidence, not a separate claim or cause of action. It is neither an independent ground for recovery nor a separate theory of liability.[3] In most states, this doctrine does not change the patient's burden of proof. It simply allows the patient to prove negligence through the use of circumstantial evidence that creates an inference, not a presumption, of negligence.[4]

Even in those circumstances in which res ipsa loquitur is applicable, the jury is not precluded from finding that the physician acted appropriately. In these circumstances the physician or health care provider has the burden of explanation, not to show he or she was free from fault but to present evidence sufficient to rebut the inference of negligence raised by the doctrine.[5] The patient must still prove the four elements of the claim of medical malpractice by a preponderance of evidence. Res ipsa loquitur is not a substitute for that proof but, rather, a tool by which to meet the burden of proof.

PROXIMATE CAUSE

The appeal of res ipsa loquitur in cases where a peripheral nerve injury is noted after anesthesia is understandable. For instance, it is indeed easy to assume that an apparent brachial plexus dysfunction after an appendectomy performed under general anesthesia must be the result of the operating room personnel's negligence in positioning the patient because such an injury is not expected to occur in this setting. All too often, patients, family members, and consulting or subsequent health care providers make this causation leap of logic without considering alternative causes.

In few other medicolegal areas does the concept of proximate cause become as important as in so-called positioning cases. Again, the burden of proof is on the patient to prove the injury he or she claims was proximately caused by the negligence of the physician. This requirement is not eliminated when res ipsa loquitur is applicable.

In fact, when it cannot be inferred that the injury of which complaint is made normally occurs only with negligence, expert testimony on that issue is probably necessary before the doctrine of res ipsa loquitur can be applied.[6] In any event, a health care defendant in such a case is clearly entitled to present competent evidence that the injury alleged did not occur as the result of negligence. This is known as a "proximate cause" defense.

After anesthesia, patients have been known to develop peripheral neuropathies. Relating that type of injury to a presumed untoward event that occurred while the patient was anesthetized is tempting. Undoubtedly, such an injury can occur if a patient is improperly positioned during the surgery, and without further thought one can easily and conveniently presume that it was caused by negligent care of the operating room personnel.

We recognize, however, that patients do awake from anesthesia and experience peripheral neuropathies when no unusual event occurred during the surgery and when the patient was appropriately positioned.[7] There is a recognized condition called neuralgic amyotrophy that, when applied to the brachial plexus, encompasses entities referred to as acute brachial neuropathy, idiopathic brachial neuritis, Parsonage-Turner syndrome, and so on.[8] In general terms, this nontraumatic condition can present in a fashion similar to a brachial plexus injury and may be inappropriately attributed to, among other things, improper positioning of the patient on the operating room table.[9] Two large studies of perioperative ulnar neuropathies have reported that more than half of the lesions were noted at least 24 hours after surgery and anesthesia.[10, 11] A condition similar to acute brachial neuritis, but which occurs in a lower extremity, has been reported and referred to as idiopathic lumbosacral plexitis.[12] The liability implications of the erroneous attribution of a peripheral nerve injury to simply operative or anesthetic misadventure are obvious. Accordingly, the physicians examining and treating patients for peripheral nerve injuries after anesthesia have the responsibility to consider explanations other than improper positioning. It would further seem important for consultants, subsequent treating physicians, and expert witnesses to explore the possibility that peripheral nerve injuries after surgery are idiopathic and not iatrogenic. Certainly the patient, for treatment reasons, as well as fellow physicians, for liability reasons, deserves this consideration.

DOCUMENTATION

A familiar admonition in the medicolegal arena holds that "the palest ink is better than the strongest memory." Pointing to a contemporaneously created written statement as proof that an order was written, an explanation given, or a treatment performed is much more persuasive than to merely testify from even the clearest memory that an event occurred but for which no documentation exists.

This concept is no less true when it comes to claims against physicians related to patient positioning. Documentation as to the patient's position, the padding involved, changes in position, the reasons for such changes, and a description of the condition of the patient at the conclusion of the anesthesia can be powerful weapons 2 or 3 years later when testimony is rendered in court.

As a general rule, more is better when it comes to documentation. Obviously, space limitations may not permit comprehensive descriptions of matters related to positioning. Even brief notes or notes made in a code developed by the writer can become extremely valuable to prove proper positioning and appropriate monitoring of positioning rather than having to rely only on memory or on a practitioner's usual course of conduct.

Documentation of abnormalities is particularly important. It may later be necessary to explain an unusual outcome because of an abnormal event or condition that occurred or was noted at surgery. Absent that documentation, details of, or even the fact of, the abnormality may be lost to memory.

One caveat applies to all charting: *Never alter a record!!* A charting error made while the document is being created is easily remedied by writing the word "error" and initialing the correction. However, to go back weeks, months, or years later and delete notes or make additions to the record is a completely different issue. More than one lawsuit, which was otherwise defensible, has become indefensible when a record was altered. If the jury believes that the physician is not truthful and candid, which is suggested by an alteration to a record, then the physician has little chance of persuading the jury about other important issues in the case.

Certain states have held that the wrongful alteration of a medical record can be grounds for an award of punitive damages. As a general rule, punitive damage awards are rare in medical malpractice cases. As one of the elements of such a claim, the patient must usually prove "actual malice" on the part of the physician. This level of conduct seldom exists in the context of medical malpractice. In one case, however, a court held that an intentional alteration, falsification, or destruction of a medical record to avoid liability for medical negligence was enough to show actual malice and supported a claim for punitive damages, regardless of whether the alteration, falsification, or destruction directly caused the patient harm.[13] Stated another way for emphasis, the mere wrongful alteration or destruction of a medical record to avoid malpractice liability, which in and of itself did not injure the patient, could still give rise to punitive damages.

EXPERT WITNESS

With few exceptions, a patient who brings a medical malpractice action will need the testimony of an expert witness to prove liability. The expert is necessary to establish the requisite standard of care under the circumstances and to opine whether the physician deviated from that standard. In most instances, an expert must also testify to the probable relationship or cause of any such deviation and the harm suffered by the patient. Without such expert testimony, the patient's case fails. By the same token, once a patient presents expert testimony on standard of care and proximate cause, the defendant physician must, in turn, present expert testimony that the standard of care was met and/or any alleged breach did not cause the patient's injury. Otherwise, the defendant physician risks the probability of being found liable for the patient's injury.

Obviously, therefore, the expert witness plays a crucial role in medical malpractice actions. In many instances, each party's case turns on the expertise, logic of thought, and perceived candor of the expert. The expert's opinions and testimony have tremendous consequences for both the patient and the physician charged with malpractice. If the expert is casual in determining that a case has merit, the patient can gain false hope and may embark on an undertaking that is lengthy, emotional, and futile. Likewise, by rendering an erroneous opinion that a physician is guilty of negligence that harmed the patient, the accused physician suffers emotional stress and possible loss of reputation from which he may never recover, but for which there is little prospect of redress against the patient or the expert.

That physicians err and patients are harmed is an unfortunate fact of medical life. If physicians have the expertise to render opinions and have thought through the issues completely, they should not be reticent to provide expert testimony in medicolegal matters. To this end, the American Society of Anesthesiologists has promulgated guidelines for the qualifications and testimony of anesthesiology experts.[14] Consistent with these guidelines, and whether testifying on behalf of the patient or the physician, potential experts should consider several factors.

First, physicians should be competent to testify. Some states have specific criteria that must be met before a physician can testify on issues of liability in a medical malpractice action. This may include a certain percentage of time presently engaged in the active practice of medicine or the teaching of medicine at an accredited institution. Consultation with the attorney for the party seeking the expert's opinion should clarify any such requirements.

Second, physicians should determine whether they are truly qualified by education, training, and experience to testify regarding some or all of the issues involved in the case. Potential experts may come to the conclusion that they are qualified to render opinions on the standard of care but not on proximate cause. The expert should make the retaining attorney aware of this, and the physician should limit testimony accordingly.

Third, physicians should request and make every effort to obtain all of the facts and medical records arguably relevant to the case. Opinions rendered on partial facts or records are likely to be limited opinions and subject to vigorous cross examination by the opposing party. This, in turn, can lead to a very embarrassing experience for the expert.

Fourth, physicians should undertake a complete and thorough analysis of the facts and records provided. Potential experts should consider all viewpoints and explanations of events, not just those most favorable to the party retaining their services. In reviewing a medicolegal case, the expert should keep in mind that in most instances the opinion must be rendered to a reasonable degree of medical probability, that is, more probable than not. Opinions to mere possibilities generally will not be permitted on direct examination to establish or refute the requisite elements of medical negligence. If the expert cannot render an opinion to a probability, either because no one could possibly express such an opinion or because it would be pure speculation to do so, the expert's testimony will be deemed inadmissible in most instances.

Fifth, if an expert renders an opinion in good faith but, after further consideration or the benefit of receiving another opinion on the subject from the other party's expert, believes that the original opinion or testimony may be in error, that expert should re-evaluate the stated position and make a determination at the earliest moment whether further testimony can be given in good conscience. Even putting aside the consideration that testimony is rendered under oath at trial or in a deposition, the expert should honestly reconsider a position if there are reasonable grounds to do so. Both sides to a medicolegal matter should have the benefit of an honest appraisal of their position. It is unfair to all concerned if litigation is perpetuated on erroneous positions no matter when determined.

Lastly, and perhaps the touchstone for the decision to offer testimony, should be the potential experts' willingness to submit their opinions to peer review. This does not mean the expert's colleagues should be expected to all agree with the opinions expressed. There are issues in medicine on which reasonable minds will differ. The expert's opinions, however, should be premised on sound scientific principles and a thorough analysis of the issues at hand. If the expert's opinions rise to this level, then peer analysis should not be resisted. More importantly, if the expert would be confident about presenting opinions for this scrutiny, those opinions are probably premised on sound medical principles in the first instance. On the other hand, if the expert would be uncomfortable with having the provided opinions reviewed by colleagues, those opinions probably should not be expressed in a courtroom.

PHYSICIAN'S RESPONSE TO SUIT NOTIFICATION

The process by which a medicolegal claim is instituted varies from state to state, as does the procedure for prosecuting the claim. Accordingly, specific advice on the response to notification of a legal action, and what follows thereafter, is not the same in all jurisdictions. There are, however, certain matters that should be considered on notification that a suit is contemplated or has been filed.

First, the applicable medical malpractice insurance carrier(s) should be notified immediately. This action of prompt notification is usually a requirement of the insurance contract, and, further, is a condition precedent to invoking insurance coverage. If the patient's care occurred over a period of several years, and various medical malpractice carriers provided insurance during that time span, in most instances all carriers should be notified. They can then sort out which company actually provides insurance for the claim or suit.

Second, *under no circumstances should the patient's medical records be altered in any respect;* however, they should be secured to assure their safety. A separate file should be maintained regarding all correspondence and documentation related to the claim or lawsuit. Such papers and letters should not be placed in the patient's chart. Correspondence between the physician and the attorney could inadvertently be disclosed if left in the patient's chart and, thus, the attorney–client privilege arguably would be waived.

Third, at the earliest opportunity, consultation should be sought with the attorney who has been assigned by the insurance carrier to handle the matter. Before that first meeting, consideration should be given to preparing a narrative of the patient's care specifically addressed to the designated attorney. The narrative serves the dual purpose of (1) helping focus the discussion with defense counsel and (2) preserving recollections of the patient's care and medical course. Those recollections will be much fresher at this point than will be the case months or years later when the trial is conducted. One should refrain from talking to any other physicians about the patient or the claim unless approved by counsel. Furthermore, a literature search should not be conducted or medical texts of journals consulted regarding medical issues involved in the patient's care without the approval of the defense attorney. Literature that is reviewed possibly can be discovered by opposing counsel and, in certain circumstances, used against the defendant physician at trial.

Some thought, however, should be given to possible expert witnesses, to be consulted or called at trial, who would be appropriate to review the treatment rendered or to deal with the proximate cause issues in the case. *Without the specific approval of counsel, the defendant physician should not contact any such experts or discuss the case with them at any time.* That task should be left to counsel.

Fourth, in the absence of a medical emergency or extraordinary circumstances, the physician against whom notice has been served should refrain from again treating or evaluating the complainant patient. If a statute of limitations issue exists regarding the claim, that is, whether the patient either filed suit or put the physician on notice of a possible lawsuit within the applicable statutory time period, any such defense may be jeopardized by again treating or evaluating the patient. An expired statute of limitations period could be rekindled and the claim period started to run anew from the time of any such further patient contact.

Lastly, the defendant physician should cooperate fully with the assigned defense attorney and the insurance company. Most insurance contracts have a specific provision that requires the cooperation of the insured physician. If the physician does not "cooperate" as defined under the policy, the company may have grounds to withdraw insurance coverage. Just as important, however, is the awareness that no one better than the physician understands the relevant facts and medical

procedures concerning the care of the patient. Defense counsel must be freely provided with the thought processes that were involved with the patient's care. That insight and knowledge will be invaluable in defending against the patient's contentions.

REFERENCES

1. Bruni v. Tatsumi (1976), 46 Ohio St2d 127, 346 NE2d 673.
2. 57B Am. Jur2d, Negligence, §2182 at 809.
3. Ibid., §2183 at 809–810.
4. Ibid., §2183 and 2184 at 810.
5. Ibid., §2185 at 814.
6. Ibid., §1864 at 531.
7. Kroll DA, Caplan RA, Posner K, et al.: Nerve injury associated with anesthesia. Anesthesiology 73:202, 1990.
8. Wilbourn AJ: Brachial plexus disorders. *In* Dyck PJ, Thomas PK (eds.): Peripheral Neuropathy, 3rd ed., vol. 2. Philadelphia, WB Saunders, 1993, pp. 911–933.
9. Ibid., p. 934.
10. Alvine FG, Schurrer ME: Postoperative ulnar nerve palsy: Are there predisposing factors? J Bone Joint Surg Am 69:255, 1987.
11. Warner MA, Warner ME, Martin JT: Ulnar neuropathy: Incidence, outcome and risk factors in sedated or anesthetized patients. Anesthesiology 81:1332, 1994.
12. Donaghy M: Lumbosacral plexus lesions. *In* Dyck PJ, Thomas PK (eds.): Peripheral Neuropathy, 3rd ed., vol. 2. Philadelphia, WB Saunders, 1993, p. 951.
13. Moskovitz v. Mt. Sinai Medical Center (1994), 69 Ohio St3d 638, 653 NE2d 331.
14. ASA Standards, Guidelines and Statements. Park Ridge, IL, American Society of Anesthesiologists, October 1994, p. 20.

Index

Note: Page numbers in *italics* refer to illustrations; those followed by t refer to tables.

Abdominal insufflation, with head-down tilt, 111
Abdominal relaxation, lawn chair position and, 43
Abrasion, corneal, 325–326
    in prone position, 181
Accessories, for operating table, *21, 21–25, 23–25*
Aerobic training, and cardiovascular response to supine position, 30
Age, and cardiovascular response to supine position, 30
Aging, 281–285. See also *Elderly*.
    problems of, 281–282
Air embolism, CNS complications with, 293
    in lateral decubitus position, 149
    in prone position, 184
    in sitting position, 74–75, 75t, *76*, 82–85
    paradoxical, 84
    with head-down tilt, 118
Airway, in lateral decubitus position, 142–143
Aldosterone, effect of supine position on, 34
Aldrete score, 319, 320t
Alertness, in postanesthesia care unit, 322
Alopecia, pressure, 228–229
    from lateral decubitus position, 146
    from supine position, 45
    occipital, following cardiopulmonary bypass, 12
Andrews frame, *161,* 171–172
Anesthesia, general, during pregnancy, 270–271
    hypotensive, with head-down tilt, 115–116
    in sitting position, 87
    obesity and, 245–246
    regional, during pregnancy, 271–275, *273*
    repositioning during, 11–12
    with head-down tilt, 97–98
Angiotensin, effect of supine position on, 34
Ankle, positioning of, 204t
Anklets, for head-down tilt, *102,* 104–105, *105*
Ankylosing spondylitis, neck in, 226, 231
Anterior scalene syndrome, 230
Aortocaval compression syndrome, 35, 45
    during pregnancy, *268,* 268–271, *269*
Arm abduction, brachial plexus injury due to, 214–215
Arm injuries, 299–302, *300–303*
    during extracorporeal shock wave lithotripsy, 239, *239, 240*
    in head-down tilt, 118–119
    in prone position, 180
    postanesthesia evaluation of, 308, *310,* 324
Arm positioning, in head-down tilt, *105,* 105–106, *106,* 120
    in lateral decubitus position, 138, *138*
    in lithotomy position, 55–56, 60

Arm positioning *(Continued)*
    in prone position, 174–175, 192
    in supine position, 312–314, *313–315*
Arm protection, 9
Arm support systems, 22, *23*
Arm toboggan, 175
Armboards, 9
    in lateral decubitus position, 138
    in supine position, 314, *315*
Arrhythmias, in head-down tilt, 109–110
    in sitting position, 85
Arterial baroreceptor reflexes, 29–30
Arterial bypass procedures, extracranial-to-intracranial, 292
Arterial oxygen pressure (PaO_2), with obesity, 246, 247, *248*
Arthralgia, from head-down tilt, 119
Arthritis, in elderly, 282
    of knees, prone position with, 193
    rheumatoid, of neck, 226, 231
Aspiration, pulmonary, in obstetrics, 271
Atelectasis, in head-down tilt, 118
    in lateral decubitus position, 144, 149
Atlantoaxial instability, with Down syndrome, 264
Atrial natriuretic peptide, effect of supine position on, 34
Augmentation mammaplasty, prone position with, 188, 192
Axillary nerve, *300, 310*
Axillary roll. See *Chest pad.*
Axonotmesis, 206, 307

Backache, from lateral decubitus position, 146
    from lithotomy position, 65–66
    from supine position, 40, 44
Bainbridge reflex, 28
Baldness. See *Alopecia.*
Bardeen pad, 167, *168*
Baroreceptors, 29–30
Bean bags (Vacu-Pac), for children, 257
    for lateral decubitus position, 137–138, *138*
    for ventral decubitus positions, 169
Bed rest, and positioning, 7–8
Bent-knee/anklet system, for head-down tilt, *102,* 104–105, *105*
Blindness, 229, 326
    from prone position, 181–182
    from sitting position, 86

ISBN 0-7216-6674-4